MW01201546

THE ART
OF SKIN HEALTH
RESTORATION
AND REJUVENATION

THE ART OF SKIN HEALTH RESTORATION AND REJUVENATION

THE SCIENCE OF CLINICAL PRACTICE

SECOND EDITION

ZEIN E. OBAGI, M.D.
Obagi Skin Health Institute
Beverly Hills, California
USA

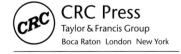

CRC Press
Taylor & Francis Group
Boca Raton London New York

CRC Press is an imprint of the
Taylor & Francis Group, an **informa** business

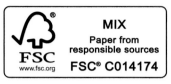

CRC Press
Taylor & Francis Group
6000 Broken Sound Parkway NW, Suite 300
Boca Raton, FL 33487-2742

© 2015 by Taylor & Francis Group, LLC
CRC Press is an imprint of Taylor & Francis Group, an Informa business

No claim to original U.S. Government works

Printed on acid-free paper
Version Date: 20140911

International Standard Book Number-13: 978-1-84214-596-8 (Pack - Book and Ebook)

This book contains information obtained from authentic and highly regarded sources. While all reasonable efforts have been made to publish reliable data and information, neither the author[s] nor the publisher can accept any legal responsibility or liability for any errors or omissions that may be made. The publishers wish to make clear that any views or opinions expressed in this book by individual editors, authors or contributors are personal to them and do not necessarily reflect the views/opinions of the publishers. The information or guidance contained in this book is intended for use by medical, scientific or health-care professionals and is provided strictly as a supplement to the medical or other professional's own judgement, their knowledge of the patient's medical history, relevant manufacturer's instructions and the appropriate best practice guidelines. Because of the rapid advances in medical science, any information or advice on dosages, procedures or diagnoses should be independently verified. The reader is strongly urged to consult the relevant national drug formulary and the drug companies' printed instructions, and their websites, before administering any of the drugs recommended in this book. This book does not indicate whether a particular treatment is appropriate or suitable for a particular individual. Ultimately it is the sole responsibility of the medical professional to make his or her own professional judgements, so as to advise and treat patients appropriately. The authors and publishers have also attempted to trace the copyright holders of all material reproduced in this publication and apologize to copyright holders if permission to publish in this form has not been obtained. If any copyright material has not been acknowledged please write and let us know so we may rectify in any future reprint.

Except as permitted under U.S. Copyright Law, no part of this book may be reprinted, reproduced, transmitted, or utilized in any form by any electronic, mechanical, or other means, now known or hereafter invented, including photocopying, microfilming, and recording, or in any information storage or retrieval system, without written permission from the publishers.

For permission to photocopy or use material electronically from this work, please access www.copyright.com (http://www.copyright.com/) or contact the Copyright Clearance Center, Inc. (CCC), 222 Rosewood Drive, Danvers, MA 01923, 978-750-8400. CCC is a not-for-profit organization that provides licenses and registration for a variety of users. For organizations that have been granted a photocopy license by the CCC, a separate system of payment has been arranged.

Trademark Notice: Product or corporate names may be trademarks or registered trademarks, and are used only for identification and explanation without intent to infringe.

Visit the Taylor & Francis Web site at
http://www.taylorandfrancis.com

and the CRC Press Web site at
http://www.crcpress.com

To my most loving and supportive wife, Samar

CONTENTS

ACKNOWLEDGMENTS

This comprehensive book represents the evolution of my philosophy of the science of skin health and clinical experience as a dermatologist for the past 35 years. It would not have been possible without the assistance, support, and contributions of a long list of many dedicated and talented individuals.

First and foremost I want to thank my wife Samar for her love and patience and all the tremendous effort she has devoted to coordinating the whole team as skillfully as a movie director. I have always been able to count on her love and support, for which I am very grateful every day.

I also want to thank my wonderful children for their love and support, especially Serene and Zaidal, who must be acknowledged for providing invaluable assistance in searching the web for me, even while he was so busy with his pre-med studies. I know that he will develop into a brilliant physician.

To my dermatologic colleagues many thanks also to my Junior Associate, Monika Kiripolsky, MD, for her monumental effort in writing the chapter entitled, "Topical Agents for Skin Health Restoration," and devoting so much of her valuable time to editing numerous chapters in the book. She raised the most intriguing questions that required answers to make the theories advanced in this book more precise. I also want to thank my esteemed colleague E. Victor Ross, MD, for his tremendous contribution. He was gracious enough to provide the chapter on lasers and energy-based systems and share his great insights and incredible knowledge. And I wish to thank Rachael Eckel, MD, for her help with editing some of the chapters and fine-tuning many ideas for clarity and accuracy, and for her excellent suggestions.

To my pharmacist colleague, Kevin Nagengast: I wish to thank him for contributing a superb chapter covering the full spectrum of supplements and their role in Skin Health Restoration.

To my editorial team: I want to thank Julia Petrauskas for her assistance in providing her expert medical writing services, quest for accuracy, and dedication. I also want to thank Wendy Lewis for her astute advice, counsel, and publishing expertise.

To the Obagi Skin Health Institute Staff: I wish to thank Angeli Lacson and the entire team for their help with research and administrative work and for tolerating all of the rewrites and edits of the chapters. I wish to thank Cynthia S. Gordon (medanimations.com) for expert illustrations and timely delivery. My special thanks go out to Albert Waisman for helping to select and compile the clinical photography with great precision and professionalism.

To the ZO Skin Health Management Team: I want to acknowledge the hard work of my longtime friend Jim Headley, as well as Deborah Tomes and Chris Kraneiss, for their never-ending dedication to helping me achieve my vision for the ZO brand, ZO Skin Health and ZO Medical. I also wish to thank Tommy Lee for his brilliant creative contributions to the cover design for the book.

To the CRC medical team: I want to thank Robert Peden and his colleagues for their patience and professionalism in helping me bring this book to fruition.

To my patients, who believed in my innovative approach to skin health, had faith in the outcomes that we could achieve together, and afforded me the honor of treating them throughout my career in dermatology.

Finally, much of the wisdom that I have gained was from my beloved mother who told me from an early age: "A blind person cannot see with his eyes, but he may acquire more knowledge better than a person who can see. Don't accept what you see as the ultimate that is etched in stone; open your mind to see and absorb."

PREFACE

"The science of skin health must be taught in medical school. Physicians must know the difference between diseased skin and healthy skin to restore skin health."

This comprehensive book represents the entirety of my philosophy of healthy skin and clinical experience as a dermatologist for the past 35 years. This is the second edition of my original book (*Obagi Skin Health Restoration and Rejuvenation*, Springer-Verlag, 2000) and serves to describe my new way of thinking about the science behind skin health. The emphasis in this text is on skin, and it covers the science of restoring skin health, cellular function, and improving the skin's ability to tolerate procedures and surgery. The range of skin conditions addressed includes diseases of pigmentation (melasma, hypopigmentation, hyperpigmentation), textural disorders (scars, rhytides, large pores), aging, photodamage, inflammatory disorders, rosacea, and acne. The modern solutions described in this book are based on the latest scientific advances coupled with my 35 years of clinical experience. It is intended to provide the reader with a wealth of original theories and information on many issues encountered in day-to-day practice when dealing with skin. Any physician can follow these principles, both students and advanced skin care professionals, and they can be adapted to treat any patient.

Health and skin care occupy a prominent place within the mind of consumers. "Looking one's best" is an innate desire shared by all. The cry for youthful, disease-free, healthy skin has been heard, as can be seen in the dramatic expansion in skin care products currently available on the market. But sadly, such formulations often lack the support of research and science. Because of their ineffectiveness and lack of long-term improvement and sustainable results, customers are repeatedly left feeling disappointed and hopeless. These self-prescribed products are not part of a comprehensive program tailored to the patient's skin needs; their use is haphazard and lacks physician guidance.

Regrettably, patients seeking a clinician's advice are often misled. An increasing number of clinicians today make recommendations based on personal enticements and nonscientific marketing pitches. They may favor a "quick fix" for their patients because of time and economic benefits. As such, they are hasty to recommend any procedure that cuts, evaporates, resurfaces, plumps, and tightens the skin. They fail to address the skin itself—its quality, integrity, vitality, and, most important, suitability for a procedure.

Having begun my career in pathology, I was regularly exposed to diseased tissue. The way in which cells function, both individually and collectively, became my principal focus. My mind was trained to think at a cellular level when addressing disease, an invaluable foundation that proved advantageous when I switched to dermatology. It soon became obvious that the generally accepted approach to treating skin was flawed. It is simply inadequate to treat a disease or its symptoms independently. Instead, the cells involved in the condition must be comprehensively and collectively addressed. The skin is not a wall that one can paint and superficially plaster; it is an organ that requires cellular activation and regulation to achieve health. It is therefore crucial that any practitioner dealing with skin—whether with incision, lasers, peels, injections, or other treatments—first respects and understands the skin's function at a cellular level in order to achieve the best possible results.

A baby's skin has always fascinated me. Microscopically, each cell is fulfilling its precise function, and this corresponds to its flawless appearance. As a physician, I wanted to offer this possibility to patients of all ages. And so, more than 35 years ago, my passion ignited, I set out to define the science underlying skin health. The fundamental principle driving my approach is that skin must be holistically restored at the cellular level. If the focus is limited to treating only the disease or its symptoms, the results will be limited and short lived.

Skin health and its science have many features that allow for a standardized method of treatment and superior overall patient outcome. Innovative products and protocols have been created in parallel, using the most novel scientific research and clinical experience. There are programs for diseased and nondiseased states, each relying on a systematic approach to holistically restore skin health.

Since my introduction of skin health science (which is the core of what this book is about), I have devoted my career to educating physicians all over the world on how to deal with skin from a different perspective. My goal has been to shift their focus away from the disease they intend to treat, which will help to calm down the symptoms and provide short-term remission, to focus mainly on the skin itself in order to bring it back to the state of optimal cellular activity and functions while treating disease. This approach will lead to better and longer lasting overall results. It is most gratifying to me to see that skin health science is currently being adapted by thousands of physicians worldwide and enabling them to obtain the best results in skin treatment and rejuvenation.

It is about time that as professionals dealing with skin, we set aside our differences on how to approach skin. We must adapt a unified approach that is proved to be the ideal one rather than follow the current individualistic, misguided, and narrow-minded approaches that focus solely on the surface of the skin and symptoms. We must address the science of skin health as the essential basis for treatment and intervention. This should be recognized as a science to be studied beginning in medical schools and residency programs, before learning about diseases of the skin. It will help to establish clear objectives when treating skin problems. It is no longer enough to say that a specific problem has been resolved, as many of us still believe. Wouldn't it be better to be able to say, "The main problem has been resolved, and skin health has been restored"?

Adapting skin health science should be the only valid approach to deal with skin because it is a comprehensive process that yields many benefits. The new definition of skin health that I have introduced will clarify the exact meaning of skin health and eliminate the use of loosely described terminology that is often used to sell products that have nothing to do with skin health. Unfortunately, clinicians have become targets for promotion of certain products and devices, and few among us have the courage to refute some of the erroneous concepts that now dominate clinical practice. My hope is to challenge traditional procedure-oriented approaches to skin care and shift the emphasis back to skin health.

My new definition of skin health science will establish a well-rounded approach to restore and maintain skin health using fundamentals that can be adopted clinically and histologically through subjective and objective criteria, applicable to any skin type. The definition helps to establish a comprehensive diagnosis, to identify the objective of the treatment required, to allow the monitoring of treatment progress, and to accurately measure results on completion of the treatment.

Skin health science will also guide the physician through novel original principles, including

- Adapting Zein Obagi Skin Classification System as a guide in planning any treatment plan, selecting procedures, and determining the safe depth for any skin type
- Insuring that the proper topical agents are used for treatment by following Zein Obagi Skin Classification System
- Simplifying the proper selection of procedures by following Zein Obagi Skin Procedure Classification System based on the mechanism of action

Those of you who joined me years ago and are familiar with my original products, including Obagi NuDerm and the Obagi Blue Peel, will find this book more exciting than my first edition and easier to follow. I have maintained the original principles of skin health that I introduced 25 years ago, and the book contains many clinical concepts I used to develop Obagi NuDerm and the Obagi Blue Peel. However, my original principles have been expanded in this book, as evidenced by a selection of patients' photographs before and after using the original Obagi NuDerm, as well as patients' photographs before and after using the new ZO Medical system. The latter program was developed to include wider indications and applications when used purely for Skin Health Restoration, for maintaining skin health, and as a skin treatment. Those patients with no medical problems were given ZO skin health for prevention and daily skin care.

The three original principles of Skin Health Restoration include correction (improving the epidermis); stimulation (improving the dermis); and bleaching and blending (correcting pigmentation problems). Recently, I added a fourth principle, stabilization. This novel concept was created to address the need for prevention. It aims to maintain skin health by preventing diseases, changes in skin texture, and cellular dysfunction. When targeting any disease, the four principles should be employed, and the disease approached within the larger context of overall skin health. Using acne as an example, my treatment plan first involves correction, followed by specific acne agents, then stimulation, and finally bleaching and blending if discoloration exists. My objective here is to remedy the skin disease by thoroughly treating it within the entire skin unit. The rationale is that disease does not affect only a single spot on the face that can be seen or touched; rather, it influences all cells and layers, and one must comprehensively treat every element to restore the skin to its optimal health. After the disease has been treated, the focus should shift to stabilization to maintain the results achieved.

The reader will notice that I address skin in a novel way. My style contrasts with the traditional, narrow approach to treating skin in which the focus is on the disease or its symptoms. This primitive method often yields limited improvement, frequent recurrences, and treatment failures. My approach is broader, yet still targets the core of the problem: the cells. The two primary objectives to my method are to restore skin health while treating the disease in parallel to achieve maximal results.

This book will provide key insights into achieving and optimizing patients' results. My extensive research and clinical experience on defining and refining the science of skin health has enabled me to provide a standard step-by-step approach to treating skin. I hope the text will prove to be an indispensable tool for practitioners dealing with skin in the following ways:

- Selecting a daily skin care program
- Providing treatment
- Rejuvenating skin
- Preventing skin problems
- Maintaining results
- Selecting the appropriate procedure based on the problem, the skin type, the mechanism of action, and the objective of such procedures
- Conditioning skin for procedures
- Managing skin after procedures

The practitioner will further learn that many currently used principles related to skin are either outdated or do not provide adequate information. This book will address these matters and set new standards for the following:

- Skin classification
- Topical agent classification
- Classification of procedures based on their mechanism of action
- Understanding and treating skin sensitivity and dryness
- Preventing and treating pigmentation disorders, aging, photodamage, and inflammatory diseases
- Selecting and performing the best procedure for a patient, from chemical peels to laser resurfacing

"Finis origine pendet"; the end depends on the beginning.

This book is intended for anyone who desires to deliver the safest, most comprehensive, current, and effective treatment results to their patients. Many of the principles I have put forth in this book are original. The ideas may challenge you and stimulate your own research, experimentation, and clinical studies. I encourage this; it is precisely what I have done and continue to do throughout my career in dermatology. I want the reader to see my principles as tools and to adapt them to create their own tour de force. Practitioners will develop their own preferences, and I encourage them to do so. But they must do so with a solid understanding of the skin's cellular function: the control of cells before and after procedures, the interaction between skin types, the safe procedure depth, and the skin's response to injury.

By being inventive, we progress as a species, in technology and in medicine. We must begin somewhere—and with imagination, inspiration, and hard work as key ingredients, it shall evolve. I often find comfort remembering that not too long ago our ancestors believed the world was flat. The pioneer who sought to change this view was ridiculed. Criticism and doubt will indeed follow whenever you seek to be inventive and change the established mindset. But we must never let this distract us from our patient's best interest.

As Aristotle said, "There is only one way to avoid criticism: do nothing, say nothing, and be nothing."

Zein E. Obagi, MD
Obagi Skin Health Institute
Beverly Hills, California 90210

Note: I have created this text for physicians and skin care professionals who want to learn about the products that we use in our clinics. Please contact ZO directly for more information about ZO Skin Health and ZO Medical protocols and standards of care.

ZO Skin Health by Zein Obagi, MD
1 Technology Drive, Suite B-123
Irvine, CA 92618
Telephone: 949-988-7524
Customer service: 888-893-1375
Fax: 949-988-7544
customerservice@zoskinhealth.com
zoskinhealth.com

Note on Terminology: In this book, *ZO* refers to the products developed by Dr. Zein Obagi in conjunction with ZO Skin Health Inc. Neither has a business connection with Obagi Medical Products.

A NEW PERSPECTIVE ON SKIN ANATOMY AND PHYSIOLOGY

Many textbooks are available on the structure and the physiology of the skin, and reading of these is recommended for a firm grounding in dermatological science. The purpose of this chapter is to connect the Skin Health Restoration program approach to the anatomical and physiological properties of the skin (Box 1.1).

The skin is the largest organ of the body, having a surface area of 1.8 m^2 and making up approximately 18% of body weight. It is readily available for inspection and can reveal health or disease. Functionally, the skin has many roles: thermal regulation, detection of sensation, immune responsiveness, energy storage, vitamin D production, and protection against environmental insults. During a lifetime, the skin undergoes numerous changes, including adapting to the change from a water to air environment at birth; adapting to hormonal influences at puberty; and, in females, adjusting to the effects of hormonal changes seen during menstruation and pregnancy and while taking contraceptive pills during the reproductive years. In addition, profound changes can occur during illness, trauma, and environmental exposures and throughout the aging process. Sun exposure, smoking, disease, scarring, and psychological factors can profoundly change the structure and appearance of the skin. Skin Health Restoration principles and treatments were developed to address many of these changes.

Some of the factors leading to deteriorative changes in the skin are controllable, whereas others, with our present state of knowledge, are not. This chapter examines the structure and function of the skin (Table 1.1), with an emphasis on defining the controllable factors of skin health. It also examines the physiological changes that accompany aging of the skin, both intrinsic biological aging and extrinsic photoaging that results from exposure to sunlight. Along the way, the chapter lays the scientific foundation on which the clinical treatments and procedures that follow are based.

Box 1.1

Skin health can be restored and maintained by directly targeting the different layers and cells of the skin involved in the processes of skin aging, dysfunction, and disease.

TABLE 1.1 Skin Functions and Activities

Function	Activity
Protection	Protect inner organs and maintain homeostasis
Barrier function	Prevent invasion of water, bacteria, irritants
	Prevent transepidermal water loss
	Build skin tolerance and reduce sensitivity
	Provide natural protection from ultraviolet radiation through melanin and keratin
Stability of body organs	Synthesize vitamin D
	Eliminate certain toxins
Immune system role	Carry out antigen processing and immune surveillance through Langerhans cells
Sensory recognition	Relay information to brain about external environment, mechanical stimulation
Temperature control	Conserve body heat through insulation, vascular constriction; cool the body through vasodilation, sweat evaporation
Sebum production	Reduce water loss, form acid mantle, discourage microbial growth

LAYERS AND COMPONENTS OF THE SKIN

SKIN STRUCTURES

The skin is stratified horizontally into three compartments—the epidermis, dermis, and subcutaneous layer—and is penetrated vertically by appendages such as hair follicles, sweat glands, and sebaceous glands (Figure 1.1). The outermost, thinnest layer, the epidermis, forms a barrier to the world (the barrier function), keeping out water, bacteria, toxins, ultraviolet light, and allergens in healthy skin. The epidermis also shows the genetic expression of skin color and reveals dryness, softness, or roughness. It can be clear or diseased, as is the case with acne, or have precancerous or cancerous lesions, pigmentation problems, psoriasis, rosacea, and a host of other conditions. Throughout the body, the epidermis is uniform in thickness, except for certain thickened areas, such as the palms and soles.

The dermis, composed of the papillary dermis and the thicker reticular dermis, lies below the epidermis. The papillary dermis contains thin, haphazardly arranged collagen fibers, abundant ground substance, and delicate elastic fibers, whereas the reticular dermis comprises thick collagen bundles and coarse elastic fibers. Upward projections of the dermis, the papillae, fit into the epidermal depressions, the rete ridges. This arrangement provides a greater interface between the epidermis and the dermis than would result from contact between two flat surfaces. A rich supply of blood vessels and

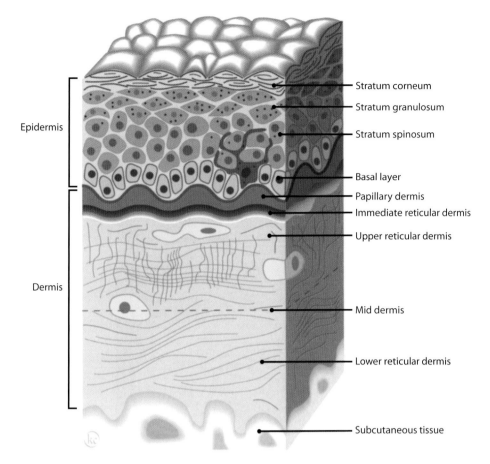

Epidermis

Dermis

Stratum corneum
Stratum granulosum
Stratum spinosum

Basal layer
Papillary dermis
Immediate reticular dermis
Upper reticular dermis

Mid dermis

Lower reticular dermis

Subcutaneous tissue

Figure 1.1   The layers of the skin (blood vessels omitted for clarity).

nerve endings can be found in the dermis. The deepest layer of the skin, the subcutaneous layer, is composed primarily of fatty tissue.

THE EPIDERMIS

Keratinocytes and the Keratinocyte Maturation Cycle
Four cell types are found in the epidermis: keratinocytes, melanocytes, Langerhans cells, and Merkel cells. Keratinocytes are the major cells of the epidermis. They originate at the basal layer, mature, lose their nucleus, and flatten as they move upward. At the uppermost level, they form a strong, flexible, dry surface known as the stratum corneum. This layer, composed of cells firmly attached to one another, continually loosens, detaches, and falls away in the natural process of exfoliation that takes 30 to 40 days in normally maturing skin. However, this transit time varies widely after mild injury or major trauma, in the presence of disease states like psoriasis, and throughout the aging process.

   Keratinocytes are involved in a steady state of cell production and cell loss. The *keratinocyte maturation cycle* is the amount of time it takes for a keratinocyte to mature and transform into a corneocyte, reach the stratum corneum, and subsequently exfoliate from the surface of the epidermis. One of the main objectives of skin health, as discussed in this book, is restoration of a normal maturation cycle through skin conditioning. It usually takes 6 weeks of skin-conditioning treatment to complete one cycle, and more than one cycle may be required in some patients (Box 1.2). Some of the factors that participate in the regulation of the keratinocyte maturation cycle are the dermis, hormones, vitamin A and its derivatives, epidermal growth factor, and cyclic nucleotides. Normal barrier function, in turn, increases skin tolerance. Skin barrier function, however, can be disrupted by overuse of moisturizers. The layers and cells of the epidermis are shown in Figure 1.2.

Melanocytes, Melanosomes, and Skin Pigmentation

Melanocytes are melanin-synthesizing cells that are found only in the basal layer where they are interspersed among the basal keratinocytes. Approximately every 10th cell of that single-cell layer is a melanocyte. Through its finger-like

---

Box 1.2

- One of the main objectives of skin health is restoration of a normal maturation cycle through skin conditioning
- It usually takes 6 weeks of skin conditioning treatment to complete one keratinocyte maturation cycle.

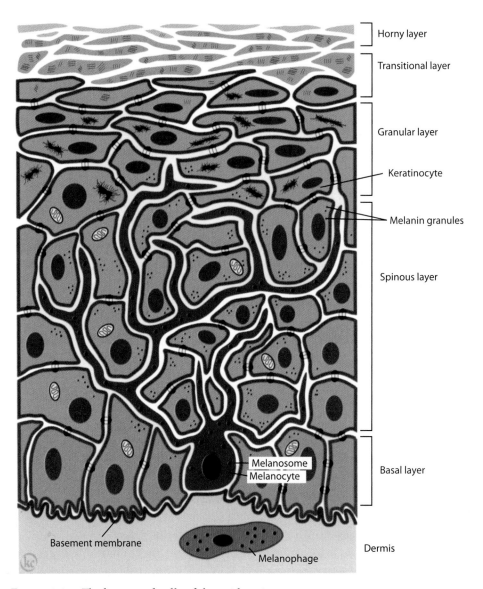

Horny layer

Transitional layer

Granular layer

Keratinocyte

Melanin granules

Spinous layer

Melanosome
Melanocyte

Basal layer

Basement membrane

Melanophage

Dermis

FIGURE 1.2 The layers and cells of the epidermis.

dendritic processes, each melanocyte is in contact with 30 to 40 keratinocytes. Inside the melanocyte, organelles known as melanosomes produce melanin pigment—the primary pigment of skin. These pigment granules migrate from the cytoplasm into the dendrites and are transferred from there into the surrounding keratinocytes, where they form a protective cap over the keratinocyte nucleus, protecting the nuclear DNA from the effects of ultraviolet (UV) radiation. Normal pigmentation of the skin depends on the efficient transfer of melanosomes to keratinocytes.

Variation in normal skin color, including that due to racial differences or the process of tanning, is not determined by the number or density of melanocytes but by the number, size, and distribution of melanosomes; the distribution of the pigment granules in the melanosomes; and the quantity of melanin produced. Melanosomes in darkly pigmented skin are large, single, and individually bound by a membrane. In lightly pigmented skin, melanosomes are smaller and clustered together in complexes enclosed by a membrane.

The main function of melanin is to protect DNA from UV light by acting as an antioxidant to reduce inflammation. Even melanin production in dark skin leads to the desirable tan, whereas in fair skin it leads to freckles, uneven color tone, and no tanning. The two types of melanin are eumelanin and pheomelanin. Eumelanin is stable, darkens when oxidized by UV light (produces a tan), and protects from UV light at a sun protection factor of 4 to 8. It is dominant in dark skin (skin types IV to VI on the Fitzpatrick scale). Pheomelanin, on the other hand, is unstable, provides little natural UV protection, and breaks down when exposed to UV light (causing DNA damage). Pheomelanin is present in all skin types (Fitzpatrick types I to VI) but is dominant in fair skin. It may be the causative factor in skin cancer in dark skin.

Melanin exists in the skin of animals and in many botanical and marine plants. Plant melanin should be included in skin care products, especially sunscreen, to offer extra protection from UV light, to protect skin melanocytes through an antioxidant effect, and to act as a shield to prevent penetration of UV light.

Tanning of the skin occurs in response to the UVA (320 to 380 nm) and UVB (290 to 320 nm) spectrums of solar radiation that reach the earth's surface. Within a few minutes of exposure to UVA, an immediate reaction occurs that then fades over 6 to 8 hours. During this time, preexisting melanin is photo-oxidized, resulting in an immediate pigment darkening, and melanocytes increase in size. A delayed reaction involving new pigment production becomes apparent only after 2 to 3 days of repeated exposure. This delayed reaction occurs in response to both UVA and UVB and involves an increase in the number of active melanocytes, enhanced melanosome production, and an increase in melanogenesis. The transfer of mature melanosomes from the melanocytes into keratinocytes increases, and keratinocyte proliferation increases. Changes also occur in the size and aggregation pattern of melanosomes, from smaller and grouped to larger and singly dispersed.

Skin can also darken in response to hormonal stimulation, such as with increased synthesis of melanocyte-stimulating hormone or adrenocorticotropic hormone, or during the poorly understood process of postinflammatory hyperpigmentation. Persons with lentigines (sun-induced dark spots) show increased numbers of melanocytes at the dermal-epidermal junction. Lentigines tend to be stable in color regardless of the length of exposure to UV light. These lesions are believed to result from an increase in metabolically active melanocytes. Ephelides (freckles), on the other hand, are not due to an increase in melanocytes but represent areas of increased melanin synthesis. Freckles appear in childhood, and their pigmentation usually increases during the summer, indicating that melanocytes respond to UV light. Melasma, a very common patchy brown, tan, or blue-gray facial skin discoloration, is almost entirely seen in women in the reproductive years. It typically appears on the upper cheeks, upper lip, forehead, and chin. Melasma is thought to be the result of stimulation of melanocytes or pigment-producing cells by the female sex hormones estrogen and progesterone to produce more melanin pigments when the skin is exposed to sun. Women with a light brown skin type who are living in regions with intense sun exposure are particularly susceptible to developing this condition. Figure 1.3 shows a woman with melasma on the cheeks and forehead.

THE DERMIS

In contrast to the epidermis, the dermis is a layer of connective tissue 500 to 1,000 μm thick that is largely acellular. It is composed of a mucopolysaccharide gel held together by a fibrous matrix of primarily collagen fibers and about 5% elastin. The dermis lies beneath the epidermis and gives it structural support. It also provides nutrition and removes waste products. The dermis is subdivided into two layers: the more superficial papillary dermis and the deeper reticular dermis (see Figure 1.1). The papillary dermis is the most active dermal layer. It is constantly repairing damaged collagen and elastin tissue and producing collagen, elastin, and glycosaminoglycans. It contains a rich supply of blood vessels that penetrate from the deeper layers, as well as numerous nerve endings, thermoreceptors, and cryoreceptors.

Below the papillary dermis is the thicker, major layer of the dermis, the reticular dermis, which is densely packed with collagen and elastic fibers. Various cell types are also present, including mast cells, fibroblasts, macrophages, and dermal dendritic cells. The transition from papillary dermis to

FIGURE 1.3 Asian patient with melasma on cheeks and forehead.

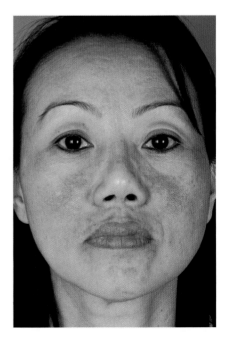

upper reticular dermis (called the *immediate reticular dermis,* or IRD) can be observed histologically. The IRD is the line where collagen fibers become thicker and more horizontal and elastic fibers become less distinct. Peels reaching the papillary dermis and the IRD lead to maximum skin tightening (Box 1.3). They are suitable for all skin types, and there is no risk for permanent effects, such as hypopigmentation skin thinning or textural changes. Complications such as keloids are rare. Healing is rapid, usually occurring in 8 to 10 days. Procedures below the IRD, such as those penetrating to the upper reticular dermis, can achieve skin leveling, but they have a higher incidence of color and texture changes and the possibility of keloids.

Collagen and Tensile Strength

Collagen is produced by fibroblast cells that lie among collagen fibers and makes up approximately 70% of the dry weight of the dermis. It has great tensile strength—a single fiber 1 mm in diameter can withstand a load of up to 20 kg (Box 1.4). It is insoluble because of chemically stabilizing intermolecular cross-linking. In young skin that has not been exposed to sun, mature collagen is cross-linked into collagen fibrils that come together into small groups of fibers, which are then organized into thin, wavy fiber bundles. The collagen fiber bundles are arranged in a mat-like orthogonal pattern, such that each layer is at right angles to the one above and the one below. These bundle formations are loosely arranged in the papillary dermis and become thicker in the deep dermis. Newly formed collagen fibrils become less soluble and more stable as they mature. Fully mature collagen fibers have a very low turnover rate compared with other body proteins.

In elderly persons, dermal collagen fibers become more heterogeneous, and the dermis becomes thinner. Reports on changes in the amount of collagen in unexposed human skin over time have been contradictory. It appears that the absolute amount of skin collagen decreases with age as skin becomes thinner, whereas the relative amount of collagen does not undergo significant change. Skin exposed to sunlight shows similar but more severe changes than normally aged skin, with less insoluble collagen than normal skin.

Box 1.3

Procedures for Skin Tightening

Peels reaching the papillary dermis and the immediate reticular dermis lead to maximum skin tightening.

Box 1.4

Collagen and Skin Tensile Strength

Collagen fibers provide the skin with its tensile strength, allowing the skin to serve as a protective organ against external trauma.

Elastic Fibers, Skin Elasticity, and Resilience

Elastic fibers are extracellular matrix protein complexes produced by fibroblasts, and they make up 2% to 4% of the total volume of the dermis. They form a network that is composed mostly of the protein elastin, which has unusual elasticity and tensile strength, and a small amount of microfibrils composed of a family of proteins. It is this network that maintains normal skin tension and provides extensibility. The integrity of the elastic fiber network in skin is very important because wrinkling, looseness, sagging, and other structural and mechanical changes in aging skin appear to be due to alterations in this network. In young skin, elastic fibers snap back quickly after stretching. Elastic fibers are continuously degraded and replaced by newly synthesized fibers in normal situations, but the turnover is slow.

The components of skin strength are shown in Box 1.5.

Extracellular Matrix and Hydration

The insoluble fibers of collagen and elastin are imbedded in the gel-like extracellular matrix of the dermis. This matrix is made up of noncollagenous glycoproteins and glycosaminoglycan-proteoglycan macromolecules. The glycoproteins facilitate cell adhesion, cell motility, and cell-matrix interactions, whereas the macromolecule complexes are important for hydration. Although the glycosaminoglycans are less than 1% of the dry weight of the skin, they are able to bind up to 1,000 times their own weight in water. Hyaluronic acid and dermatan sulfate are the major glycosaminoglycans in adult skin. As part of innate cutaneous aging, the content of hyaluronic acid diminishes with age; this may in part explain the reduced turgor of aged skin. Because of their high water-binding capacity, glycosaminoglycans allow some movement in dermal structures.

Fibroblasts and the Synthesis and Degradation of Connective Tissue

Fibroblasts, the "master" cells of the dermis, are responsible for synthesizing the connective tissue elements (the dermal-extracellular matrix) of the dermis, including collagen, elastic fibers, and the proteoglycan-glycosaminoglycan macromolecules. They are more numerous and larger in the papillary dermis than in the reticular dermis. Fibroblasts also control the turnover of connective tissue by secreting enzymes that degrade collagens (collagenases), elastin (elastases), and proteoglycans and glycosaminoglycans. With advancing age,

---

Box 1.5

Components of Skin Strength

Skin strength is the combination of:

- Skin firmness: resistance to shearing forces, which is related to quantity and quality of *collagen*
- Skin tightness: ability of skin to snap back after pulling or stretching, which is related to quantity and quality of *elastin*, especially in the papillary dermis

fibroblasts become smaller and less active. In photodamaged skin, they are often hypertrophied.

Mast Cells and the Inflammatory Response

A second cell type of the dermis is the mast cell. These cells are found close to blood vessels, nerves, and appendages and are present in greater numbers in the subpapillary dermis. Mast cells are distinguished primarily by the presence of numerous, large cytoplasmic granules that contain histamine, enzymes, and other mediators. During an allergic reaction, mast cells bind to immunoglobulin E, and the granules discharge their contents as part of the inflammatory response.

THE SUBCUTANEOUS LAYER

The subcutaneous layer, composed of lobules of fatty tissue, functions as a buffer against blunt trauma and gives the skin its appealing full and plump appearance (Box 1.6). It also provides "gliding ability" to both the dermis and epidermis, which helps to make skin more flexible. Areas with abundant subcutaneous tissue heal better and have less severe scarring than areas with a very thin or no subcutaneous layer. This can explain why certain areas of the face, such as the upper lip, jawline, and neck, where the dermis is in contact with the underlying muscles with little or no fat in between, have an increased tendency for fibrosis and scarring after procedures. It is very important to avoid deep dermal penetration in these areas.

SEBACEOUS GLANDS

Sebaceous glands are found on all parts of the body except the palms and soles, but they are small and relatively inactive in hairless areas. They are formed from epidermally derived cells that bud out from the side of a hair follicle. The purpose of the sebaceous glands is to form oil, sebum, which lubricates and thus protects the hair and skin. The dominant pathological condition of the sebaceous glands is acne.

There are several misconceptions about sebum and aging. Skin aging involves changes to collagen and elastin and does not depend on the amount of sebum production or skin dryness. Thus, oily skin does not age at a slower rate. Dryness is in fact related to the loss of glycosaminoglycans and abnormal barrier function (Box 1.7). Sebum helps to keep the skin at a slightly acidic pH (between 6 and 7).

Box 1.6

Fatty Tissue

The subcutaneous layer, composed of lobules of fatty tissue, gives the skin its appealing full and plump appearance.

Box 1.7

Sebum and Skin Dryness

Dryness is related to the loss of glycosaminoglycans and abnormal barrier function, not to a decrease in sebum.

THE AGING PROCESS

In any discussion of skin aging, it is important to differentiate between biological aging (chronological aging) and photoaging that is a direct result of exposure to sunlight. Clinically, the appearance of photoaged skin is distinctly different from biologically aged, sun-protected skin (Table 1.2). The most visible signs of biological aging include laxity, paleness, smooth-to-fine wrinkling, deepening of expression lines, dryness, and general thinning. Bruising is more common, and healing is slower. In contrast, visibly photoaged skin is more yellowish in pigmentation with marked areas of hyperpigmentation, coarser and roughened in texture, more lax, and more deeply wrinkled. These differences are readily evident when comparing skin areas of elderly persons that are usually covered, and thus photoprotected, with areas that have not been photoprotected. As a general rule, individuals with biologically aged, photoprotected skin appear younger than individuals with photodamaged skin who are of the same chronological age. In biological aging, most skin functions are slowed, and there is atrophy of tissues, whereas in photoaging, there is an increase in irregular activity with hypertrophy of certain tissues. Although exposure to UV radiation is the most important extrinsic factor in skin aging, other external factors, such as environmental toxins and infectious agents, may also play a role. Figure 1.4 shows a patient with skin atrophy, laxity, and wrinkles (intrinsic aging). Figure 1.5 shows a patient with classical signs of photodamage.

BIOLOGICAL AGING

Biological aging is characterized by a decrease in functional capacity and increased susceptibility to certain diseases and environmental insults. The

TABLE 1.2	Clinical Appearance of Biologically Aged and Photoaged Skin
Biologically Aged Skin	*Photoaged Skin*
Lax	Leathery
Deepened expression lines	Dry
Dry	Nodular and hypertrophied
Overall thinning	Yellow
	Telangiectasia
	Deep wrinkles
	Accentuated skin furrows
	Sags and bags
	Variety of benign, premalignant, and malignant neoplasms

most pronounced changes in biologically aged skin occur within the epidermis, affecting primarily the basal cell layer. The aging process takes place within all organs of the body and can be seen visibly in the skin. Skin aging is influenced by several factors, including genetics, environmental exposure, hormonal changes, and metabolic processes. Together, these factors lead to cumulative alterations of skin structure, function, and appearance. The functioning of the central nervous, immune, endocrine, and cardiovascular systems, as well as of the skin, is also impaired with age. Chronologically aged skin is thin, relatively flattened, dry, and unblemished, with some loss of elasticity and age-related loss of architectural regularity. General atrophy of the extracellular matrix is reflected by a decrease in the number of fibroblasts. Reduced levels of collagen and elastin, with impaired organization, are primarily due to decreased protein synthesis affecting types I and III collagen in the dermis, with an increased breakdown of extracellular matrix proteins. Oxidative stress is considered of primary importance in driving the aging process. The original

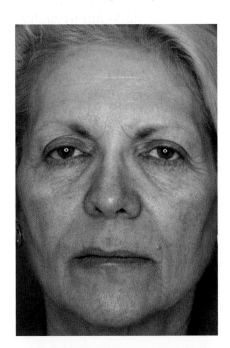

FIGURE 1.4 Patient with intrinsic aging. Notice skin atrophy, laxity, and wrinkles.

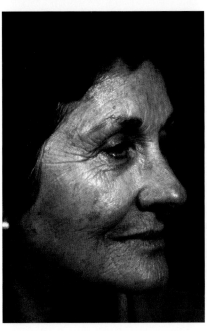

FIGURE 1.5 Patient with classical signs of photodamage (extrinsic aging).

free radical theory of aging purported that the molecular basis of aging was derived from a lifetime accumulation of oxidative damage to cells resulting from excess reactive oxygen species (ROS) produced as a consequence of aerobic metabolism. Although the skin possesses extremely efficient antioxidant activities, ROS levels rise, and antioxidant activities decline during aging.

A flattening of the dermal-epidermal interface is one of the more profound structural changes that occur with age. Because of this and the other aged-related structural and morphological changes that occur at both the tissue and cellular levels, normal skin functions progressively deteriorate, and skin becomes more susceptible to the development of various benign and malignant diseases. Hereditary factors, hormone levels, and various metabolic substances modulate the structural and physiological changes inherent in the aging process. Skin barrier functioning, permeability, thermoregulatory mechanisms, response to injury, sensory perception, metabolism, and immune function are all altered as we age. Several theories have been proposed over the years to explain the changes that occur, but it is likely that multiple pathways are involved. Alterations occurring during biological aging are shown in Box 1.8.

Changes to the Epidermis

With age, corneocytes become bigger and adhere less to one another, the rete pegs of the epidermis disappear, and, along with a decrease in the number and size of dermal papillae, the lower surface loses its undulating contour. As a result, the epidermis flattens and has less surface contact with the dermis (with less nutrient and waste transfer). In this way, the skin becomes less resistant to shearing forces and more vulnerable to insult, leading to an increased risk for epidermal peeling. Although this flattening of the dermal-epidermal junction may give the appearance that the epidermis thins substantially with age, the actual thickness of the epidermis decreases only 20% over the human lifespan. It is the dermal layer that thins markedly during the biological aging process. Along with the various structural changes that occur, there is a progressive decline in active melanocytes. In addition, keratinocytes change shape, becoming shorter and fatter.

Changes in Histology of the Dermis and the Appearance of the Skin following Biological Aging

Alterations in the dermal structural network of elastic fibers, collagen, proteins, and glycosaminoglycans lead to changes in the resilience and strength of aging skin. One of the most prominent changes occurring in biological

---

Box 1.8

Alterations during Biological Aging

Skin barrier functioning, permeability, thermoregulatory mechanisms, response to injury, sensory perception, metabolism, and immune function are all altered as we age.

aging is the decrease and increasingly abnormal structure of the elastic fibers, which may cause skin laxity and the loss of resiliency after stretching. Loss of elastic microfibrils and the appearance of cavities are also highly characteristic of biological aging. Collagen is a tougher, more stable material and does not show the well-defined aging changes that are seen with elastic fibers. However, there is less collagen per surface area in aging skin, and it is less dense and stiffer, probably owing to progressive cross-linking. Also, the fibers of collagen appear thickened and stain differently. The three-dimensional meshwork of collagen becomes distorted from many years of mechanical stress and, in this way, contributes to the laxity, sagging, and wrinkling of older skin.

One of the marked differences between the sexes is that men have a thicker dermis than women across all age groups. Similarly, collagen density is greater in men than women, although the rate of collagen loss is similar in both sexes. These differences may explain why facial skin of women appears to show greater deterioration with age.

Additional age-related dermal changes affect fibroblasts, which become smaller and show decreased metabolic activity and a decreased proliferation rate. The concentrations of glycosaminoglycans—an important factor in the water-holding capacity of the dermis—are stable until about 40 years of age and then fall continuously. This decrease of glycosaminoglycans that is observed in later years may be due to decreased synthesis and might have explained the dry and wrinkled appearance of aged skin. However, biological aging does not appear to alter the water structure significantly.

Other Changes

With age, lipid content of the skin decreases, and lipid composition changes. And, although the fat content of the subcutaneous layer is greater in women than in men, the distribution of subcutaneous fat changes and the volume decreases in both sexes as they age. Androgen-dependent production of sebum by the sebaceous glands begins to decrease in postmenopausal women and declines steadily thereafter. The clinical consequences are a 40% to 50% decrease in sebum output, which may account for the prevalence of dry skin in older women. Excessive use of soaps and cosmetics and actinic damage may be even more important. In men, the output of sebum does not begin to decline until about their early 70s. The secretions of sweat glands are also diminished. Table 1.3 shows skin changes in biological aging.

TABLE 1.3   Skin Changes in Biological Aging

Skin Component	Histological Change	Clinical Change
Elastic fibers	• Decreased amount • Abnormal structure	• Skin laxity • Loss of resiliency
Collagen	• Less per surface area • Less dense and stiffer • Three-dimensional meshwork becomes distorted	• Laxity • Sagging • Wrinkling
Glycosaminoglycans	Decreased synthesis	• Dryness • Wrinkling
Subcutaneous fat	Decreased volume	• Loss of full and plump skin appearance

PHOTOAGING

Ongoing photoaging results in marked changes to both the epidermal and dermal layers that are distinct from those observed with biological aging (see Table 1.2). Photoaging of the skin is broadly characterized by hypertrophy. Sebaceous glands become enlarged, and neoplastic growths are frequent. In marked contrast to biologically aging skin, the dermis of photodamaged aging skin thickens, and small blood vessels become dilated and deranged. The microvasculature collapses, showing only a few dilated, thickened, tortuous vessels. In addition, the number of hair follicles is reduced, and hair thinning is more prominent than in biologically aged skin. Figure 1.4 shows a patient with photoaging and fine wrinkles.

Epidermal Damage

Excessive sun exposure causes significant changes in the epidermis. Melanocytes increase, enlarge, and become more branched. Keratinocytes may become vacuolated and necrotic or show variation in size, shape, and staining properties. The thickness of the photodamaged epidermis is variable, with alternating areas of atrophy and hyperplasia. It is thought that atrophy may result from depletion of cells from the basal layer, whereas areas of hyperplasia may reflect compensatory overgrowth of UV-damaged tissue.

Not surprisingly, many of these morphological changes are associated with clinical changes in the appearance of the skin. Melanocyte hyperplasia causes irregular pigmentation interspersed with more severely damaged areas in which melanocytes are depleted or unable to transfer pigment to keratinocytes. Hyperplastic melanocytes that produce great amounts of pigment give rise to solar lentigines. Also known as liver spots, solar lentigines are benign lesions that occur on photodamaged skin. Most lightly pigmented persons develop solar lentigines on sun-exposed hands, wrists, arms, neck, and face in middle age. Injury to basal keratinocytes results in a scaly stratum corneum and actinic keratoses.

Dermal Damage

Many of the visible signs of deterioration in photoaged skin reflect major structural changes in the dermis. The dominant change to the dermis is hyperplasia of the elastic tissue, ending in complete disorganization. Compared with biologically aged skin, new apparently abnormal elastin accumulates, whereas elastin degradation is slowed. The degree of elastosis correlates with the amount of sun exposure. Histologically, large quantities of thickened, tangled, disorganized, and degraded elastic fibers are seen, and with extreme damage, an amorphous mass of what once was elastic tissue is present. In sun-protected skin, elastosis this extensive is never seen, even in people of advanced age.

Together with hyperplasia of the elastic tissue, collagen fibers become fragmented, thickened, and more soluble in sun-damaged skin, whereas glycosaminoglycans increase. Collagen is degraded as a result of the upregulation of collagen-degrading enzymes that occurs in response to UVB radiation. In contrast, mature collagen appears to become more stable and resistant to enzymatic degradation with biological age.

Box 1.9

Maintaining Proper Skin Functioning

Despite the effects of aging, it is theoretically possible to keep the skin functioning properly throughout life so that it overcomes damage from the environment and remains in a healthy state.

MAINTAINING SKIN HEALTH AND FUNCTION THROUGHOUT LIFE

Facial skin is remarkable for its ability to reveal health or disease of the skin, as well as that of the other organs of the body. Genetics, environmental exposure, hormonal changes, and metabolic processes, alone or together, lead to changes in skin structure, function, tolerance, and appearance. Moisturizers, so popular in over-the-counter products, cannot slow the progress of these intricate and inter-related changes. In fact, moisturizers slow down the rate of natural exfoliation, causing decreased skin tolerance, dullness, dryness, and actual moisturizer addiction. Yet consumers continue to purchase moisturizers in the hope that "this one will be different." For profound beneficial clinical changes, skin must be treated on the cellular level with agents that target different layers and cells of the skin. The restoration and maintenance of skin health should be based on many of the anatomical and physiological properties of the skin reviewed in this chapter. This volume presents the advances in Skin Health Restoration that allow the maintenance of skin health and function throughout life. The principles of skin health are defined and described, skin-conditioning processes are presented, and simple, standardized programs are explained. It is time to end patients' moisturizer addiction and give them the solutions that lead to fundamental and lasting changes. Box 1.9 discusses a view on maintaining proper skin functioning throughout life.

REFERENCES

1. McGrath JA, Uitto J. Anatomy and organization of human skin. In: Burns T, Breathnach S, Cox N, Griffiths C, eds. *Rook's Textbook of Dermatology.* 8th ed. Oxford: Wiley-Blackwell; 2010:Ch 3.
2. Bergstresser PR, Costner MI. Anatomy and physiology. In: Bolognia J, Jorizzo JK, Rapini RP, eds. *Dermatology.* 2nd ed. Edinburgh: Elsevier; 2007:25-35.
3. Piérard GE, Paquet P, Xhauflaire-Uhoda E, Quatresooz P. Physiological variations during aging. In: Farage MA, Miller KW, Maibach HI, eds. *Textbook of Aging Skin.* Berlin: Springer-Verlag; 2010:45-54.
4. Glogau RG. Systematic evaluation of the aging face. In: Bolognia J, Jorizzo JK, Rapini RP, eds. *Dermatology.* 2nd ed. Edinburgh: Elsevier; 2007:2295-2299.
5. Piérard GE, Paquet P, Xhauflaire-Uhoda E, Quatresooz P. Physiological variations during aging. In: Farage MA, Miller KW, Maibach HI, eds. *Textbook of Aging Skin.* Berlin: Springer-Verlag; 2010:45-54.

6. Raschke C, Elsner R. Skin aging: a brief summary of characteristic changes. In: Farage MA, Miller KW, Maibach HI, eds. *Textbook of Aging Skin.* Berlin: Springer-Verlag; 2010:37-43.

7. Elsner P, Fluhr JW, Gehring W, et al. Anti-aging data and support claims: consensus statement. *J Dtsch Dermatol Ges.* 2011;9(Suppl 3):S1-S32.

8. Makrantonaki E, Zouboulis CC. Skin alterations and diseases in advanced age. *Drug Discov Today Dis Mec.* 2008;5:e153-e162.

9. Farage MA, Miller KW, Maibach HI. Degenerative changes in aging skin. In: Farage MA, Miller KW, Maibach HI, eds. *Textbook of Aging Skin.* Berlin: Springer-Verlag; 2010:25-35.

10. Kanitakis J. Anatomy, histology and immunohistochemistry of normal human skin. *Eur J Dermatol.* 2002;12:390-401.

11. Stanley JR. Synergy of understanding dermatologic disease and epidermal biology. *J Clin Invest.* 2012;122:436-439.

12. Gilchrest BA. Aging of differentiated cells (excluding the fibroblast) in skin: *in vitro* studies. In: Kligman AM, Balin AK, eds. *Aging and the Skin.* New York: Raven Press; 1993:77-92.

13. Arin MJ, Roop DR, Koch PJ, Koster MI. Biology of keratinocytes. In: Bolognia J, Jorizzo JK, Rapini RP, eds. *Dermatology.* 2nd ed. Edinburgh: Elsevier; 2007:731-742.

14. Balin AK, Lin AN. Skin changes as a biological marker for measuring the rate of human aging. In: Kligman AM, Balin AK, eds. *Aging and the Skin.* New York: Raven Press; 1993:43-75.

15. Kligman AM, Balin AK. Aging of human skin. In: Kligman AM, Balin AK, eds. *Aging and the Skin.* New York: Raven Press; 1993:1-42.

16. Grove GL. Age-associated changes in human epidermal cell renewal and repair. In: Kligman AM, Balin AK, eds. *Aging and the Skin.* New York: Raven Press; 1993:193-204.

17. Bolognia JL, Orlow SJ. Melanocyte biology. In: Bolognia J, Jorizzo JK, Rapini RP, eds. *Dermatology.* 2nd ed. Edinburgh: Elsevier; 2007:901-911.

18. Bolognia JL, Pawelek JM. Biology of hypopigmentation. *J Am Acad Dermatol.* 1988;19:217-255.

19. Thody AJ. Skin pigmentation and its regulation. In: Priestley GC, ed. *Molecular Aspects of Dermatology.* Chichester, UK: John Wiley & Sons; 1993:55-73.

20. Schwartz T. Immunology. In: Bolognia J, Jorizzo JK, Rapini RP, eds. *Dermatology.* 2nd ed. Edinburgh: Elsevier; 2007:63-79.

21. Krieg T, Aumailley M. The extracellular matrix of the dermis: flexible structures with dynamic functions. *Exp Dermatol.* 2011;20:689-695.

22. Matsuoka LY, Uitto J. Alterations in the elastic fibers in cutaneous aging and solar elastosis. In: Kligman AM, Balin AK, eds. *Aging and the Skin.* New York: Raven Press; 1993:141-151.

23. Ghersetich I, Lotti T, Campanile G, et al. Hyaluronic acid in cutaneous intrinsic aging. *Int J Dermatol.* 1994;33:119-122.

24. Kamell JM, Maibach HI. A quantitative approach to anatomy and physiology of aging skin: barrier, dermal structure, and perfusion. In: Baran R, Maibach HI, eds. *Textbook of Cosmetic Dermatology.* 4th ed. London: Informa Healthcare; 2010:14-27.

25. Tur E. Skin physiology and gender. In: Baran R, Maibach HI, eds. *Textbook of Cosmetic Dermatology.* 4th ed. London: Informa Healthcare; 2010:1-13.

26. Assaf H, Adly MA, Hussein MR. Aging and intrinsic aging: pathogenesis and manifestations. In: Farage MA, Miller KW, Maibach HI, eds. *Textbook of Aging Skin.* Berlin: Springer-Verlag; 2010:129-138.

27. Kligman L. Skin changes in photoaging: characteristics, prevention, and repair. In: Kligman AM, Balin AK, eds. *Aging and the Skin.* New York: Raven Press; 1993:331-346.

28. Yaar M, Gilchrest BA. Biochemical and molecular changes in photoaged skin. In: Gilchrest BA, ed. *Photodamage.* Cambridge, UK: Blackwell Scientific; 1995:168-184.

PRINCIPLES AND OBJECTIVES OF SKIN HEALTH RESTORATION

A LIFETIME OF HEALTHY SKIN

This chapter presents the original principles and objectives of the Skin Health Restoration program that were developed over the past 30 years. These comprehensive solutions defy the traditional narrow focus on skin *disease* and aim to provide truly healthy skin for the lifetime of any individual, regardless of age, sex, race, or skin condition. Current dermatology training, published literature, and clinical practice focus mostly on the treatment of skin disease and do not address overall skin health. This situation gives rise to a number of questions, including the following: 1) If a patient has no active skin *disease,* is his or her skin healthy? 2) Is skin health restored when a skin disease has been treated and cleared? 3) Is it advisable to wait for a disease to appear, or should we intervene to prevent its appearance? 4) Is maintenance of skin integrity and function not as important as resolving a disease or performing a procedure to improve the appearance of skin? Our answers to these questions may reveal deficiencies in the current mainstream attitude toward skin health.

HEALTHY SKIN: DEFINITION AND MODEL

Skin health does not have a widely accepted definition or model—it means different things to different people throughout the world. Healthy skin is frequently described as beautiful, flawless, glowing, and young, but these terms are imprecise and reflect subjective and nonquantifiable characteristics. The definition of skin health introduced in 1983 and expanded in 2008 provides specific, easily recognized physiological, histological, and clinical characteristics. Specifically, healthy skin is smooth, even in color tone, firm and tight, well hydrated, tolerant to external factors, contour rich, and free

> **Box 2.1**
>
> **Skin Health Defined**
>
> - Smooth
> - Even in color
> - Firm and tight
> - Well hydrated
> - Tolerant
> - Contour rich
> - Free of active disease

from underlying disease (Box 2.1). Skin treatments must correct any abnormalities in skin health that deviate from this definition so that the skin attains desirable attributes.

The definition of healthy skin has many applications. The first is in establishing a comprehensive patient diagnosis by listing the common characteristics of healthy skin and then determining which of these are lacking in the skin of the patient being evaluated (Table 2.1). The practitioner must then create a treatment plan that corrects any abnormalities (based on the definition) by treating the patient's skin disease. The definition also improves the physician's ability to monitor the progress of a topical product regimen aimed at Skin Health Restoration and for judging treatment results and success rates. Figure 2.1 highlights characteristics of a baby's skin, which illustrate the goals for achieving success in any comprehensive topical Skin Health Restoration treatment regimen. Table 2.2 delineates each of the main characteristics of healthy skin as seen in a baby and identifies the etiology behind each of these characteristics.

SKIN PHASES OVER A LIFETIME

Most of us begin life with healthy, unflawed skin. However, environmental/external and internal factors, hereditary factors, and the natural,

TABLE 2.1 Definition of Skin Health: Attribute Presence versus Absence

Attribute Present (Optimized Skin Health)	*Attribute Absence (Sub-Optimal Skin Health)*
Smooth	Rough
Evenly colored	Dyschromic
Firm	Weak (little to no resistance to shearing force)
Tight	Lax
Hydrated	Dry
Tolerant	Intolerant
Contour rich	Hollow, sunken
Free of underlying disease(s)	Underlying disease present

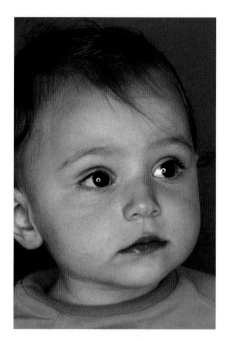

FIGURE 2.1 Healthy skin. This 1-year-old girl has skin that embodies each major skin health attribute.

TABLE 2.2 Factors Underlying Skin Health Characteristics

Characteristic	Factors
Smooth	Soft, compact stratum corneum and minimal basket-weaving (histology)
	Continuous epidermal cell renewal and repair owing to balanced and regulated keratinocyte maturation cycles (KMCs). (Each cycle is approximately 6 weeks; KMCs are described later in this chapter.)
Firm	Abundant, optimally functioning collagen
Tight	Abundant, optimally functioning collagen and elastin
Evenly colored	Properly functioning melanocytes
Well hydrated	Abundance of glycosaminoglycans (thus, no need for external moisturization)
Intact barrier function	Smooth stratum corneum with little to no basket-weaving.
	Multiple layers of corneocytes that are bound well together
	Overlying stratum granulosum and stratum lucidum below the numerous layers of well-defined, pink keratinocytes arising from the basal layer
Heals rapidly and properly	Effective renewal of keratinocytes
	Good circulation
Contour rich	Optimal volume of collagen, elastin, and subcutaneous tissue
Free of clinically active disease	Normal skin histology

chronological changes associated with aging proceed to undo what was ours at birth. With the passage of time, activities promoting skin health decrease, and a deterioration of skin quality begins. The skin is not diseased, but intrinsic aging and photoaging have caused anatomical, physiological, and clinical changes. These range from a sensation of dryness and the appearance of dull, weathered skin, to the appearance of wrinkling, jowling, laxity, hypertrophy, and easy bruising. Although these changes (phases) may not be clinically detectable at an early stage, they are occurring and will become detectable at a later age. It may be surprising to learn that skin reaches a relatively inactive phase at age 30, with decreased cellular function and the appearance of wrinkles. The phases skin passes through in a lifetime are shown in Box 2.2; they are divided into one of the following three categories: a healthy (optimally active) phase, an altered (deteriorated) phase, and an inactive phase. Some of the most common causes of skin deterioration may be controllable, whereas others are not (Table 2.3). Of note, many of the individual factors leading to skin deterioration have inflammation as an underlying cause.

SIGNIFICANT FACTORS IN ACHIEVING SKIN HEALTH

The skin health definition presented previously described the external characteristics of healthy skin, whereas the baby skin model specified the

Box 2.2

Skin Phases over a Lifetime

HEALTHY (OPTIMALLY ACTIVE) SKIN PHASE

- From birth to age 9 or 10 years
- Embodies the definition of optimal skin health
- Optimized epidermal and dermal cellular function and continuous, regular cell renewal and repair (normal KMC*)
- No sebum production
- No chronic inflammation
- No dryness or sensitivity

ALTERED (DETERIORATED) SKIN PHASE

- From age 10 to 30 years
- Begins to diverge from the main characteristics that define optimal skin health
- Irregular cellular functions, including impaired epidermal cell renewal (abnormal KMC*)
- Impaired skin barrier function
- Sebum produced at varying levels
- Chronic inflammation
- Textural irregularities
- Enlarged pores, dyschromia, atrophy, sebaceous gland hyperplasia, and a "dull" appearance
- Skin disease may be present or beginning to appear

INACTIVE SKIN PHASE

- Begins at age 30 years
- Progressively greater deviation from the characteristics that define optimal skin health (compared with the previous two phases)
- Irregular epidermal cellular function (abnormalities in KMCs*)
- Weakened, impaired barrier function
- Chronic inflammation
- Advanced textural changes and irregularity
- Conspicuous signs of extrinsic and intrinsic aging (e.g., hypertrophy, atrophy)
- Laxity and wrinkles (due to damaged existing collagen and elastin in combination with an overall decrease in the production of collagen and elastin)
- Increased likelihood of concurrent skin disease

*The keratinocyte maturation cycle (KMC) is described later in this chapter.

TABLE 2.3	Common Causes of Skin Deterioration
Controllable	**Uncontrollable**
Excess sebum production (abnormality of pilosebaceous units)	Genetic factors and skin type
Dysfunctional melanocytes	Intrinsic and chronological aging changes
Sun exposure	Abnormalities in the skin caused by an underlying, incurable, systemic disease (including immunological disorders); many of these can have an unpredictable course*
Unhealthy diet (e.g., high glycemic index and/or excessive hormonal exposure through the consumption of nonorganic dairy products), lifestyle, unsuitable topically applied products	
Medications (some systemic medications have effects on the skin)	
Complications of surgical and nonsurgical rejuvenation procedures	
Exposure to irritants and allergens	
Prolonged use of certain medical and nonmedical topical agents (i.e., topical steroid–induced skin atrophy)	
Chronic inflammation	

*Some chronic, incurable, systemic disorders and their associated skin inflammation (e.g., lupus erythematosus) can be controlled with medications; however, regardless of periods of control with medications, many are associated with an unpredictable course.

physiological, histological, and clinical characteristics of such skin. The next step was to determine the factors and processes that negatively influence skin health so that treatment programs could be created to help restore it. Investigations and clinical experience have revealed that the areas of most concern in skin health include the following: the integrity of the skin barrier function, duration of the KMC, and presence of chronic inflammation (Box 2.3).

SKIN BARRIER FUNCTION

It would be hard to overstate the importance of an intact barrier function in skin health. As a physical, chemical, and immunological barrier, it prevents penetration of harmful substances and excessive transepidermal water loss. We do not currently know all of the intricate mechanisms of the barrier function, but we do know that the barrier function can be repaired by following the ZO Skin Health Restoration principles using topical regimens.

Box 2.3

Factors Responsible for Skin Health

- Skin barrier function
- Keratinocyte maturation cycle (KMC)
- Chronic inflammation

The barrier function acts as a protective skin envelope consisting of 1) a matrix of water, lipids, and proteins that surrounds keratinocytes and corneocytes and 2) stratum corneum cells (corneocytes), which are keratinocytes that have completed their differentiation process, having lost their nuclei and cytoplasmic organelles. As new corneocytes appear, the older cells are shed through desquamation. The normal/healthy barrier function relies on a 40-day cycle of epidermal renewal (the KMC); this entails the production of new cells through mitosis within the basal cell layer, which subsequently mature to become corneocytes. Corneocytes are arranged in multiple layers, enveloped by the natural matrix of water, lipids, and proteins. These two components need to be in balance and work together to maintain the integrity of the barrier function. Disturbances of either component result in a compromised barrier function.

Moisturizers, which contain approximately the same components (water, lipids, and proteins) as the skin's natural elements, impair the skin's barrier function. Specifically, when a moisturizer is applied to the skin surface, cells on the surface detect a large amount of moisture and send a message to the body to stop delivering water to the skin (essentially, a feedback loop). To clarify, externally applied moisturizers alter the balance of water, lipids, and proteins in the skin, which leads to a compromised barrier function and to an acquired skin sensitivity.

Externally applied moisturizers are also detrimental in that they interfere with the natural exfoliation and desquamation of corneocytes (dead keratinocytes). Under normal circumstances, the KMC regulates natural skin exfoliation in a proper manner. But when moisturizers are applied, corneocytes within the stratum corneum do not exfoliate in the usual fashion but accumulate on the surface instead. This accumulation sends a message to the basal cell layer to terminate mitosis and slow down or end the creation of new keratinocytes. With repeated application of moisturizers, new epidermal cells stop being created in the basal cell layer. Subsequently, with repeated application of moisturizers, the epidermis thins, the barrier function is compromised, and skin becomes more sensitive. Box 2.4 shows barrier function activities.

Box 2.4

Barrier Function Activities

- Transmission of messages from superficial to deeper layers of the skin, which is intended to elicit appropriate responses following exposure to external stimuli
- Maintenance of proper natural epidermal hydration (e.g., minimization of transepidermal water loss)
- Enhancement of epidermal renewal and repair, which is responsible for building and maintaining skin tolerance

THE KERATINOCYTE MATURATION CYCLE

As briefly mentioned previously, the skin's normal barrier function depends on a 40-day cycle of epidermal renewal, the KMC. This cycle is the foundation of Skin Health Restoration because without adequate epidermal exfoliation and subsequent replacement with fresh, active cells, skin health is compromised. A properly regulated KMC is essential for the production of skin that is naturally hydrated and tolerant of detrimental external stimuli. In this text, the term KMC is synonymous with the process of natural skin exfoliation because each can be measured in time. The term KMC describes the amount of time it takes for a keratinocyte to mature and transform into a corneocyte, reach the stratum corneum, and subsequently exfoliate from the surface of the epidermis (Figure 2.2). This normal 40-day cycle is shortened in certain diseases such as psoriasis, malignant tumors, and verruca. The cycle can be lengthened as a result of intrinsic aging, photoaging, and the use of moisturizers and topical corticosteroids. The main objective of Skin Health Restoration regimens is to restore normal maturation cycles, which restores optimal skin barrier functions. Normal barrier function, in turn, increases skin tolerance. Skin should have developed a good level of tolerance before undergoing any rejuvenation procedure.

Benefits of Regulating the Keratinocyte Maturation Cycle

Completion of two to three KMCs while using Skin Health Restoration principles and certain topical agents will establish sufficient skin tolerance and produce a number of clinical benefits (Box 2.5). The stratum corneum becomes smooth, soft, and compact, with a minimal basket-weave pattern. Mitosis in the basal layer, as well as within adnexal structures, proceeds at an optimal rate, producing a population of healthy keratinocytes and a thicker epidermis. Bacterial flora are reduced, and comedones and enlarged pores decrease in size and number. The skin becomes properly hydrated and does not need externally applied moisturizers. With restoration of the skin's barrier function, the skin's tolerance to cosmetics, dermatological treatments, and other external or environmental factors increases, and the pigmentary system is effectively controlled.

In general, one to two maturation cycles produce a good level of tolerance; three maturation cycles (5 months) are needed to renew most of the epidermis. Renewal of the epidermis entails repairing damaged DNA, producing and maintaining adequate amounts of soft keratin, fully restoring hydration, and regulating natural skin exfoliation. With an aggressive Skin Health Restoration program, tolerance (to the initial expected amount of erythema,

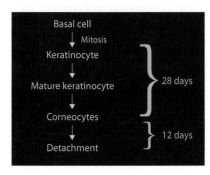

Figure 2.2 The keratin maturation cycle (KMC) describes the amount of time it takes for a keratinocyte to fully mature as it rises upward from the basal cell layer and is eventually shed from the surface of the epidermis. Specifically, the KMC describes the transformation of keratinocytes to corneocytes as they reach the stratum corneum, continue to rise upward from the basal cell layer, and ultimately exfoliate from the surface of the epidermis.

> ### Box 2.5
>
> **Benefits of Regulating Keratinocyte Maturation Cycles**
>
> - Skin surface is smooth and soft.
> - Epidermis is thicker.
> - Bacterial flora, comedones, and enlarged pores are reduced.
> - Skin is properly hydrated and does not need externally applied moisturizers.
> - Tolerance to cosmetics, dermatological treatments, and other external or environmental factors is increased.
> - Skin tone is uniform from control of the pigmentary system.

TABLE 2.4   Treatment Strength and Number of Keratinocyte Maturation Cycles for Epidermal Renewal and Restoration of Barrier Function

Treatment Strength	Number of Keratinocyte Maturation Cycles
Aggressive	1 (6 weeks)
Standard	2-3 (12-18 weeks)
Mild	4-6 (23-34 weeks)

dryness, and peeling of the treated skin) can usually be attained after one KMC (6 weeks). With less aggressive approaches, tolerance takes longer to achieve: 2 to 3 months with a moderately aggressive approach, 4 to 6 months with a standard approach, and up to 8 months with a mild approach. The duration of treatment time (as quantified by the number of KMCs) necessary for optimal epidermal renewal and barrier function restoration is correlated to the intensity and strength of the topical regimen (as shown in Table 2.4).

SKIN INFLAMMATION

We have reviewed skin barrier function and regulation of the KMC as two of the three significant factors that must be addressed in Skin Health Restoration. The third significant factor is inflammation. Humans are at risk for invasion and destruction by agents that penetrate or damage skin, including disease, bacteria, viruses, fungi, irritants, heat, and ultraviolet (UV) light. When any of these invaders strike, the skin mounts a defense in the form of acute inflammation. Acute inflammation, manifested by pain, erythema, exfoliation, and swelling, is beneficial in that it is a natural defense against the invader and an attempt to limit its spread. With proper treatment, acute inflammation can be corrected in 2 to 3 weeks. If acute inflammation is not promptly and adequately treated, the inflammation becomes chronic, more destructive, and difficult to treat.

Chronic inflammation can also occur without a preceding acute phase, as is seen with chronic sun exposure, glycation, diabetes, lupus, and exposure to photosensitizing agents. Chronic inflammation can manifest as skin sensitivity, dryness, impaired healing, eruptions, and erythema and is highly prevalent among dermatology patients. It is because of chronic inflammation that skin deteriorates rapidly after the age of 10 years. This is the age at which one's sebaceous glands begin to become active and produce sebum (excessive sebum induces inflammation).

Chronic inflammation, seen in various conditions including seborrhea, rosacea, acne, sensitivity, and dryness, is frequently observed in clinical practice and is responsible for patient discomfort and treatment failure. Despite its importance, many dermatologists do not recognize the need for addressing chronic inflammation when treating skin and instead focus mostly on treating symptoms and specific diseases. Such symptomatic treatment often fails if the factors causing the chronic inflammation are not identified and eliminated. For example, if sebum, a strong inflammatory agent responsible for acne, seborrhea, and rosacea, is not reduced, treatment of these conditions either fails or provides only short-term symptomatic relief.

One 5-month course of *low-dose* isotretinoin (20 mg per day) can eliminate sebum and facilitate the elimination of chronic inflammation. As a side note, both acute and chronic inflammatory acneiform conditions tend to be localized in small areas (e.g., face, neck, back, and chest) where sebaceous glands are present that produce excessive sebum and a localized immune response in the affected area. This same focal response to excessive sebum can be seen in patients with melasma and postinflammatory hyperpigmentation where the localized response is the face. Box 2.6 highlights important aspects of acute versus chronic inflammation. Box 2.7 highlights the most common manifestations of acute skin inflammation. Table 2.5 shows the manifestations of chronic inflammation.

Box 2.6

Acute versus Chronic Skin Inflammation

Acute inflammation is a protective repair process that is triggered by exposure of the skin to various insults (e.g., excess sebum). Chronic inflammation is destructive and gradually damages both skin texture and cellular function.

Box 2.7

Manifestations of Acute Skin Inflammation

- Erythema
- Dryness
- Edema
- Pain
- Irritability and sensitivity
- Exfoliation

TABLE 2.5   Manifestations of Chronic Skin Inflammation

Condition	Clinical Manifestations
Textural abnormalities	Solar elastosis; sebaceous gland hyperplasia
Skin sensitivity and dryness	Impaired barrier function
Dyschromia	Melanocyte instability leading to hyperactivity
Impaired healing	Cellular dysfunction
Accelerated signs of aging	Thinning of dermis, melanocyte instability, solar elastosis, etc.
Treatment failure	Offending insults to skin not adequately eliminated

Box 2.8

Halting Chronic Inflammation

The key to halting chronic inflammation is to induce a limited amount (about 2 to 4 weeks) of acute inflammation.

Treatment of Skin Inflammation

If acute inflammation in the skin is left untreated, chronic inflammation will follow. Eliminating the triggering factors easily terminates acute inflammation. This repairs and restores the barrier function, the normal renewal cycle of the epidermis, and offers symptomatic relief. In contrast, treating or eliminating chronic inflammation is more difficult in that detecting the offending factor may be more complex. Chronic inflammation may be difficult to diagnose in certain patients. Furthermore, physicians should know that chronic inflammation does not have a specific and effective treatment.

Observing the distinctly different processes involved in acute and chronic inflammation led to development of a unique treatment approach that involves the *induction of acute inflammation* to ultimately *treat* chronic inflammation. This approach restores the skin's innate ability to renew itself, while also reestablishing a strong barrier function and eliminating any inciting triggers. In short, chronic inflammation is fought by activating defense mechanisms induced by acute inflammation (Box 2.8).

In short, to eliminate chronic skin inflammation, we need to induce a limited (2- to 4-week) phase of acute inflammation through use of specific topical agents. This will enable the skin to generate its own natural mechanism to stop acute inflammation and simultaneously eliminate the existing chronic inflammation. The phases of Skin Health Restoration and the corresponding topical agents used for the elimination of chronic inflammation are presented later in this chapter.

SKIN HEALTH RESTORATION PRINCIPLES

For many years, dermatologists have focused on treating signs and symptoms of a patient's skin disease without identifying and subsequently correcting the

> **Box 2.9**
>
> **Skin Health Restoration Principles**
>
> 1. Preparation
> 2. Correction
> 3. Stabilization
> 4. Stimulation and pigmentation control
>   a. Bleaching by use of hydroquinone (HQ) or blending (topical retinoid + HQ)
>   b. Melanocyte stabilization by use of non-HQ agents
> 5. Hydration and calming
> 6. Ultraviolet light protection

cellular dysfunction underlying the condition. Frequently, these physicians administer a procedure as a first line of treatment. This approach may initially improve the appearance of the skin condition, but because the underlying source of the problem was not directly addressed, any or all improvement is typically limited and short-lived. In the long run, results of these treatments are often variable, with some patients improving greatly, others less, and some not at all. If the patient subsequently complains that the condition has failed to improve or resolve completely, he or she is often told that the recommended treatment is the current standard of care and that no other effective treatment options are currently available.

An unwillingness to simply accept this restrained and superficial approach led to many years spent studying and developing the science of skin health, which ultimately resulted in the generation of the six key principles of Skin Health Restoration (Box 2.9). These principles standardize the treatment approaches to both medical and nonmedical skin problems and eliminate variables that typically cause treatments to fail. (Nonmedical skin problems are skin changes without an underlying disease; examples include acquired sensitivity, acquired dryness, textural irregularities, and nonspecific dyschromia.) By following these six key principles, physicians are able not only to improve a patient's disease but also to restore overall skin health.

SKIN PREPARATION

The skin preparation process entails normalizing the skin surface to prepare it for the steps that follow. It involves cleansing, scrubbing (mechanical exfoliation), toning (if skin is dry and/or the pH is imbalanced), and oil and sebum control (Table 2.6). The wash, scrub, and sebum control steps are essential for preparing skin to become a "clean slate" for subsequent correction, stabilization, and stimulation. Minimizing excess sebum by use of an astringent (often containing salicylic acid as one of its active ingredients) is essential to correct abnormalities related to the pilosebaceous units, such as acne (including rosacea), seborrheic dermatitis, sebaceous gland hyperplasia, or simply the sebum in patients with oily skin.

TABLE 2.6   Skin Preparation: Processes and Purposes

Process	Purpose
Wash/cleanse	Removal of surface impurities
Scrub	Mechanical exfoliation
	Stimulation of epidermal renewal
	Regulation of surface keratin
	Elimination of microcomedone formation
	Stimulation of circulation
	Restoration of normal skin pH
Tone	Restoration of pH balance when a patient's skin is dry or thin; in these patients, a scrub is needed only twice a week (vs. every day, as recommended for all other patients)
Sebum control	Prevention of induction and progression of chronic inflammation from excessive sebum production
	Provision of antibacterial benefit
	Prevention of microcomedone formation and progression
	Tightening of enlarged pores
	Enhanced penetration of subsequently applied therapeutic topical agents

CORRECTION OF THE SKIN

The objective of the correction principle is to repair and enhance epidermal renewal, to restore and maintain proper skin barrier function, and to normalize skin color and pigmentation. Epidermal repair involves regular application of specific essential topical agents such as tretinoin (retinoic acid), alpha-hydroxy acids (AHAs), and hydroquinone (HQ), as well as the concurrent application of disease-specific agents (if necessary). In relatively uncomplicated cases, correction may be the only principle necessary for skin health maintenance, treatment and prevention of acne, and correction of nonspecific epidermal dyspigmentation in children and teenagers.

STABILIZATION

Stabilization, a new principle in Skin Health Restoration, is a process to regulate, stimulate, and repair and control cellular functions in both the epidermis and dermis. The effects of stabilization are shown in Box 2.10.

Certain topical agents are needed for stabilization, such as tretinoin/retinol, antioxidants, anti-inflammatory agents, and DNA repair agents, which are an essential part of ZOSH and ZOMD formulations. The goals of epidermal and dermal stabilization are shown in Table 2.7.

After successful correction and stabilization, the epidermis and dermis appear thicker in each layer on histologic examination, with both the epidermis and the dermis having more mucinous material (specifically, glycosaminoglycans). Melanocytes exhibit more uniform activity, with fewer melanosomes. The main histologic changes associated with successful correction and stabilization of the epidermis are shown in Table 2.8.

Box 2.10

Effects of Stabilization

1. DNA is repaired, and sun-damaged atypical keratinocytes are gradually shed—to be replaced by a healthier cell population.
2. Barrier function is restored.
3. Soft keratin production increases.
4. Epidermis becomes thicker.
5. Pores are unclogged, reducing the chance of acne or folliculitis.
6. Melanocytes become resistant to activation on exposure to ultraviolet light, drugs, irritants, epidermal injury, procedures, and acute and chronic inflammation (prevents melanin overproduction).
7. Prevents and treats dyschromia when bleaching with hydroquinone is contraindicated.
8. When a procedure is to be performed on the skin, adequate preprocedure stabilization as part of skin conditioning shortens the healing phase and reduces certain complications (e.g., postinflammatory hyperpigmentation).

Clinically, correction and stabilization of the epidermis are manifested by a softer, more resilient (spongy-feeling), uniformly pigmented, and well-hydrated epidermis that is optimally tolerant to negative external stimuli and free of underlying medical problems. Similarly, clinical examination of the dermis reveals significantly firmer, resilient, and more youthful skin.

STIMULATION

Stimulation is the process of improving both the epidermis and the dermis through use of tretinoin. When the combination of correction, stabilization, stimulation, and bleaching and blending principles is used to treat a disease, the objective is general skin repair, which is usually accomplished within

TABLE 2.7	Objectives of Epidermal and Dermal Stabilization
Epidermal stabilization	Strengthen barrier function (improves tolerance to detrimental stimuli, e.g., ultraviolet light, contact irritants, certain topical agents) to render skin more tolerant and able to resist the negative effects of external and internal stimuli
	Optimize natural exfoliation by regulation of keratinocyte maturation cycles
	Repair damaged DNA
	Restore adequate hydration
	Control melanin production and prevent melanocyte activation
Dermal stabilization	Optimize fibroblast production of collagen and elastin
	Improve repair of preexisting, damaged collagen and elastin
	Increase glycosaminoglycans
	Improve circulation*

*By optimizing dermal stabilization, the epidermis also improves through improved perfusion of oxygen and nutrients to the basal cell layer.

TABLE 2.8   Histologic Findings associated with Dermal and Epidermal Correction and Stabilization

Epidermis	Finding
Stratum corneum	Compact with minimal basket-weaving
Stratum granulosum	Thicker with coarse granules
Stratum spinosum	More uniform keratinocytes, no atypia
Stratum basalis	Increased, controlled mitosis
Dermis	Finding
Papillary dermis	Intact collagen and elastin
	No inflammatory cellular infiltrate
	Abundance of glycosaminoglycans

three KMCs. After completion of any medical treatment, general repair ends, and the objective becomes specific repair through dermal stabilization with retinol because patients without underlying medical conditions need only specific repair as a basic, daily preventative and anti-aging skin care regimen. Specifically, stimulation involves improving the papillary dermis in one of two ways. First, in skin without pigmentation abnormalities, "general repair" is accomplished through application of tretinoin, which stimulates the production of collagen, elastin, and glycosaminoglycans. It also improves circulation (nutrient and oxygen delivery to individual cells). In skin with pigmentation abnormalities, optimal stimulation is achieved through the process of blending, which entails application of a mixture of tretinoin and HQ. This ultimately restores a uniformly even color tone (Table 2.9).

Of note, when used alone, topically applied HQ bleaches the skin ("bleaching"). However, when used concurrently with tretinoin (by mixing), HQ forces an even distribution of melanin to all neighboring keratinocytes ("blending"). To clarify, when used in combination with tretinoin, HQ does not bleach the skin as it does when HQ is used alone. Also note that the stimulation mentioned previously affects only the papillary dermis and not the reticular

TABLE 2.9   Tretinoin and Hydroquinone Use in Skin Stimulation

Baseline Skin Condition	Process	Purpose (General Repair)
Dyschromia absent	Tretinoin applied alone	Dermal stimulation: Upregulates angioblast function, which improves circulation with associated increased oxygen and nutrient delivery Further optimizes the activities of fibrocytes and fibroblasts to increase the production of new and the repair of damaged collagen (firmness), elastin (tightness), glycosaminoglycans (hydration)
Dyschromia present	Tretinoin applied after being mixed with hydroquinone ("blending")	Restores normal/even color tone by blending action (decreases dyschromia) Optimizes the activities of fibrocytes and fibroblasts to increase production and repair of damaged collagen (firmness), elastin (tightness), and glycosaminoglycans (hydration) Upregulates angioblast function, which improves circulation, with associated increased oxygen and nutrient delivery

dermis. This is because fibroblastic activity in the reticular dermis responds and is activated only by deep injury (e.g., ablative lasers, deep chemical peels, full-thickness cuts or lacerations).

Stimulation produces remarkable changes in the dermis by 1) increasing and stimulating fibroblast activity and collagen synthesis (improves skin firmness); 2) decreasing collagenase activity (reduces collagen degradation); 3) increasing elastin production (increased skin tightness and resilience); 4) increasing glycosaminoglycan production (increased ability for moisture retention); and 5) creating new anchoring fibrils that subsequently strengthen the basement membrane.

The physician must keep in mind that after completion of *general repair*, in any medical treatment and Skin Health Restoration program, stimulation should be continued using appropriate concentrations of retinol. *Specific repair* is needed for the continuation of dermal stimulation and stabilization, which is required to produce lifelong benefits, especially after the age of 30, when normal skin functions begin to rapidly deteriorate.

In the past, bleaching and blending were considered appropriate for *every* patient, regardless of whether the patient had a concurrent pigmentary abnormality. However, based on the observation that melanin elimination leads to increased photosensitivity and a tendency to build resistance to HQ, which can lead to rebound hyperpigmentation, toxicity to melanocytes, and the potential for exogenous ochronosis, especially when HQ is used for longer than 4 or 5 months or in concentrations higher than 4%, bleaching and blending are now used *only* when a particular patient presents with a concurrent pigmentation problem or potential for one.

Delivering Stimulation

Stimulation of the skin can be administered with tretinoin through three strengths: mild, moderate, and aggressive (Table 2.10). In the aggressive approach, skin improvement and tolerance are quickly achieved and reach an optimal level. Anticipated reactions peak during the initial 6 weeks and then decline regardless of the strength of the topical program used (e.g., mild versus aggressive). With both the mild and the moderate approaches, benefits of skin stimulation and tolerance are reached more slowly and are less intense (Figure 2.3). Despite the decreased benefits associated with a less intense treatment approach, some patients prefer to have fewer associated reactions for professional or social reasons.

TABLE 2.10   Skin Stimulation through Three Strengths of Tretinoin

Stimulation Strength	Frequency of Application	Amount of Tretinoin Applied*
Mild	Once daily or two times weekly	0.5 gram
Moderate	Once daily	0.5 or 1 gram
Aggressive	Twice daily	1 gram

*Each reference to tretinoin in this table refers specifically to tretinoin at a concentration of 0.1%. A more mild approach to each category can be achieved by using a tretinoin concentration of 0.05% instead of 0.1%. However, use of tretinoin at 0.1% strength yields a deeper benefit and faster repair (as well as a stronger reaction) than that seen with use of 0.05%.

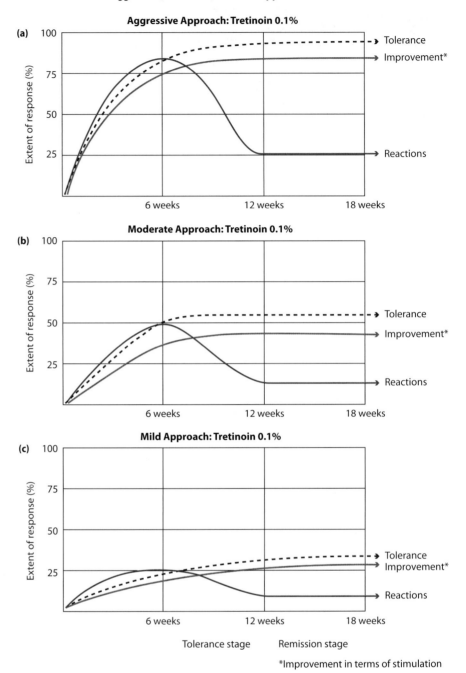

Delivering Stimulation with 0.1% Tretinoin Using the Aggressive, Moderate, and Mild Approaches

FIGURE 2.3 Keratin maturation cycle. Tretinoin 0.1% can deliver stimulation through a mild, moderate, or aggressive approach. Initially, reactions are lower with the moderate and mild approaches, but tolerance and improvement are reached more slowly, and the benefits are more superficial (epidermal).

Tretinoin is the best agent for stimulation and building skin tolerance. The aggressive program with twice-daily use of 1 gram of 0.1% tretinoin produces the most effective stimulation and correction in a Skin Health Restoration program. The moderate program of once-daily use is less effective, whereas the mild program of once-daily use of 0.5 gram is the least effective. Regardless of which program strength is chosen, some stimulation and correction are attained in 6 weeks (Figure 2.4).

Objectives of dermal stimulation in various skin types are shown in Table 2.11.

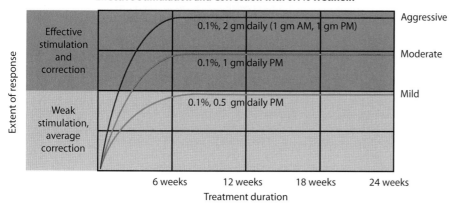

Relationship of Treatment Strength and Attainment of Effective Stimulation and Correction with 0.1% Tretinoin

0.1%, 2 gm daily (1 gm AM, 1 gm PM)   Aggressive

0.1%, 1 gm daily PM   Moderate

0.1%, 0.5 gm daily PM   Mild

Effective stimulation and correction

Weak stimulation, average correction

Extent of response

6 weeks   12 weeks   18 weeks   24 weeks

Treatment duration

FIGURE 2.4   Treatment strength and stimulation. With the aggressive or moderate approach (1 or 2 grams of 0.1% tretinoin applied daily), effective stimulation and correction are attained in 6 weeks. With the mild approach, stimulation is weak, and correction is only partially achieved at 6 weeks.

CORRECTING SKIN DYSCHROMIA IN MEDICAL TREATMENT

Concepts of Bleaching and Blending

Dyschromia can arise from multiple causes, including hyperpigmentation from increased melanin production by hyperactive melanocytes and from uneven distribution of melanin to surrounding keratinocytes. Increased melanin production by hyperactive melanocytes can be corrected by the use of HQ alone (bleaching), whereas uneven distribution of melanin to the surrounding keratinocytes can be corrected by the use of HQ in combination with tretinoin or retinol (blending). Bleaching and blending must be performed in a specific order to achieve optimal cosmesis. Bleaching should be performed first, followed by blending. The formulation in which the HQ is applied for bleaching (used alone) should be designed to prevent HQ oxidation, whereas the formulation of HQ when used for blending should be more acidic to allow stable mixing with an acidic substance (tretinoin or other retinoid). It is preferable for patients to apply the HQ alone, morning and evening, and in combination with tretinoin or another retinoid, evening only or morning and evening.

TABLE 2.11   Benefits of Stimulation with Various Skin Types and Characteristics

Skin Type or Characteristic	Objective
Thin	Increased thickness of epidermis and papillary dermis
Rough or irregular texture	Smoother, more uniform texture
Enlarged pores	Tightening and shrinkage of enlarged pores
Scars (atrophic, flat, hypertrophic keloids (e.g., at skin graft donor and recipient sites and on areas of prior burns, lacerations, cuts, or other trauma)	Reduced fibrosis, softened scar, correction of unevenly pigmented skin
	Smoother, more uniform texture
	Additional treatment modalities (intralesional steroid injections, laser procedures, chemical peels, and steroid-impregnated tape), when necessary, become easier to perform and yield better results

> ### Box 2.11
>
> ### Correcting Dyschromia
>
> | | |
> |---|---|
> | Correct the increased melanin production by hyperactive melanocytes | Hydroquinone alone (bleaching) |
> | Correct the uneven distribution of melanin to the surrounding keratinocytes | Hydroquinone in combination with tretinoin or retinol (blending) |

The bleaching step must be applied before the blending step. The products to correct dyschromia are shown in Box 2.11.

In general, the use of HQ for bleaching should be limited to a 4- to 5-month treatment course (about three full KMCs) to avoid HQ resistance, excessive photosensitivity, melanocyte toxicity, and exogenous ochronosis. Physicians should be especially cautious when treating dark or black skin. After a break lasting about 2 to 3 months, the use of HQ for bleaching can be resumed, if necessary; this is referred to as "pulse" therapy. In contrast, the use of HQ as part of the blending step (when mixed with a topical retinoid or tretinoin) can be continued for two to three additional KMCs because there are fewer side effects associated with the blending step. Blending should be discontinued sooner than noted previously if no further improvement is being seen with its use; this suggests the patient has developed resistance to HQ. Recommended HQ pulse treatment is shown in Box 2.12.

Blending is associated with anticipated reactions (redness, dryness, and exfoliation), which are induced by the tretinoin/retinol component. These initial anticipated reactions distress some patients. It is imperative that the physician inform each patient—before initiation of the topical regimen—that the redness, dryness, and peeling are *expected* and *necessary*, and will last for about 6 to 8 weeks. These unpleasant—though necessary—effects will persist for longer than 6 to 8 weeks (occasionally for up to 8 months) if the patient is not compliant with daily application of the blending step. After the dyschromia has been adequately corrected or when no further

> ### Box 2.12
>
> ### Hydroquinone Pulse Treatment
>
> - **Bleaching with hydroquinone should be discontinued after about 4 to 5 months and only restarted—if necessary—after a 2- to 3-month "break" from its use.**
> - **Blending can be discontinued two to three additional full KMCs following discontinuation of bleaching and/or observation of no further improvement with its use.**

improvement is being seen, both the beaching and the blending steps should be discontinued, and the patient should be switched to a non-HQ melanocyte-stabilizing agent.

Concept of Melanocyte Stabilization

Melanocyte stabilization, a new approach, is the process of preventing melanocyte activation or hyperactivity by making these cells more tolerant to various types of negative stimuli (e.g., irritation, inflammation, UV light, skin injury). Melanocyte stabilization (part of epidermal stabilization) can be used in combination with bleaching and blending and is accomplished through use of a topical regimen that contains proper concentrations of retinol, antioxidants, anti-inflammatory, and DNA-repair agents. Melanocyte stabilization is to be used by all patients as part of a daily skin and preventative program, regardless of whether the patient is prone to pigmentation problems. Furthermore, melanocyte stabilization is an essential maintenance step to be continued even after completion of a full course of bleaching and blending. The topical product aimed at stabilizing the melanocytes is best applied in the morning, although it can be applied twice per day for added benefit, when needed. Melanocyte stabilization is also used in medical pigmentation treatment (general repair) when bleaching and blending are being used.

HYDRATION AND CALMING

The objective of the principle of hydration and calming is to reduce skin dryness (as needed), irritation, and the severity of anticipated reactions, which include skin redness, dryness, and peeling. Integrating a product with hydration and calming benefits into a patient's daily topical skin care regimen makes the process of Skin Health Restoration more tolerable, which results in increased overall compliance. This is particularly important during the first phase of treatment (the first and second KMCs), when the patient's skin has not yet reached full tolerance to the program and is still experiencing redness, dryness, and peeling associated with use of the topical retinoid. Hydration and calming are accomplished by using a formulation that is distinct from standard moisturizers. The latter agents contain water, lipids, and protein. In contrast, the hydrating and calming formulation contains anti-inflammatory, antioxidant, hydrating, and DNA repair and protection ingredients. Hydration and calming agents are to be applied after the correction, stimulation, pigmentation control, and melanocyte stabilization steps. Although it can ultimately lead to increased patient compliance with the full therapeutic topical skin care regimen, regular use of hydrating and calming agents in Skin Health Restoration is optional. Table 2.12 summarizes the benefits of the hydration and calming step.

Ultraviolet Light Protection

The objective of the UV light protection principle is to protect the skin from UV light damage through the use of sunscreens with chemical and/or physical

TABLE 2.12 Hydration and Calming: Components and Benefits

Components	Benefits
Anti-inflammatory, antioxidant, and DNA repair agents, as well as those with hydration properties, such as hyaluronic acid	Increase skin tolerance (synergistic effects when used with melanocyte stabilizing agents)
	Reduce irritation from topical retinoids (tretinoin and retinol), alpha-hydroxy acids, and beta-hydroxy acids
	Help patients with true skin dryness* (not related to effects of topical products)

*Less than 1% of the population has true, genetically determined xerosis.

blockers. Without such protection, acute and chronic exposure to UV light induces numerous detrimental molecular effects, which can be seen histologically and clinically. Early changes associated with UV-induced photodamage include dullness, redness, roughness, and dyspigmentation. Later changes that appear after prolonged UV exposure include the formation of deep wrinkles, leathery texture, lax skin, solar lentigines (age spots), actinic keratoses, and cutaneous malignancies.

The approach to UV protection was refined after finding that all broadspectrum sunscreens (containing both chemical and physical blockers)—regardless of SPF rating—offer only 1 to 2 hours of protection. This is likely the reason for the high incidence of skin cancer and the frequently seen clinical signs of sun damage. This new approach to sun protection consists of two steps. The first step, increasing the skin's tolerance and natural resistance to UV light, is accomplished through epidermal stabilization. The second step, providing both short-term and longer-term UV protection, involves the use of a product that contains both physical and chemical blockers, as well as externally applied plant-derived melanin. The physical and chemical blockers provide short-term protection (about 2 hours), and the externally applied melanin provides more long-term protection (about 6 to 8 hours). Melanin is not sweated, washed, or rubbed off as readily as other ingredients common in over-the-counter sunscreens.

EMPHASIZING CERTAIN PRINCIPLES

Various, differing skin conditions require that an emphasis be placed on one or more of the previously mentioned principles and steps. A topical regimen formulated for a teenager with acne is not the same as that which would be used for a postmenopausal woman with melasma and lentigines. For example, in teenagers, the correction step is most important and is thus emphasized. In patients with mainly dyschromia, the bleaching and blending steps are emphasized. Furthermore, in patients at risk for developing postinflammatory hyperpigmentation, emphasis should be placed on the blending step. In contrast, in older patients with photodamage and severe textural problems (without concurrent dyschromia), an anti-aging regimen that emphasizes stimulation and dermal stabilization should be used.

TOPICAL AGENTS FOR SKIN HEALTH RESTORATION IN MEDICAL TREATMENT AND GENERAL REPAIR

Many of the topical agents used for Skin Health Restoration in a medical treatment are the same as those used for skin conditioning before procedures (details on skin conditioning appear later in this chapter); the steps for performing each process are also the same. Agents used for medical Skin Health Restoration include tretinoin (0.5% to 1%), HQ (4%), AHAs (6% to 10%), and certain disease-specific agents. Each of these agents has been carefully chosen, and the program for how they are to be used (order of application and amount used) has been designed to eliminate variables that often make traditional treatments fail (Table 2.13). See Chapter 3 for an in-depth discussion of the major classes of topical agents.

PHASES OF SKIN HEALTH RESTORATION

Skin Health Restoration, with an ultimate goal of eliminating chronic inflammation, can be divided into three phases or stages, corresponding to three KMCs: the repair phase, the tolerance phase, and the completion phase, which is followed by maintenance (Box 2.13). *Each phase takes about 6 weeks to complete*

Table 2.13 Variables Linked to Traditional Treatment Failure	
Variable	*Reason for Treatment Failure*
Patient education	Patients are inadequately educated on the nature of their skin condition and are thus less likely to comply with treatments. They do not understand the importance of each topical or oral agent, chemical peel, or laser procedure in the overall treatment approach.
Emphasis on comfort	Patient comfort is erroneously given more weight than overall efficacy of the treatment.
Skin color (as sole focus)	Color is the *only* consideration in treatment choice, and all other factors, as presented in the skin classification principles, are ignored.
Focusing on the disease	Specific disease is the *main* consideration in treatment choice. Importance of restoring and maintaining a patient's overall skin health while treating the disease is ignored.
Formulation properties of topical agents (penetration and concentration)	No standard protocol is available when selecting certain topical agents in regard to penetration or concentration. The vehicle used to deliver the active ingredient may counteract the effects of another ingredient.
Amount of agent to be applied	Patients are given little to no guidance on how much of the topical agent to use at each application.
Agent synergy	The synergistic benefits of combining certain topical agents are not considered.
Duration of treatment	Adequate timetables for treating various skin conditions and for establishing and maintaining overall skin health are not well defined.

Box 2.13

Phases of Skin Health Restoration

- Phase 1. Repair: when most anticipated reactions—redness, dryness, peeling—occur.
- Phase 2. Tolerance: when anticipated reactions start to subside and the overall improvement of the skin's appearance becomes noticeable.
- Phase 3. Completion: when minimal to no redness, dryness, or peeling persists and the skin's appearance is optimized (skin health is restored).

(one KMC), assuming that the aggressive approach is chosen and the patient is compliant with treatment. Each phase can be lengthened to last several months if the patient is not consistent with treatment and continually starts and stops use of the products. The main objectives of the repair phase include repairing the skin's barrier function, restoring hydration, stimulating cellular functions, and inducing acute inflammation. During the tolerance phase, general repair continues while the skin's barrier function is restored and epidermal renewal is optimized. After the patient completes the general repair phase, skin health has been restored, and a maintenance program is to be started.

CORRELATION OF TREATMENT BENEFITS WITH REGIMEN STRENGTH

Skin Health Restoration treatments are offered at three levels of strength: mild, moderate, and aggressive. Program strength is determined by the concentration of tretinoin used as well as by the amount and frequency of product application. The benefits of the treatment correlate well with the treatment strength. Specifically, the more aggressive the treatment, the better the results that can be achieved within a given amount of time (Box 2.14). With the aggressive approach, full Skin Health Restoration is achieved in the time it takes to complete three KMCs (about 18 weeks total). This approach is ideal for all pigmentation problems, severe textural irregularities, severe photodamage, thick skin with moderate to severe acne, rosacea, enlarged pores, and numerous areas of sebaceous gland hyperplasia. The moderate approach is good for all skin problems and all skin types. The mild approach is suitable for thin skin, mild skin abnormalities, and unmotivated patients. The correlation of treatment benefits with the strength of

---

Box 2.14

The stronger the treatment approach, the greater the benefits and the faster the repair phase is completed.

TABLE 2.14 Characteristics of Skin Health Restoration Treatment Strength

Treatment Strength*	Characteristics
Mild	Comfortable for the patient; minimal to no skin reactions
	Appropriate for patients with sensitive skin or for unmotivated patients who desire minimal reactions
	Strength is not intense enough to adequately correct pigmentary disorders or severe textural irregularities (can start at this level but must ultimately increase strength to a more aggressive level)
Moderate	Initially uncomfortable (variable intensity of skin reactions—redness, dryness, peeling)
	Good level of intensity for all patients to treat any skin condition
	For motivated and compliant patients who seek faster results
	Good for skin conditioning before procedures (chemical peels and laser treatments), but the aggressive strength is better
Aggressive	Uncomfortable; intense reactions (redness, dryness, peeling)
	Ideal for severe pigmentary and textural abnormalities
	For motivated and compliant patients
	Best for skin conditioning before procedures (chemical peels and laser treatments)

*The more aggressive the treatment strength, the greater and deeper the overall benefits and the faster these benefits become apparent.

the treatment regimen was also discussed previously under the Stimulation section and was shown in Figure 2.4.

When a mild treatment approach is followed without gradual progression to a stronger treatment approach, the benefits of Skin Health Restoration are mostly superficial (epidermal) and incomplete. Furthermore, in a small subsection of patients, anticipated reactions can be continuous and not subside throughout the phases. These patients are most likely unable to build an effective and strong barrier function and suffer from extreme sensitivity, manifested as an inability to tolerate the irritating properties of agents such as tretinoin and AHAs. In such cases, skin sensitivity should be treated first and nonirritating topical agents used with gradual introduction (e.g., once a week) of a strong topical agent to slowly strengthen barrier function.

In rare cases of severe reactions, such as extreme redness, dryness, and peeling that the patient is unable to tolerate, low-potency topical corticosteroids can be used. However, topical steroids should never be used for longer than 5 to 6 days. Longer use of corticosteroids can suppress cellular functions. Table 2.14 shows the most common characteristics associated with each of the three levels of intensity of treatment strength (mild, moderate, and aggressive) for Skin Health Restoration.

Table 2.15 shows the strength of the Skin Health Restoration approach and the corresponding time to reach skin tolerance.

For clinical examples of patients using a moderate-strength topical treatment approach, see Figures 2.5, 2.6, and 2.7. For clinical examples of patients using an aggressive strength topical treatment approach, see Figures 2.8 and 2.9.

TABLE 2.15 Skin Health Restoration Strength and Related Time to Reach Tolerance

Strength of Approach	Time to Reach Skin Tolerance*
Mild	>10 weeks
Moderate	8 to 10 weeks
Aggressive	6 weeks

*Improved tolerance = stronger barrier function

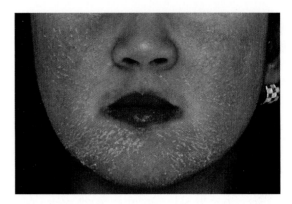

Figure 2.5 A patient shown after the moderate-strength topical treatment approach. Notice the extent of her skin's redness, dryness, and exfoliation. These are *anticipated* reactions necessary to achieve full Skin Health Restoration.

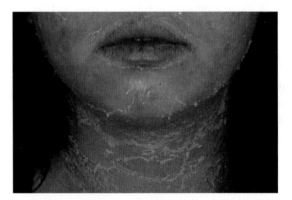

Figure 2.6 A patient shown after the moderate- or aggressive-strength treatment approach (face and neck). Notice the anticipated reactions (redness, dryness, and exfoliation) on both her face and neck. Of note, the skin on the neck is thinner and more sensitive. As such, the physician may want to recommend that, for the neck, the patient initially start the full regimen but limit use of the retinoic acid/retinol to only two to three times per week for the first few weeks. When tolerance is achieved, the goal is to have the patient increase application of the retinoic acid/retinol to every day.

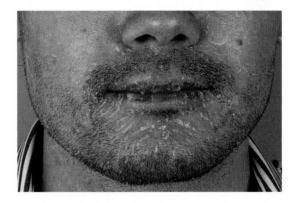

Figure 2.7 A male patient shown after the moderate- or aggressive-strength treatment approach. Notice the anticipated reactions to Skin Health Restoration (increased erythema and peeling, especially in the perioral area). The lower face typically peels/reacts more than the upper face regardless of the treatment strength, and the patient should be made aware of this at the start of treatment to limit confusion on initiation of the regimen.

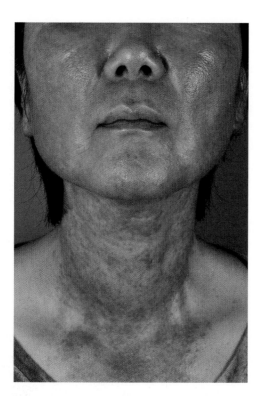

FIGURE 2.8   A patient using the moderate- to aggressive-strength topical treatment approach to achieve Skin Health Restoration of her face and neck. Notice the intense, blotchy erythema and mild diffuse edema, which are anticipated reactions in some patients in the beginning of the treatment course.

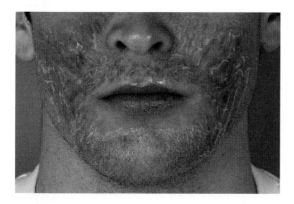

FIGURE 2.9   A patient shown after the aggressive-strength topical treatment approach. Notice the intense exfoliation and erythema. It is important to educate the patient that this is not an "allergic reaction" but an expected, anticipated reaction, and that its intensity will fade over time assuming the patient is compliant with daily application of the Skin Health Restoration topical program.

Exceptions to Skin Health Restoration Principles and Programs

In certain cases, exceptions may need to be made to the strength or duration of the recommended Skin Health Restoration program.

> **Exception 1: Duration of treatment.** Treatment may need to last longer than 5 months if the patient started with a mild approach, did not comply with daily use of products as directed, or used a smaller than recommended amount of one or more of the topical agents.

Exception 2: Inherited defect in skin barrier function. In such cases (atopic dermatitis, diseases associated with suppression or dysfunction of the immune system, and congenital syndromes), reactions can be severe even with the mild approach. In these rare cases, a very mild treatment approach is recommended, using a lower amount of certain agents and a less frequent application of the products (e.g., only once or twice weekly). Treatment regimens in these patients can be increased gradually as tolerance is restored.

Exception 3: Continuous reactions to tretinoin. In a few patients, reactions are continuous and not limited to the repair phase. The exact etiology has yet to be elucidated. However, this phenomenon may be due to a genetic deficiency in a patient's skin's barrier function. Strengthening the barrier function should be addressed first, followed by addition of a low concentration of retinol that can be increased in strength and frequency; later, the tretinoin can be added in the same fashion. Unlike the situation with tretinoin, all patients can build complete tolerance to topically applied retinol.

Exception 4: Continuous reactions to tretinoin. Continuous reactions to tretinoin indicate that its irritating properties are dominant. For that reason, after 5 months of treatment (general repair), tretinoin can be discontinued (pulse treatment). For example, in this scenario, the patient can be switched to another topical retinoid or switched to a topical retinol preparation. After this "vacation" period, the tretinoin can be restarted, if needed, and skin weakness will most likely have resolved.

SKIN CONDITIONING VERSUS SKIN HEALTH RESTORATION

Skin conditioning is a standardized program that has been carefully developed for the following purposes: to prepare skin to best tolerate a procedure, to hydrate skin and optimize skin healing after a procedure, and to further expedite the return of skin to a normal, healthy state. The principles of correction, stabilization, stimulation, and bleaching and blending are used in *both* medical Skin Health Restoration and skin conditioning. The difference is that Skin Health Restoration is a program to restore skin health and treat any existing disease with or without a procedure, whereas skin conditioning is designed to prepare skin for a procedure and manage skin after a procedure (Box 2.15).

Patients with very young and healthy skin should follow a nonmedical maintenance or preventive program to maintain the best skin quality and tolerance. Patients with more damaged and deteriorated or aged skin, however, are best suited to start a Skin Health Restoration program, during which some procedures can be performed. Studies have shown that skin preconditioning can enhance wound healing after a procedure, yield overall more uniform

Box 2.15

Skin Health Restoration versus Skin Conditioning

- Skin Health Restoration entails restoring a patient's skin to its healthiest baseline state (the main objective).
- Skin Conditioning entails preparing skin for a procedure and managing skin following the procedure (the procedure is the main objective).
- The principles of correction, stabilization, stimulation, and bleaching and blending are used in both Skin Health Restoration and Skin Conditioning.

and reliable depths of penetration of the chemical peel or laser procedure, and lengthen the beneficial effects of a rejuvenation procedure.

THE ZO SKIN HEALTH CIRCLE

Physicians see a wide variety of patients in their offices. Some need only a basic skin care program, whereas others need a prevention program. Still others need medical treatment and Skin Health Restoration, whereas others need a procedure that requires skin conditioning. All of these patients should join the ZO Skin Health Circle (like a "members-only" club) to receive continuous observation and services. The concept of the ZO Skin Health Circle is the continuum of care in both the medical and the nonmedical approaches to achieve optimal Skin Health Restoration and preservation (Figure 2.10, Box 2.16).

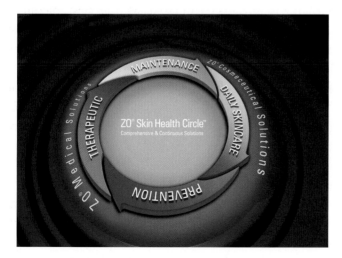

FIGURE 2.10   The ZO Skin Health Circle represents the comprehensive continuum of skin care.

Box 2.16

The ZO Skin Health Circle

The ZO Skin Health Circle represents the continuum of care in both the medical and nonmedical approaches to achieve optimal Skin Health Restoration and preservation.

REFERENCES

1. Goldsmith LA. *Biochemistry and Physiology of the Skin.* 2nd ed. New York: Oxford University Press; 1991:873-909.
2. Montagna W, Parakkal PF. *The Structure and Function of Skin.* 3rd ed. New York: Academic Press; 1974:2-39.
3. Zelickson AS. *Ultrastructure of Normal and Abnormal Skin.* Philadelphia: Lea and Febiger; 1967:202-227.
4. Sparr E, Millecamps D, Isoir M, et al. Controlling the hydration of the skin through the application of occluding barrier creams. *J R Soc Interface.* 2012;26;10:788.
5. Pierard GE. What does "dry skin" mean? *Int J Dermatol.* 1987;26:167-169.
6. Draelos Z. Facial moisturizers and eczema. In: Draelos Z, ed. *Cosmetic and Dermatological Problems and Solutions.* London: Informa Healthcare; 2011:18-26.
7. Held E, Sveinsdóttir S, Agner T. Effect of long-term use of moisturizer on skin hydration, barrier function and susceptibility to irritants. *Acta Derm Venereol.* 1999;79:49-51.
8. Lodén M. Effect of moisturizers on epidermal barrier function. *Clin Dermatol.* 2012;30:286-296.
9. Kraft JN, Lynde CW. Moisturizers: what they are and a practical approach to product selection. *Skin Ther Lett.* 2005;10:1-8
10. Wildnauer RH, Bothwell JW, Douglass AB. Stratum corneum biomechanical properties. I. Influence of relative humidity on normal and extracted human stratum corneum. *J Invest Dermatol.* 1971;56:72-78.
11. Baroni A, Buommino E, De Gregorio V, et al. Structure and function of the epidermis related to barrier properties. *Clin Dermatol.* 2012;30:257-262.
12. Levin J, Momin SB. How much do we really know about our favorite cosmeceutical ingredients? *J Clin Aesthet Dermatol.* 2010;3:22-41.
13. Davis EC, Callender VD. Postinflammatory hyperpigmentation: a review of the epidemiology, clinical features, and treatment options in skin of color. *J Clin Aesthet Dermatol.* 2010;3:20-31.

TOPICAL AGENTS FOR SKIN HEALTH RESTORATION

Monika G. Kiripolsky, MD, FAAD

INTRODUCTION TO TOPICAL AGENTS

Dermatologists and others who consider themselves experts in skin care may not be recommending to patients the most essential, scientifically proven, and beneficial topical products. Several reasons underlie this problem. Because there are no standardized Skin Health Restoration and maintenance treatment guidelines, doctors are left to promote topical products based on their own variable beliefs and the influence of heavy industry marketing. Practitioners are also guided by patient comfort and their ill-advised desires. Clinicians therefore do not recommend products that may cause irritation and subsequent patient complaints (e.g., retinoids, astringents).

When assessing the value of a topical agent, physicians must distinguish between scientifically proven claims and those that are of only theoretical benefit. Furthermore, if a topical agent is not delivering beneficial effects within a relatively "limited" amount of time (e.g., 2 to 3 months, which correlates to approximately two full keratinocyte maturation cycles), its use should be discontinued. Box 3.1 gives an overview on how to effectively assess topical agents.

Guidelines that categorize topical agents based on their therapeutic values could greatly aid physicians in making evidence-based decisions on topical products. The active ingredients within the product formulations should be classified into one of three categories: essential, supportive, or questionable (Table 3.1). Essential agents are therapeutic, and they primarily work intracellularly. Their contribution to overall Skin Health Restoration is undeniable and scientifically justified. Supportive agents, on the other hand, are only mildly therapeutic. They often have extracellular mechanisms of action and should therefore be used in combination with essential agents. Questionable agents have not shown any scientifically proven benefit. These should only be used, if at all, after essential and supportive topical agents have been employed. Of note, approximately 80% of all cosmeceuticals currently available on the market use active ingredients that fall into the questionable category. Whether

Box 3.1

Assessing Topical Agents

In assessing the value of topical agents, physicians must distinguish between scientifically proven claims and those that are of only theoretical benefit.

TABLE 3.1   Classification of Topical Agents for Skin Conditioning

Agent Classification	Characterization
Essential	Enhance natural epidermal exfoliation
	Ensure proper epidermal barrier function by restoring the correct balance of water, lipids, and proteins
	Stabilize melanin production by melanocytes
	Ensure even distribution of melanin to surrounding keratinocytes
	Enhance skin vitality through constant stimulation of collagen and elastin repair/production
	Ensure adequate hydration through glycosaminoglycan production
	Minimize chronic inflammation (e.g., through the reduction of sebum) and free radical generation
	Repair damaged DNA
Supportive	Mildly therapeutic and should be used in combination with essential agents
Questionable	Have not shown any scientifically proven therapeutic benefit
	Value in skin conditioning is questionable

classified as essential, supportive, or questionable, each topical formulation can further be categorized by the mechanism of action of its active ingredients.

Examples of essential and supportive changes are shown in Table 3.2. Questionable agents, which are optional, include the following: gold, platinum, caviar, silk, ursolic acid, Planifolia PFA, and Imperiale Orchidee molecular extract. A seemingly endless array of questionable agents are being used in various skin care products currently available on the market. A complete list of these agents would not only fail to fit within the confines of this book but would also be irrelevant because these have shown no scientific benefit in either Skin Health Restoration or maintenance processes.

TABLE 3.2   Examples of Essential and Supportive Topical Agents

Essential Agents	Supportive Agents
Vitamin A derivatives (tretinoin and retinol)	Alpha-hydroxy acids (glycolic, lactic, and malic acids)
Hydroquinone	Beta-hydroxy acids (salicylic acid)
Antioxidants (α-lipoic acid, glutathione, ubiquinone, idebenone, vitamin C, vitamin E, vitamin B_3)	Nonhydroquinone pigment-stabilizing agents (kojic acid, azelaic acid, arbutin, resorcinol)
DNA repair agents (oxo-guanine glycosylase, ultraviolet endonuclease, photolyase, and natural DNA precursors including Unirepair T-43)	Disease-specific agents (5-fluorouracil, imiquimod, benzoyl peroxide, topical antibiotics, and topical antifungals)
Anti-inflammatory agents	
Growth factors	

CHOOSING TOPICAL AGENTS

Physicians and other skin care professionals often recommend topical agents with active ingredients that are inert but that provide comfort and quick gratification to patients. With demanding schedules, practitioners prefer not to deal with unwanted reactions from topical agents, even if these expected reactions are necessary to achieve Skin Health Restoration. Furthermore, dermatologists are often recruited by skin care companies to promote their products. Hence the term *dermatologist tested*. Each year, many meaningless studies are performed in this fashion, with the principal investigating physicians paid handsomely by pharmaceutical companies for these tasks.

Patients tend to seek a skin care program based on recommendations from their dermatologists and aestheticians. Pharmaceutical company marketing and promotional activity is also influential. This approach is laced with bias and often oriented toward products that generate the most instant gratification for patients and profit for pharmaceutical companies.

Ideally, before commencing any skin care program, patients should themselves research and analyze the component ingredients. This could ensure that only products proved to be beneficial, therapeutic, and specifically matched to a patient's particular skin type and needs are used. But with so much unclear and misleading information, this task can be overwhelming. To assist patients with their choices and be able to discourage them from using unproven products with inert active ingredients, practitioners must be able to step in and offer scientifically based advice. Explanation should be given that these products provide quick gratification (through looking, smelling, and feeling good) but yield no visible or lasting benefit. It must further be emphasized that pleasant properties do not necessarily correlate with skin improvement. These comfortable products are ultimately counterproductive; skin is weakened through barrier function disruption, and the innate proliferative properties are hampered. Furthermore, patients should be made aware that most currently marketed anti-aging products are useless and do not live up to their claims because their active ingredient (or "hero" molecule) is ineffective, too low in concentration, or too large of a molecule to penetrate the skin and reach the intended target.

ESSENTIAL AGENTS

Essential agents are fundamental for restoring skin health. These have been scientifically validated as having beneficial activity, and they are the only known substances that can return the skin to its best possible original state. A comprehensive overview of their characteristics is given in Table 3.1.

Topical agents in the essential category must offer one or more of the following features: intracellular activity, therapeutic effect, anti-inflammatory benefit, activation of cellular function, or improvement of the barrier function. These products, which are crucial to achieving Skin Health Restoration and successful maintenance, include vitamin A derivatives (tretinoin and retinol), hydroquinone (HQ), antioxidants, DNA repair agents, anti-inflammatory agents, and growth factors (Table 3.2).

TRETINOIN (RETINOIC ACID)

Tretinoin (retinoic acid) has profoundly beneficial effects on the stratum corneum and the deeper layers of the skin. It has an intracellular mechanism of action, with direct effects on the nuclear receptors. By stimulating gene expression and regulating cellular functions, it ultimately provides strong therapeutic benefit for a myriad of skin conditions. Most notably, keratin is made softer and more gelatinous, and the stratum corneum becomes smooth and compact. These effects last for up to 4 months, even after application has ceased. This is in contrast to the shorter-lasting, smoothening effects of alpha-hydroxy acids (AHAs).

Initially, tretinoin dehydrates the outer surface of the stratum corneum while keeping the desmosomes intact. This leads to a rapid, coarse exfoliation and the shedding of an attached group of cells. This is in opposition to the shedding of individual cells, as occurs with AHAs when the desmosomes are disbanded. Tretinoin is the preferred agent for treating the stratum corneum and disorders focused within deeper layers of the epidermis because it repairs damaged keratinocytes, increases basal cell mitosis, and restores adequate hydration.

Tretinoin has been extensively used as an effective topical treatment for a number of dermatological conditions, including photoaging. Its efficacy in improving this condition was first demonstrated by Kligman and colleagues in 1984 using an animal model of photoaging.[1] The authors observed that treatment of photoaged mouse skin with tretinoin for 10 weeks resulted in a significant repair zone of new collagen in the papillary dermis. This further correlated with wrinkle effacement.

Topical tretinoin has further shown efficacy in improving signs of aging (both intrinsic and extrinsic), including fine lines, hyperpigmentation, and wrinkles.[2-18] Effectiveness has also been histologically documented.[2,17-19] A study with 0.025% tretinoin applied to intrinsically aged skin showed an increase in epidermal thickness and a more uniform keratinocyte density.[3] Dermal changes included an increase in glycosaminoglycan deposition, elastic fibers, and angiogenesis.[2] The vehicle comparison study showed similar clinical and histological changes when tretinoin 0.1% and 0.025% were used in patients with photoaging.[17] Histological changes included epidermal thickening, increased granular layer thickness, stratum corneum compaction, increased vascularity, and decreased melanin content. A further study showed alterations in dermal matrix components including neocollagenesis. Here, treatment was continued beyond 24 months, and collagen organization only continued to improve while elastosis further decreased. Ongoing increases in epidermal and dermal mucin production and decreases in epidermal melanin formation were also consistent throughout the treatment period.[18]

The concentration of tretinoin has a direct correlation with its beneficial activity; the higher the concentration, the deeper and more potent its effects. Lower concentrations (≤0.025%) have mainly epidermal benefit, whereas higher concentrations (0.05% to 0.1%) have both epidermal and dermal effects. The vehicle in which tretinoin is delivered also affects its potency. Vehicles that add moisturizing components to the formulation weaken the action and the benefits of tretinoin, regardless of the concentration.

Retinoid use (tretinoin and retinol) is associated with skin dryness, erythema, and exfoliation. These factors can sometimes limit patient compliance. The anticipated "retinoid reaction" varies with concentration and frequency of application; the higher the concentration and the greater the application frequency, the more irritation that is expected to occur.[10,11,17,18] These reactions generally manifest within the first few weeks of treatment, and they are thought to be initiated by the release of pro-inflammatory cytokines.[20] As the treated skin begins to accommodate product application, the associated signs and symptoms subside. Photosensitivity is another notable side effect associated with retinoid therapy, and typically, it is most pronounced at the start of treatment. To counteract this, patients using topical retinoids are advised to avoid excessive sun exposure, use broad-spectrum sunblock, and wear sun-protective clothing. Box 3.2 shows the effects of tretinoin.

A patient may continue using topical tretinoin for maintenance purposes. In that case, tretinoin is to be applied two to three times weekly and a retinol-based product used on the remaining days. Alternatively, the patient may switch to daily application of a retinol agent for maintenance and specific repair. The first option is occasionally recommended to maintain skin free from active medical disease (e.g., melasma, acne, rosacea). The second option is preferred, however, especially in patients without underlying medical conditions, for daily prevention and anti-aging benefits.

The reason for these suggestions is that tretinoin serves two functions: therapeutic and irritative. The former is fulfilled after 18 weeks of product use, and then the latter predominates. Patients are unable to build tolerance to the tretinoin, and their skin remains red, dry, and exfoliating long-term. This state of irritation is unfavorable, so tretinoin use should be discontinued after the 18-week time frame. Retinol should instead be used for maintenance purposes; it is not associated with long-term irritation because skin is able to successfully build tolerance to this agent.

Box 3.2

Effects of Tretinoin

- Tretinoin has profoundly beneficial effects on the stratum corneum and on the deeper layers of the skin.
- In the epidermis, tretinoin:
  - Repairs damaged keratinocytes, increases basal cell mitosis, restores natural hydration, and increases epidermal thickness.
- In the dermis, tretinoin:
  - Increases angiogenesis, elastic fibers, and glycosaminoglycan deposition.
- Lower concentrations (<0.025%) of tretinoin have mainly epidermal effect, whereas higher concentrations (0.05% to 0.1%) produce both epidermal and dermal benefit.

RETINOL

Retinol, like tretinoin, is a vitamin A derivative. Both are among the most common ingredients found in prescription and over-the-counter skin care products. They are frequently studied ingredients and have the most data supporting their efficacy in skin care.

Within the skin, retinol is first oxidized to retinaldehyde and then to tretinoin, the biologically active form of vitamin A.[21,22] Topical retinol (at concentrations up to 1.6%) has been shown to induce the same beneficial effects as those associated with tretinoin (at a concentration of 0.025%).[23] In particular, topical retinol leads to a decrease in the appearance of wrinkles through the increased production of glycosaminoglycans (which retain substantial amounts of water) and collagen.[24] However, despite demonstrating the same beneficial effects as tretinoin, topical retinol produces only minimal signs of irritation and erythema.[23] More specifically, retinol has been shown to induce less scaling, transepidermal water loss, and erythema compared to tretinoin.[25]

Retinol, although ultimately converted within the skin to tretinoin (a prescription product), is available over the counter. However, concentration strengths of retinol and tretinoin are not comparable. Topical retinol products typically contain strengths of 1% or higher, yet tretinoin is rarely available above 0.1%. It is important to note that retinol is approximately 20 times less potent than tretinoin (Box 3.3).[23,26] Thus, a concentration of 1% retinol is approximately equivalent to a 0.05% concentration of tretinoin. Furthermore, when determining efficacy, the vessel and the vehicle in which the topical retinol is delivered must be considered. Retinol is extremely unstable for it is degraded to biologically inactive forms on exposure to air and light.[27]

HYDROQUINONE

HQ is a skin-lightening agent derived from phenol. It is commonly used in dermatology practice to treat conditions of hyperpigmentation, including melasma, ephelides, lentigines, and postinflammatory hyperpigmentation (PIH). HQ works by inhibiting the tyrosinase enzyme, which is necessary for converting dihydroxyphenylalanine (DOPA) to melanin.[28,29] Tyrosinase activity can be reduced by as much as 90% with the use of HQ.[30] HQ may also degrade melanosomes and be selectively toxic to melanocytes. It achieves this through structurally altering the melanocyte's organelles, thereby decreasing the production of melanosomes and increasing their breakdown.[31] Because HQ only prevents the formation of new melanin (from melanocytes located within or near the basal cell layer), skin brightening is not seen immediately.

Box 3.3

Potency of Retinol

Retinol at a 1% concentration is approximately equal to a 0% to .05% concentration of tretinoin.

HQ is available in a lotion, cream, liquid, or gel formulation. The lotion and cream vehicles are preferable because the liquid and gel forms result in uneven application. It is important to note that after the HQ formulation has been oxidized and turns brown, it has little to no activity.

HQ is available over the counter at a concentration of 2% and in prescription topicals at concentrations of 3% to 5%. Higher concentrations (6% to 8%) have not been shown to be more effective and carry the increased risk for inducing an idiosyncratic reaction during or after discontinuation of treatment (similar to ochronosis). Occasionally, pharmacies will compound topical HQ to concentrations as high as 20% for specifically treating conditions such as vitiligo universalis. However, the use of HQ in strengths greater than 4% is not generally condoned because these are associated with an increased risk for paradoxical skin darkening (exogenous ochronosis), which can be permanent. Exogenous ochronosis presents as patches of bluish-black skin color, and it is more common in black-skinned people of certain tribal origins. It can occur, however, in any skin color or type.

The recommended use of HQ is limited to a 4- or 5-month period. Prolonged use of even lower strengths of HQ can be toxic to cells and is associated with an increased risk for exogenous ochronosis. In patients who do present with exogenous ochronosis, effective results can usually be obtained by having the patient use HQ for bleaching and blending, along with a papillary dermal peel and a series of Nd:YAG laser treatments.

Other rare side effects associated with the use of HQ are stinging, burning, irritation, rash-like reaction, and allergic contact dermatitis. Systemic absorption or toxicity from prolonged use of topical HQ (at concentrations of 2% to 4%) has not been reported. Even if accidentally ingested, HQ seldom produces systemic toxicity. This contrasts to depigmenting agents used in the past, such as mercurial compounds, which caused renal damage, and monobenzone, which causes permanent melanocyte destruction. An increased risk for skin cancer has not been documented with the use of HQ. Also, HQ does not directly cause increased photosensitivity. However, a resulting decreased amount of melanin will allow the skin to absorb more ultraviolet (UV) rays. This in turn leads to chronic sun damage. Broad-spectrum sunblocks, preferably those containing physical blockers, are therefore recommended while HQ is being used.

For optimal results, with each application, patients should saturate the epidermis with approximately 1.5 grams of HQ (similar to the amount in 1 inch of toothpaste). This quantity should be massaged fully into the skin. After HQ has been applied, the pH of the skin will shift toward neutral, thereby facilitating the product's oxidation. Because of this phenomenon, the activity of HQ is relatively short lived, and it should therefore be used twice daily. When an even skin color becomes apparent, the frequency of application can be gradually reduced. Application should not be stopped abruptly.

Although HQ is a powerful depigmenting agent, its efficacy can be further enhanced when it is used in combination with AHAs, tretinoin, or both. The presence of AHAs in products containing HQ also prevents oxidation of the latter, thus preserving its activity. Because HQ is relatively unstable, when compounding it with tretinoin, the two products should be freshly combined just before topical application. Penetration of HQ can also be increased by coupling it with other key agents (e.g., azelaic acid) and by adjusting the pH of the skin before treatment. Of note, the aforementioned process of enhanced penetration is entirely different from a state of increased permeability. The penetration of a product's active ingredients can be enhanced by using it in conjunction with another topical agent (as when we are treating a disease). In contrast, an increase in epidermal permeability is a disorder characterized by a damaged epidermal barrier function. This leads to skin dryness, sensitivity, irritation, and impaired healing. Moreover, when using HQ, the presence of oily skin must be noted and reduced. Oily skin requires proper washing and the use of additional topical or systemic agents. These both aid in reducing sebum and allow for the increased penetration of HQ.

The combined use of HQ and tretinoin for at least 6 weeks is essential before performing a procedure like the ZO Controlled Depth Peel (20% or 26% to 28% trichloroacetic acid [TCA]). This prior conditioning decreases the skin's ability to produce melanin and therefore reduces the risk for developing PIH. The HQ and tretinoin combination further evens the skin's hydration, yielding more uniform results because water is the chromophore for the peeling agent.

Melamin (HQ 4%, ZO Medical), when used alone, can mitigate most hyperpigmentation problems attributed to the increased activity of melanocytes and their overproduction of melanin. In this instance, the suppression of melanin hyperproduction is referred to as *bleaching*. However, when HQ is mixed with tretinoin or AHAs, the bleaching effect becomes less important, and another effect takes preference. The term *blending* refers to this process, which constitutes a more even distribution of melanin to surrounding keratinocytes.

For faster, more effective results, the two steps should be combined. The bleaching step should be performed first, followed by blending. When a product containing HQ (Melamix, 4% HQ, ZO Medical) is intended for combination with another containing tretinoin (for blending purposes), the HQ vehicle must have a more acidic pH to allow for effective mixing with tretinoin. This contrasts to products containing HQ alone, which are more basic, and intended for bleaching purposes. Because of their suppression of bleaching and blending effects, topical HQ products that contain steroids should also be avoided. Box 3.4 shows a summary of hydroquinone properties and effects.

ANTIOXIDANTS

Antioxidants are molecules that inhibit the oxidation of surrounding molecules. Oxidation involves the transfer of electrons or hydrogen from one molecule to another, the oxidizing agent. This chemical reaction leads to the production of free radicals. These trigger intracellular chain reactions and ultimately, cell damage or cell death ensues. Antioxidants, through their preferential oxidation, stop these adverse chain reactions. Free radicals are therefore removed, and further oxidation reactions are terminated.

Inflammation causes the depletion of collagen, and antioxidants help to inhibit this process. They also protect against acute and chronic photodamage and skin cancer. The most common topically applied antioxidants include the following: alpha-lipoic acid, glutathione, idebenone, ubiquinone, vitamin C (L-ascorbic acid), vitamin E (tocopherol), and vitamin B_3 (niacinamide).

Box 3.4

Hydroquinone Summary

- Hydroquinone (HQ) prevents the formation of new melanin by inhibiting the tyrosinase enzyme.
- HQ is available over the counter at a concentration of 2% and in prescription topicals at concentrations between 3% and 5%.
- In strengths above 4%, HQ may cause paradoxical skin darkening (exogenous ochronosis), which can be permanent.
- The efficacy of HQ can be enhanced when used in combination with alpha-hydroxy acid (AHA), tretinoin, or both.
- Bleaching is the use of HQ to suppress the overproduction of melanin.
- Blending is HQ mixed with tretinoin or AHAs to obtain a more even distribution of melanin to surrounding keratinocytes.
- Bleaching and blending should be combined for faster, more effective results.
- To decrease the risk for postinflammatory hyperpigmentation, HQ and tretinoin should be applied for approximately 6 weeks before a procedure is performed.

Alpha-Lipoic Acid

Alpha-lipoic acid (ALA), created in the mitochondria of animals and plants, acts as a potent antioxidant. It protects cells from UV and other environmentally generated free radical damage. Because of its solubility in both aqueous and lipid layers, ALA penetrates rapidly through the epidermis to reach the dermis and subcutaneous layers of the skin. Although most free ALA is rapidly converted (reduced) to dihydro-lipoic acid (DHLA), both ALA and DHLA are highly effective antioxidants. Like ALA, DHLA acts as a scavenger of reactive oxygen species (ROS). DHLA has also been shown to repair oxidatively damaged proteins and to regenerate endogenous antioxidants such as glutathione, ubiquinol, vitamin E, and vitamin C.[32,33] Furthermore, both ALA and DHLA act as anti-inflammatory mediators through the scavenging of ROS secreted by macrophages and leukocytes at sites of inflammation.

Glutathione

A cysteine-containing peptide found in most forms of aerobic life, glutathione is a strong intracellular antioxidant because of its thiol group (within the cysteine moiety). This compound acts primarily as a reducing agent, mopping up ROS.[34] Glutathione also serves as a co-antioxidant, in that it supports vitamin E and L-ascorbic acid.[35,36] Furthermore, topically applied glutathione reduces UV-induced erythema.[37]

Ubiquinone (Coenzyme Q$_{10}$)

Ubiquinone, which functions both as an antioxidant and an energy generator, is ubiquitous and present in almost all living cells (with the exception of some fungi and bacteria). Ubiquinone has been shown to reduce UV-induced oxidative DNA damage within keratinocytes. It has also been shown to impair UV-generated collagen degradation through its ability to suppress fibroblast production of collagenase. Moreover, topically applied ubiquinone decreases the loss of hyaluronic acid (a glycosaminoglycan produced by fibroblasts) and the slowing of cell division, both of which contribute to intrinsic aging.[33] Thus, ubiquinone is an important topical antioxidant because it protects the dermis from both extrinsic and intrinsic related aging.

Idebenone

Idebenone, an engineered analog of ubiquinone, acts as a potent primary antioxidant. Clinical research evaluating its topical benefits suggests a more well-rounded free radical scavenging capability compared with other traditional antioxidants (ALA, tocopherol, and ascorbic acid).[38] *In vivo* studies of topically applied idebenone have shown decreased lipid peroxidation and inhibited UVB-induced DNA damage and erythema.[38] Research has also suggested that idebenone is best used in combination with other antioxidants. This is because of its lack of photoprotective benefits, which are present in several other topical antioxidants.[39,40]

Vitamin C (L-Ascorbic Acid)

The only truly bioavailable form of vitamin C, L-ascorbic acid, is also the only form that provides the molecule's antioxidant benefits. When applied topically, L-ascorbic acid serves as a multifunctional antioxidant, quenching ROS generated in the skin's aqueous environment.[41] Proper stabilization (through encapsulation and anhydrous vehicles or esterification) of a topical containing vitamin C is crucial because L-ascorbic acid is easily oxidized.[42] When formulated in an aqueous base, the preferred method, topical products containing L-ascorbic acid should have a pH of 3.5 or lower.[43] Although ester versions of vitamin C (such as magnesium ascorbyl phosphate and ascorbyl palmitate) have shown some of the antioxidant capabilities in clinical studies, they do not provide the collagen synthesis, anti-inflammatory, and photoprotective activities.[44] Thus, esterification is not the preferred method of stabilization compared with encapsulated or anhydrous preparations.

Vitamin E (α-Tocopherol)

Vitamin E is the most abundant, lipophilic antioxidant found in the skin. Tocopherols, which consist of four different subtypes (alpha-, beta-, gamma-, and delta-tocopherol), are the most abundant form of vitamin E in the body. Alpha-tocopherol is the primary form of vitamin E present in the skin; topical preparations permeate both the epidermis and the dermis. After application, vitamin E accumulates in cell membranes and within the extracellular lipid matrix of the stratum corneum. It is here that it contributes its antioxidant benefits. Because it reduces ROS and thereby protects cellular membranes from lipid peroxidation by free radicals, vitamin E is classified as an antioxidant. In addition, vitamin E can absorb energy from UV light. This enables it to be named a photoprotective agent because ultimately it prevents UV-induced free radical skin damage.[45]

Alpha-tocopherol is also available as an ester derivative, which increases its stability on exposure to air, light, and heat. Vitamin E content in the skin is decreased with exposure to UV light, ozone, and advancing age.[46-52] Topically applied vitamin E has been studied in varying concentrations, typically between 0.1% and 1%. Even with solutions containing concentrations as low as 0.1%, increased vitamin E levels have been observed in the skin.[53] However, studies comparing the dose-dependent accumulation of vitamin E and its effectiveness in terms of antioxidant benefits are lacking.

Vitamin B₃ (Niacinamide)

Vitamin B$_3$, a potent antioxidant, reduces transepidermal water loss, thereby improving the lipid barrier function of the epidermis. Interestingly, vitamin B$_3$ also reduces the appearance of hyperpigmentation by inhibiting the transfer of melanosomes. Studies evaluating the effects of topically applied vitamin B$_3$ have also found a significant improvement in fine lines, wrinkles, and skin elasticity.[54-56] Properties of antioxidants are displayed in Box 3.5.

DNA Repair Agents

Repeated exposure to UVA and UVB induces skin thinning, acute erythema, wrinkling, and chronic discoloration. These external manifestations reflect internal, molecular damage to the DNA double helix that lays within the cell's nucleus.[57] An example of UVB-related DNA damage is the formation of cyclobutane pyrimidine dimers (CPDs). These are mutations formed between adjacent pyrimidine bases on the same DNA strand.[58] CPDs alter the function of DNA and cause transformational, tumorigenic, and lethal cellular events.[59-61] Moreover, with chronological aging, one's innate DNA repair mechanisms decrease, conferring a heightened mutational risk.[62,63] UV exposure further induces the formation of ROS. Proteins are one of the main targets for this ROS-mediated oxidation.[64,65] No longer functional, oxidized proteins are either repaired, eliminated by exocytosis, or broken down by proteolysis into amino acids and peptides.[66]

In addition to the cellular DNA damage, chronic exposure to UVA and UVB results in increased expression of matrix metalloproteinases (MMPs) typically associated with intrinsic cutaneous aging. Extrinsic aging therefore yields both damaged DNA and increased MMP production. The factors

---

Box 3.5

Antioxidants

- Oxidation involves the transfer of electrons or hydrogen from one molecule to another, the oxidizing agent. This chemical reaction leads to the production of free radicals. These trigger intracellular chain reactions that produce cell damage.
- Antioxidants, through being oxidized themselves, remove free radicals. Further oxidation reactions are thereby terminated.
- Alpha-lipoic acid, glutathione, idebenone, ubiquinone, vitamin C, vitamin E, and vitamin B$_3$ are all potent topical antioxidants in human skin.

involved in generating these changes include oxidative stress (nuclear and mitochondrial), UV exposure, glycation, and alkylation. Topically applied, DNA repair enzymes complex, excise, extract, and repair DNA damaged by a variety of insults.

Oxo-Guanine Glycosylase-1 (OGG-1)

Oxo-guanine glycosylase-1 (OGG-1) is an enzyme that repairs DNA damaged by oxidative stress. To effectively penetrate the epidermis, OGG-1 can be encapsulated within pH-sensitive liposomes. The inflammatory response induced by exposure to UVB leads to the formation of oxidative DNA byproducts such as 8-hydroxy-2-deoxyguanine (8-oxo-dG). These have been linked to the development of skin cancer. The OGG-1 enzyme repairs 8-oxo-dG adducts, suggesting that supplementing its activity through topical application might increase repair of 8-oxo-dG and subsequently prevent skin cancer development.[67]

Ultraviolet Endonuclease

UV endonuclease is also best delivered through liposomal encapsulation. It acts to recognize distorted DNA molecules (e.g., UV-induced thymine dimers), break the DNA chain near the dimer, excise the small damaged region, and patch up the strand with the complementary bases to the bases on the intact strand. Exposing skin to UV endonuclease also helps to reduce cytokines regularly released during stress (e.g., interleukin-1 [IL-1], IL-6, IL-8, IL-10, and tumor necrosis factor-α [TNF-α]). UV endonuclease further downregulates UV-induced elevated levels of MMP's (e.g., MMP-1, also called collagenase-1, which cleaves collagen I, the major subtype of collagen in the extracellular matrix of the dermis). A subtype of UV endonuclease, T4 endonuclease V, is a DNA repair enzyme specific for pyrimidine-dimers. When administered through liposomal encapsulation to UV-irradiated human cells, this form increases the incision of UV-irradiated DNA, the survival of these cells, and the DNA repair replication process.[68] Therefore, application of this DNA repair enzyme topically to human skin can potentially prevent skin cancer formation.

Photolyase

Photolyase is also best delivered when encapsulated within liposomes. It cleaves and reverses DNA damage specifically in relation to CPDs caused by UV with shorter wavelengths. This process, known as photoreactivation, cleaves the UV-induced cyclobutane. Photolyase also reduces UV radiation-induced cellular apoptosis.[69]

Natural DNA Repair Precursors

Natural DNA repair precursors such as acetyl tyrosine, proline, hydrolyzed vegetable protein, and adenosine triphosphate (ATP) can be delivered to areas of damaged DNA for additional benefit. A recent study demonstrated the safety and efficacy of a topical product regimen containing both biologically stable DNA repair enzymes (OGG-1, UV endonuclease, and photolyase) and natural precursor proteins (a mixture of acetyl tyrosine, proline, hydrolyzed vegetable protein, and ATP). The study's outcome was measured via improvement in the most common signs of photoaging. These variables included the following: fine and deep rhytides, skin texture, color, suppleness, brightness, roughness, elasticity, mottled pigmentation, pore prominence, and overall photodamage. The study investigators concluded that twice daily use of a topical skincare regimen containing DNA repair enzyme complexes and natural repair protein precursors was well-tolerated and effective with respect to improvement of the most common signs of facial photoaging.[70]

Unirepair T-43, a product of Induchem (Switzerland), is a DNA-repairing bioactive complex that boosts cutaneous cells' natural DNA repair mechanism through its supplementation of amino acids like proline and acetyl tyrosine.[71] Both proline and acetyl tyrosine have shown redox properties.[72] In the DNA repair pathway, proline and acetyl tyrosine are targets for protein kinases, which are involved in repairing damaged DNA.[73] Several studies have found a strong association between erythema formation and repair of DNA damage. Protection or repair from UV-induced DNA damage is linked to reduced erythema development.[74-78] Interestingly, patients pre-treated with topical Unirepair T-43 showed reduced erythema following UV exposure. This was thought to be due to ability of Unirepair T-43 to hasten the repair of CPDs, thereby reducing DNA damage and the subsequent triggering of an inflammatory response.[79] Box 3.6 shows known DNA repair agents.

Anti-inflammatory Agents

Cutaneous inflammation weakens the epidermal barrier function by altering the skin's permeability. It induces cellular dysfunction and causes textural irregularity. Until relatively recently, inflammation (both acute and chronic) was not considered an important factor that required control. Now it is increasingly evident that inflammation is a destructive process in both diseased and nondiseased skin. For example, inflammation is the main cause of scarring (as seen in acne), induction of skin cancer (as seen following UV-induced damage to DNA), accelerated skin aging (extrinsic), and both hyperpigmentation and hypopigmentation (after chronic UV-induced melanocytic dysfunction or damage).

Inflammation is the immune system's defense against an insult to its integrity. In certain conditions, such as wound healing, inflammation can be constructive because it is necessary for injury repair. This is an example of acute inflammation, which is a beneficial process and should be facilitated for faster

---

Box 3.6

DNA Repair Agents

- ■ Aging is believed to be a consequence of an accumulation of unrepaired naturally occurring DNA damage.
- ■ Known DNA repair agents include:
  - ■ Oxo-guanine glycosylase-1
  - ■ Ultraviolet endonuclease
  - ■ Photolyase
  - ■ Natural DNA repair precursors

injury resolution. Therapeutic, acute inflammation usually subsides in 8 to 20 days following adequate treatment. Resolution of acute inflammation is marked by re-epithelialization, increased basal cell mitosis, and repair of the extracellular matrix. After an acute injury, supportive and beneficial dermal modulation may last 4 to 6 months. Conversely, when inflammation becomes chronic, it can lead to a destructive state, with permanent and adverse sequelae (e.g., scars).

The wound healing process attracts neutrophils and macrophages that are eventually replaced by lymphocytes and histiocytes. The release of MMPs ensues, and these trigger several inflammatory pathways. Ultimately, this results in destructive processes such as scarring and textural irregularities. When an insult to the stratum corneum fails to permit renewal to a normal stratum corneum, and therefore an active barrier function, said destruction occurs. If such acute inflammation is not accordingly treated, chronic inflammation will result.

Chronic inflammation can also occur from three other processes: glycation, formation of ROS, and induction of the arachidonic acid cascade. Glycation is characterized by saccharides (sugar) in the circulation that are deposited within the blood vessels. This results in vascular insufficiency. Activation of the arachidonic acid cascade, however, commonly induced by UV exposure, results in the impairment of the lipid bilayer (barrier function). It also leads to the activation of prostaglandins, the inhibition of apoptosis, increased angiogenesis (to feed oxygen and nutrients to tumors), proliferation of tumor cells, and their eventual local invasion and metastases.

Acute inflammation can be easily treated through the application of specific topical ingredients, leading to a quick restoration of the skin's inherently strong barrier function. Treatment of chronic inflammation, on the other hand, requires a more methodical and long-term approach. This may be accomplished through the use of a combination of topical antioxidants that will target chronic inflammation through multiple avenues. To clarify, the use of one antioxidant or anti-inflammatory agent is not enough to adequately treat chronic inflammation. When applied, the single agent may convert through inflammation to a damaging oxidizing agent; a combination approach in which the second agent acts as an antioxidant is therefore suggested instead. Features of chronic inflammation are shown in Box 3.7.

Box 3.7

Chronic Inflammation

- Chronic inflammation leads to destructive processes, such as scarring and textural irregularities.
- Chronic inflammation can be treated by inducing a controlled, therapeutic period of acute inflammation.
- One antioxidant or anti-inflammatory agent is not enough to adequately treat chronic inflammation because the agent may convert to a damaging oxidizing agent.
- A combination of antioxidants must be used to treat chronic inflammation.

An effective approach to arresting and eliminating chronic inflammation is through the induction of controlled, therapeutic, acute inflammation. Using the proper volume and concentration of select topical agents, a 2-week phase of controlled acute inflammation is generated. The skin will respond to this and, through innate mechanisms, will overcome both the acute and chronic inflammation. This process will in turn fortify the barrier function, restore the skin's renewal ability, eliminate the offending agent, and return skin to a healthy state.

In addition to their primary function, many topical antioxidants (e.g., vitamin E) and topical antibiotics (e.g., metronidazole) provide anti-inflammatory benefits. Similarly, certain topically applied botanical agents, including green tea and *Ginko biloba,* also produce anti-inflammatory effects.[80]

Ginkgo Biloba
Ginkgo biloba is a plant with leaves containing flavonoids, flavonol glycosides, and polyphenols (such as terpenoids). These decrease inflammation through antilipoperoxidant and antiradical properties. Controlled clinical studies evaluating anti-inflammatory and other beneficial effects of topical Ginkgo biloba are currently lacking.

Green Tea
Topically applied green tea extract contains epigallocatechin-3-gallate, a polyphenol shown to decrease UVB-induced inflammation.[81] These findings were confirmed through skin-fold thickness measurements in mice both before and after UVB exposure. This measurement reflects the amount of tissue edema (a sign of inflammation) and is the current cosmeceutical industry standard for quantifying inflammation. Although this is the current industry standard, it is a difficult test to replicate, and the murine model findings may not necessarily correlate with similar findings in humans.

Growth Factors
Growth factors are chemical messengers between cells to turn on or off specific cellular activities such as cell proliferation, chemotaxis, and extracellular matrix formation.[82] Topical application of growth factors also reduces signs of photoaging; they promote fibroblast and keratinocyte proliferation and induce extracellular matrix formation.[83-86] Growth factors can be derived from several sources, including epidermal cells, human foreskin, placental cells, colostrum, recombinant bacteria, yeast, and plants.[87] Growth factors can also be produced synthetically. A partial list of human growth factors and their corresponding functions in the skin is shown in Table 3.3.[88-90]

The use of human-derived growth factors in topical skin care products is controversial. Although human growth factors have been shown to repair photodamage through the induction of cell proliferation and differentiation, the associated increase in angiogenesis (secondary to excessive VEGF exposure) has also been shown to be a critical step in the transition of dormant tumors to malignancies (Box 3.8). Furthermore, various types of melanomas have receptors for growth factors (e.g., VEGF).[91-93] Thus, alternate, nonhuman sources of growth factors have been sought to offer the same cutaneous benefits as the human-derived growth factors, but without the potential for stimulating skin cancers. Animal-derived growth factors, such as one derived from a mollusk, have been shown to be effective substitutes in repairing

TABLE 3.3 Human Growth Factors and Their Respective Functions in the Skin

Growth Factor	Function in Skin
Fibroblast growth factor (bFGF [FGF-2], FGF-4, FGF-6, KGF [FGF-7], FGF-9)	Angiogenic and fibroblast mitogen*
Transforming growth factor (TGF-β1, TGF-β2, TGF-β3)	Keratinocyte migration; chemotactic for macrophages and fibroblasts
Platelet-derived growth factor (PDGF AA, PDGF BB, PDGF Rb)	Chemotactic for macrophages and fibroblasts; fibroblast mitogen and matrix production; macrophage activation
Vascular endothelial growth factor (VEGF)	Influences angiogenesis and vascular permeability to improve tissue nutrition
Placental growth factor (PGF)	Promotes endothelial cell growth (member of VEGF family)
Insulin-like growth factors (IGF-1, IGF-BP1, IGF-BP2, IGF-BP3, IGF-BP6)	Endothelial cell and fibroblast mitogen
Hepatocyte growth factor (HGF)	Strong mitogen; wound healing and three-dimensional tissue regeneration

*Mitogen induces cell mitosis (replication) and transformation and differentiation.

Adapted from Mehta RC, Smith SR, Grove GL, et al. Reduction in facial photodamage by a topical growth factor product. *J Drugs Dermatol.* 2008;7:864-871; and Sundaram H, Mehta R, Norine J, et al. Role of physiologically balanced growth factors in skin rejuvenation. *J Drugs Dermatol.* 2009;8(5 Suppl):1-13.

Box 3.8

Growth Factors

- The use of human-derived growth factors in topical skin care products is controversial.
- Growth factors have been shown to repair photodamage, but there is concern that dormant tumors may be transformed into malignancies.
- Nonhuman and synthetically sourced growth factor variants are preferable because of their enhanced safety profile.
- Ossential Advanced Growth Factor Serum contains synthetic lipopeptides.

---

photodamage.[94] Kinetin, a plant-derived topical growth factor, has similarly shown promise in repairing photodamage. Synthetically produced growth factor, composed of lipopeptides (the main active portions of growth factors, composed of small-chain amino acid sequences), has shown great potential in terms of providing the necessary building blocks for fibroblasts to produce collagen and elastin. These synthetic lipopeptides are one of the main ingredients in Ossential Advanced Growth Factor Serum. Because no human or animal product is directly applied to the skin when synthetic growth factors are used, their safety profile is enhanced.

SUPPORTIVE AGENTS

Because they often have only extracellular mechanisms of action and offer only mildly therapeutic benefit, supportive agents should be used in combination with essential agents. Topical products considered to be supportive agents include AHAs, beta-hydroxy acids (BHAs), non-HQ pigment-stabilizing agents (kojic acid, azelaic acid, and arbutin), resorcinol, and disease-specific agents (5-fluorouracil, imiquimod, benzoyl peroxide, topical antibiotics, and topical antifungals).

Alpha-Hydroxy Acids

The exact mechanism of action of AHAs, such as glycolic, lactic, and malic acid, is not known. Dermatologic effects, however, are believed to be primarily limited to the epidermis. AHAs, also referred to as fruit acids, are weakly hydroscopic (i.e., they draw water into dry skin cells). AHAs are characterized as having an alcohol (hydroxyl) function in the alpha position relative to the carbon atom bearing the carboxyl function. Skin feels rough when there is an accumulation of partially attached surface stratum corneum cells. Forced exfoliation with topical agents, such as the AHAs, can restore a smoother texture. The concentration of the AHA agent is critical. At low concentrations (2% to 8%), only a few layers of the stratum corneum are removed, and enough cells remain to keep the skin's barrier function intact. Conversely, concentrations higher than 12% may lead to a total loss of stratum corneum (affecting 10 to 20 layers of cells) and cause irritation of the skin. This is especially true if AHAs are used more than once daily.

Although the exact mechanism of action of AHA is unknown, it is hypothesized that AHAs act as chelating agents for calcium and reduce the calcium ion epidermal concentration. Removing calcium ions from intercellular keratinocyte adhesions disrupts their function and results in desquamation. Moreover, these reduced ion levels promote cell growth and slow differentiation, giving the skin a more youthful appearance.[95] AHA-induced effects are temporary, however, because they do not regulate the keratinization process, nor do they produce softer keratin as tretinoin does. Thus, when the use of AHAs is discontinued, the condition being treated often returns within 2 or 3 weeks.

In an attempt to create a more potent product, a recent trend has been to increase the concentration of AHAs, thereby decreasing their overall pH. This, however, is not wholly beneficial. Using glycolic acid as an example, when the pH is increased, so too is the efficacy (to a mild extent), but the irritation and adverse effects also increase (Table 3.4).[96] Acidity alone does not predict acantholytic efficacy. Hydrogen bonding, electrostatic, inductive, and steric effects are also

TABLE 3.4 Glycolic Acid Concentrations and Their Different pH Values

Concentration (%)	pH
5	1.7
10	1.6
20	1.5
30	1.4
40	1.4
40	1.3
50	1.2
60	1.0

involved.[97] Cutaneous surface pH changes induced by AHAs should be seriously noted because these changes can persist for up to 4 hours following application.

The acidic pH of glycolic acid is buffered to approximately 2.8 to 3.5 for facial application.[97] Many cosmetic products on the market claim to be "neutralized" or "buffered," thereby yielding less irritation. It should be noted, however, that neutralized products would have little cutaneous efficacy.[98]

Glycolic and lactic acids are the AHAs most commonly used in skin care products. As the molecular sizes of AHAs vary, so do their respective efficacies. Glycolic acid is the smallest and thus has the best penetrating activity. Glycolic acid is hydroscopic and binds to water in the skin. It also decreases the bonds between keratinocytes. At higher concentrations, glycolic acid detaches the epidermis from the dermis (epidermolysis) through lysis of hemidesmosomes. It can be used alone or in combination with other chemicals in facial peels.[96,99-102]

Mild to moderate concentrations (≤30%) of glycolic acid have been used for "lunch-time" peels. These remove epidermal corneocytes and produce exfoliation at the lower levels of the stratum corneum.[103,104] Because they have no dermal effects, lunch-time peels are not true peels. Indeed, they may yield temporarily smoother skin and improve acneic comedones, but they have no effect on wrinkles, scars, or skin tightening. The effects of AHAs are shown in Box 3.9.

Beta-Hydroxy Acids

BHAs induce smoothness of the stratum corneum surface through their keratolytic action. BHAs, such as salicylic acid, however, are irritating and increase skin sensitivity. They are not recommended for daily use on normal skin because of the potential for causing allergic reactions. Typically, BHAs are used to increase the efficacy of a chemical peel or treat warts and acne. They may also be used independently (as in a salicylic acid "peel"). It is worth

---

Box 3.9

Effects of Alpha-Hydroxy Acids

- Alpha-hydroxy acids (AHAs) cause stratum corneum exfoliation that can restore skin smoothness.
- At low concentrations (2% to 8%), AHAs remove only a few layers of the stratum corneum, leaving enough cells to keep the skin's barrier function intact.
- Concentrations higher than 12% may lead to a total loss of stratum corneum (10 to 20 layers of cells) and cause skin irritation and adverse effects.
- Glycolic acid has the smallest molecule size and therefore shows the best penetration of skin.
- "Lunch-time" peels with AHAs are exfoliations and not true peels; they do not reach the dermis, have no effect on wrinkles or scars, and cannot tighten skin.

noting here that the use of the term *peel* to describe the effects of topically applied salicylic acid is incorrect because it has no dermal effects. Thus, BHAs are not recommended as the primary treatment for wrinkles, scars, or skin tightening.

Nonhydroquinone Pigment Stabilizers
Kojic Acid
Kojic acid is a skin-lightening agent that inhibits the tyrosinase enzyme involved in melanogenesis. It is derived from several fungal species such as *Penicillium* and *Aspergillus*. Kojic acid is often used in concentrations between 1% and 4%, and it is usually more effective at lightening the skin when used in combination with other agents (e.g., vitamin C, arbutin, glycolic acid, hydroxy acids, gamma-aminobutyric acid, licorice extract).[105] Kojic acid is a good skin-lightening option for patients who cannot tolerate HQ. Products containing kojic acid are recommended to be used twice daily for approximately 2 months, or until the desired amount of skin lightening is achieved. However, because of its high potential for sensitization, it often induces irritant contact dermatitis and is thus poorly tolerated.

Azelaic Acid
A dicarboxylic acid sourced from *Pityrosporum ovale*, azelaic acid acts as a tyrosinase inhibitor to lighten the skin. Optimal stabilization of melanocyte activity, and thus correction of hyperpigmentation, is achieved when azelaic acid is used concomitantly with a product that enhances its penetration (e.g., glycolic acid, retinol).

Arbutin
Arbutin, a glycoside derived from the bearberry fruit, has skin-lightening effects through the inhibition of tyrosinase. In general, arbutin is believed to be less potent than kojic and azelaic acid. Therefore, it is best used in combination with other skin-lightening agents to achieve optimal correction of hyperpigmentation.

Resorcinol
Resorcinol (*m*-dihydroxybenzene) has keratolytic activity and may be used as a superficial peeling agent to decrease microcomedone formation. When used in conditions such as acne, it can enhance the penetration of concomitantly used essential topical agents. In low concentrations (1% to 2%), resorcinol is a component in many keratolytic and antiseptic topical products. Higher concentrations (up to 40%) in a paste vehicle can be used as a peeling agent for a stronger acne treatment option. The use of higher strengths of resorcinol is not advised because they can cause methemoglobinemia and other systemic central nervous system side effects that are similar to those seen with phenol use.[106]

5-Fluorouracil
5-Fluorouracil (5-FU), a fluorinated pyrimidine analog, has cytotoxic effects. Interestingly, it penetrates areas of abnormal skin (e.g., actinically damaged) more thoroughly than areas of normal skin. Topically applied, a 5% concentration of 5-FU is approved by the U.S. Food and Drug Administration (FDA) for

the treatment of multiple actinic keratoses and basal cell carcinoma.[107] When treating patients with actinic keratoses, a cream containing 5% 5-FU is recommended to be applied twice daily for 2 to 4 weeks. For treatment of superficial basal cell carcinoma, a cream containing 5% 5-FU is also recommended twice daily, but for a longer duration (3 to 6 weeks). The most common side effects, which are limited to the treatment site, include inflammation (redness, swelling, and exfoliation) and occasionally superficial erosions. Alternative treatments for actinic keratoses include cryotherapy, electrodessication with curettage, chemical peels, and photodynamic therapy.

Imiquimod

A non-nucleoside heterocyclic amine and synthetic member of the imidazoquinolone family, imiquimod (Aldara) acts as an immunomodulating medication. It is FDA approved for the topical treatment of actinic keratoses, superficial basal cell carcinoma, and external genital warts. A 5% concentration of imiquimod in a cream vehicle is recommended for use two times per week for 16 weeks for actinic keratosis and five times per week for 6 weeks for superficial basal cell carcinoma. For external genital warts, it is recommended that imiquimod be applied three times per week for 16 weeks. Imiquimod binds to toll-like receptor-7 (TLR-7) on macrophages, monocytes, and dendritic cells.[108] Stimulation of these cells through TLR-7 causes various pro-inflammatory cytokines to be released (TNF-α, IFN-α, IL-1, IL-6, IL-8, IL-10, and IL-12), which subsequently activate the helper T-cell type 1 (Th-1) cell-mediated immune response. The TH-2 pathway is in turn inhibited.[109] In addition to this immune system modulation, imiquimod upregulates natural killer cell activity by inducing the production of 2′5′-oligoadenylate synthetase.[110] Together, these actions inhibit the growth of tumors and viruses. Common, expected side effects include itching, redness, swelling, peeling, and occasionally the formation of erosions at the application site.

Benzoyl Peroxide

Topically applied benzoyl peroxide, a powerful oxidizing and bactericidal agent against *Propionibacterium acnes*, *Pityrosporum ovale*, and several strains of *Staphylococcus*,[111] is indicated for the treatment of mild to moderate acne. It also has comedolytic and keratolytic activity.[112] Topical benzoyl peroxide is available in a variety of concentrations (2.5% to 20%) and in numerous vehicles (gel, cream, and lotion).[113]

TOPICAL ANTIBIOTICS

An extensive list of all topical antibiotics used in dermatology would be long and beyond the scope of this chapter. Most topical antibiotics used in dermatology, however, can be simply categorized into one (or both) of the two following categories: those used to treat acne or rosacea, and those used to treat healing wounds.

For the treatment of acne or rosacea, the most commonly prescribed topical antibiotics are erythromycin (from the macrolide class), clindamycin (from the lincosamide class), and metronidazole (from the nitroimidazole class). For the treatment of cutaneous wounds, the most frequently used topical antibiotics are mupirocin, bacitracin, neomycin, gentamicin, polymyxin B, and silver sulfadiazine.

Acne and Rosacea Treatment

Erythromycin, a macrolide antibiotic, is bactericidal. It inhibits protein synthesis by irreversibly binding to the 50S subunit of the bacterial ribosome. Erythromycin is effective against the following bacteria: gram-positive cocci, *Legionella pneumophila*, *Chlamydia*, *Corynebacterium diphtheriae*, *Haemophilus influenzae*, *Treponema pallidum*, *Ureaplasma urealyticum*, and *Mycoplasma pneumoniae*.[114] Improvement in acne is induced by erythromycin's further activity against *Propionibacterium acnes*. Erythromycin is poorly soluble in water. Therefore, vehicles composed of liposomal and conventional emulsions are more effective at delivering this medication than hydroalcoholic vehicles.[115,116] Topical concentrations of erythromycin typically range between 1% and 4%.

Clindamycin, a synthetic lincomycin derivative, has the same mechanism of action as erythromycin (irreversible bacterial 50S subunit binding). Clindamycin is effective against anaerobic gram-positive and gram-negative bacteria, as well as most aerobic gram-positive cocci.[117] As with erythromycin, clindamycin improves acne through its bactericidal effects on *P. acnes*. Topical clindamycin is available as a 1% concentration in a lotion, gel, or solution (alcohol based).

Metronidazole, a synthetic nitroimidazole antibiotic, is also bactericidal. It inhibits the synthesis of nucleic acid and disrupts the DNA in susceptible bacteria (which include most anaerobic bacteria and protozoa).[118] But unlike erythromycin and clindamycin, metronidazole is not active against *P. acnes*. It is also inactive against *Demodex folliculorum*, streptococci, and staphylococci.[119] Because the microflora of the skin in rosacea patients does not change significantly with topical metronidazole use, the beneficial effects are most likely due to the agent's anti-inflammatory effects.[120] Inflammation is decreased through the suppression of cell-mediated immunity and by limiting leukocyte chemotaxis.[121]

Wound Treatment

Mupirocin, a metabolite of *Pseudomonas fluorescens*, is bactericidal when applied topically. Mupirocin interrupts bacterial protein synthesis, RNA synthesis, and cell wall synthesis through the inhibition of bacterial isoleucyl-tRNA synthetase.[122] Mupirocin is active against *Staphylococcus epidermidis*, *Staphylococcus aureus*, *Streptococcus pyogenes*, beta-hemolytic streptococci, and some strains of methicillin-resistant *S. aureus* (MRSA).[123] Interestingly, because of the heightened use of mupirocin, one study found that up to 65% of the MRSA strains tested were resistant to mupirocin.[124] Mupirocin is available in a 2% ointment or cream. Because very little of the mupirocin is metabolized by the skin, most of the medication applied remains on the surface to fight bacteria.

Bacitracin is bacteriostatic. It is sourced from a strain of *Bacillus subtilis*, and it inhibits bacterial cell wall synthesis. Bacitracin is active against *Streptococcus pneumoniae*, *S. aureus*, *H. influenzae*, *T. pallidum*, and *Neisseria* strains. Bacitracin is indicated for short-term use on minor wounds because patients can otherwise become sensitized to the medication and subsequently develop allergic contact dermatitis. This is especially common when it is applied to nonintact skin and used for prolonged periods.

Derived from *Streptomyces fradiae*, neomycin is a bactericidal aminoglycoside that inhibits protein synthesis by binding to the 30s subunit of the bacterial ribosome. Neomycin may additionally inhibit DNA polymerase enzymes within the bacteria.[125] It is effective against most gram-negative and some gram-positive bacteria, including *H. influenzae*, *Escherichia coli*, *S. aureus*, *Proteus*, *Klebsiella*, and *Serratia*. To reduce the potential for bacterial resistance and compensate for neomycin's relatively weak streptococcal coverage, bacitracin is commonly combined with neomycin and occasionally with polymyxin B. The latter improves gram-negative coverage to include *Pseudomonas*. As seen with bacitracin, when neomycin is used for prolonged periods, the potential for developing allergic contact dermatitis increases. Treatment therefore is typically limited to one week.

Gentamicin, derived from *Micromonospora purpurea*, is a bacteriostatic aminoglycoside. It irreversibly binds the bacterial 30s ribosomal subunit and is effective against gram-negative bacteria such as *Proteus*, *Pseudomonas aeruginosa*, and *E. coli*. Gentamicin also has some gram-positive effect against organisms such as *S. aureus*. Of note, gentamicin does not cover streptococci.[126] Although allergic contact dermatitis to gentamicin is rare, approximately 40% of patients who have a neomycin allergy (with no prior exposure to gentamicin) also demonstrate positive patch testing to gentamicin.[127]

Polymyxin B is bactericidal and derived from *Bacillus polymyxa*. It destroys bacterial cell membranes through a detergent-like mechanism.[126] Polymyxin B is especially effective against gram-negative bacteria, such as *P. aeruginosa*, *Serratia marcescens*, and *Proteus mirabilis*.[127] Because of its inability to cover gram-positive bacteria, polymyxin B is usually combined with bacitracin and neomycin to broaden its coverage.

Silver sulfadiazine is commonly used for the topical treatment of burns. It is formulated through a reaction between silver nitrate and sodium sulfadiazine. Silver sulfadiazine inhibits bacterial replication by binding to bacterial DNA. It covers both gram-positive and gram-negative bacteria, including MRSA and *P. aeruginosa*.[128]

Topical Antifungals

Cutaneous fungal infections are among the most common conditions encountered by dermatologists. Topical agents used to treat dermatomycoses typically fall within one of the following categories: azoles, polyenes, and allylamines-benzylamines. These three main antifungal classes are further detailed later. Less commonly used topical antimycotic agents, which do not fall into these three categories, include selenium sulfide, hydroxypyridone (ciclopirox olamine), and thiocarbonate (tolnaftate).[129]

Azoles

Azoles, effective against *Candida*, dermatophytes, and *Malassezia furfur* (also known as *Pityrosporum ovale*), work by blocking the production of ergosterol, a primary component of the fungal cell membrane.[130,131] More specifically, the azoles block synthesis of ergosterol by inhibiting lanosterol 14α-demethylase, a cytochrome P-450–dependent enzyme that converts lanosterol to ergosterol. After the fungal cell membrane is compromised (by decreased ergosterol and accumulation of intracellular 14α-methylsterols), its increased rigidity and altered permeability prevent the fungi from growing and surviving.[130,132-134] The most commonly prescribed topical azoles include ketoconazole, clotrimazole, miconazole, and econazole.

Ketoconazole is a water-soluble imidazole derivative. It has a broad spectrum of activity against *Candida albicans*, *M. furfur*, and dermatophytes. In one study, ketoconazole 2% cream, when applied twice daily for 4 weeks, showed marked clinical improvement in approximately 82% of patients with tinea corporis, tinea pedis, and tinea cruris.[135] In another study, approximately 80% of infants with seborrheic dermatitis treated with topical ketoconazole for 10 days demonstrated a good to excellent degree of disease clearance.[136] Similar efficacy has been observed in adults with the condition, who were treated with ketoconazole cream, ketoconazole 2% shampoo, or both. These effects are largely due to its activity against *M. furfur*.[136-145] Tinea versicolor and cutaneous candidiasis have also shown excellent clearance rates with ketoconazole cream.[146-151]

Clotrimazole exhibits the same mechanism of action as the other azole antifungals. It is effective against most strains of *Epidermophyton*, *Trichophyton*, *Microsporum*, gram-positive bacteria, and *Candida*.[152,153] When used twice daily, clotrimazole is an effective treatment for tinea corporis, tinea pedis, tinea versicolor, tinea cruris, and cutaneous candidiasis.[152-160] It comes in lotion, cream, and solution formulations.

Although exhibiting the same mechanism of action as the other azole antifungals, miconazole is unique. After a single application, it can be detected within the stratum corneum for up to 4 days. This is a significantly longer duration compared with the other topicals in its class. Miconazole is active against the following common dermatophytes: *Trichophyton mentagrophytes*, *Trichophyton rubrum*, and *Epidermophyton floccosum*. It also inhibits the growth of *M. furfur* and *C. albicans*.[161,162] The cream formulation of miconazole has shown efficacy in the treatment of tinea cruris, tinea pedis, tinea corporis, tinea versicolor, and cutaneous candidiasis.[162-166] Twice-daily application is recommended for each condition with the exception of tinea versicolor, for which a once-daily application is effective.

Econazole, exhibiting the same mechanism of action as the other azole antifungals, is notable for its depth of penetration. Its minimal inhibitory concentrations for dermatophytes extend as deep as the mid-dermis.[168,169] Econazole inhibits most strains of *Microsporum*, *Trichophyton*, and *Epidermophyton* species, as well as *M. furfur* and *C. albicans*.[168] Topical econazole effectively treats tinea cruris, tinea pedis, and tinea corporis caused by dermatophytes, cutaneous candidiasis from *C. albicans*, and tinea versicolor from *Malassezia* organisms.[168,170-175] Interestingly, with respect to the treatment of cutaneous candidiasis and tinea infections, econazole 1% cream has been shown to be just as effective as clotrimazole 1% cream. However, econazole-treated patients show a more rapid onset of improvement.[175]

Polyenes

Identified through their molecular structure, polyene antifungals are composed of carbon atoms with conjugated double bonds in a macrolide ring. The macrolide ring is closed by lactose or by an internal ester.[176] Although two clinically significant polyene antifungals exist, nystatin and amphotericin B, the latter is rarely used in the United States.

Nystatin, produced by *Streptomyces albidus* and *Streptomyces noursei*, demonstrates both fungistatic and fungicidal properties.[177] Nystatin's mechanism of action involves irreversible binding to sterols within the cell membrane of certain species of *Candida*. This leads to increased cell membrane permeability and the subsequent leakage of intracellular elements.[176-179] Nystatin is not water soluble and so is not absorbed by intact skin. Although nystatin is ineffective against dermatophytes that cause cutaneous infections, it is effective in treating cutaneous as well as mucosal infections due to *C. albicans*, *Candida krusei*, *Candida tropicalis*, and *Candida parapsilosis*.[128,175] Recommended treatment involves twice-daily application of nystatin to the affected areas. A cream, powder, or ointment formulation is available for use. For oral mucosal thrush, the suspension form is more appropriate, and the recommended use is four to five times daily.

Allylamines and Benzylamines

Allylamines, which include naftifine and terbinafine, and benzylamines, which include butenafine, share a similar structure and mechanism of action. Both allylamines and benzylamines exhibit a comparable mechanism of action to the azole class of antifungal agents. They all inhibit the synthesis of ergosterol, an essential element within the fungal cell membrane. This results in increased fungal cell membrane permeability, allowing important intracellular elements to escape from within. An intracellular accumulation of sterol precursors additionally occurs.

Allylamines and benzylamines differ from azoles in that the former two agents inhibit ergosterol synthesis independent of cytochrome P-450 (an enzyme involved in drug metabolism and bioactivation). In opposition, azoles work in a cytochrome P-450 dependent manner. Furthermore, allylamines and benzylamines block ergosterol synthesis at an earlier stage in the production pathway compared with azoles.[180-182]

Naftifine is a synthetic allylamine with both fungicidal and fungistatic behavior.[183,184] It is strongly lipophilic, which leads to its effective penetration and the subsequent accumulation of large concentrations within the stratum corneum.[185-187] Naftifine specifically inhibits squalene epoxidase, an enzyme necessary for the conversion of squalene to squalene oxide in the production of ergosterol. Naftifine is effective against a broad spectrum of dermatophytes (including *T. mentagrophytes*), saprophytes (including *Sporothrix schenckii*), and yeasts.[183,184,188] One study evaluated the treatment of tinea corporis and tinea cruris by comparing naftifine 1% cream with econazole 1% cream.[189] Although they were both similar in efficacy, naftifine displayed a faster onset of action. When compared with clotrimazole, naftifine was just as effective at treating tinea cruris, tinea corporis, tinea pedis, and candidiasis, but it had an earlier onset of action compared with clotrimazole.[189-194] Available in both gel and cream formulations, naftifine's recommended application frequency is once to twice daily in each of the aforementioned conditions.

Terbinafine, like naftifine, is a synthetic allylamine antifungal agent. Through a cytochrome P-450–independent mechanism, it compromises the integrity of fungal cell membranes. Terbinafine halts ergosterol synthesis by inhibiting squalene epoxidase. Similar to naftifine, terbinafine has both fungistatic and fungicidal capabilities. It is also highly lipophilic, which allows for high concentrations to accumulate within the stratum corneum.[183,195] Interestingly, persistent concentrations above the mean inhibitory concentrations for common dermatophytes were detected 7 days after topical application of terbinafine.[184,196] Terbinafine was created through structural modifications to naftifine, which makes the former 10 to 100 times more potent (in terms of antifungal activity) than the latter.[180,197,198] Terbinafine is fungicidal against numerous dermatophytes, *C. albicans*, and several dimorphic fungi, including *S. schenckii*, *Histoplasma capsulatum*, and *Blastomyces dermatitidis*.[195,199] Terbinafine 1% cream is effective in treating tinea cruris, tinea corporis, tinea pedis, tinea versicolor, and intertriginous candidiasis.[200] One study found the overall efficacy of terbinafine in treating all tinea infections to be approximately 70% to 90%, with the greatest efficacy seen in the treatment of tinea cruris and tinea corporis.[201]

Butenafine, a benzylamine antifungal, is structurally similar to the allylamines, with the exception of a butylbenzyl group in the former, replacing the allylamine group in the latter.[202,203] An impressive characteristic of butenafine is that fungicidal concentrations of this agent can be detected within the stratum corneum for at least 72 hours after topical application.[204,205] The mechanism of action of butenafine is the same as that of naftifine and terbinafine. Butenafine is fungicidal against aspergilli, dermatophytes, and dimorphic fungi, including *S. schenckii*.[202,203] Its inhibitory capabilities have been found to be equal to or greater than those of naftifine and terbinafine. Cure rates for tinea cruris treated with butenafine range between 84% and 100%. Topical butenafine is also an effective treatment against tinea corporis, tinea pedis, tinea versicolor, and cutaneous candidiasis.[206-213] In general, for each of the previously mentioned conditions, once- to twice-daily application of butenafine for approximately 2 weeks is recommended. Notably, after ceasing application of the butenafine, clinical and mycological cure rates continue for up to 2 weeks. This is likely because of its strong keratin-binding capacity.

Wound Healing

Biafine

Biafine (OrthoNeutrogena), a water-based topical emulsion, is used to hasten healing after radiation dermatitis, burns, wounds, and ablative laser treatments. Biafine contains the following ingredients within its aqueous phase: alginate of sodium salts, demineralized water, and triethanolamine. Within the lipid state, the following exist: ethylene glycol stearic acid, paraffin liquid, propylene glycol, paraffin wax, squalene, cetyl palmitate, avocado oil, and fragrance.[214] Biafine is a chemotactic agent for macrophages and works at the level of the dermis (within granulation tissue).[215] Biafine also reduces the secretion of IL-6, thereby increasing the IL-1/IL-6 ratio.[216] The formation of granulation tissue is thus enhanced, as is the production of collagen.[216]

QUESTIONABLE AGENTS

Questionable agents have not shown any scientifically proven therapeutic benefit. These should therefore only be used, if at all, after essential or supportive topical agents are already employed. A seemingly endless array of questionable agents are added to various skin care products currently on the market. A complete list of these agents not only would fail to fit within the confines of this book but would also be irrelevant because they have shown no scientific benefit in either Skin Health Restoration or maintenance processes. Many of the most expensive over-the-counter skin care creams (ranging in price from $200 to $1,000 per small container) contain only questionable agents as their active ingredients. Examples of these include gold, platinum, caviar, silk, ursolic acid, Planifolia PFA, and Imperiale Orchidee molecular extract. Randomized, controlled clinical studies demonstrating the efficacy of the following popular questionable agents do not currently exist: gold (found in Chantecaille's Nano Gold Energizing Cream and Orlane's Creme Royale), platinum (found in La Prairie's Cellular Radiance Cream), caviar (found in La Prairie's White Caviar Illuminating Cream), silk (found in Kanebo's Sensai Collection Premier The Cream), ursolic acid (found in Sisley's Sisleya Global Anti-Age Cream), Planifolia PFA (found in Chanel's Precision Sublimage Serum Essential Regenerating Cream), and Imperiale Orchidee Molecular Extract (found in Guerlain's Orchidee Imperiale Cream Next Generation). Correspondence to the previously mentioned companies requesting clinical data to support product efficacy went largely unanswered. The few companies that did reply, however, offered only anecdotal reports of efficacy. Thus, the high price of many popular skin care products does not necessarily reflect effectiveness. It is therefore more appropriate to eat caviar, wear silk clothing, adorn ourselves with gold and platinum jewelry, and visually admire orchids than to apply products containing these questionable ingredients onto our skin.

REFERENCES

1. Kligman LH, Chen HD, Kligman AM. Topical retinoic acid enhances the repair of ultraviolet damaged dermal connective tissue. *Connect Tissue Res.* 1984;12: 139-150.

2. Kligman AM, Dogadkina D, Lavker RM. Effects of topical tretinoin on the non-sun exposed protected skin of the elderly. *J Am Acad Dermatol.* 1993;29:25-33.

3. Kligman DE, Sadiq I, Pagnoni A, et al. High-strength tretinoin: a method for rapid retinization of facial skin. *J Am Acad Dermatol.* 1998;39:S93-97.

4. Kligman AM. Cosmeceuticals. *Dermatol Clin.* 2000;18:1-7.

5. Goldfarb MT, Ellis CN, Weiss JS, et al. Topical tretinoin therapy: its use in photoaged skin. *J Am Acad Dermatol.* 1989;21:654-650.

6. Ellis CN, Weiss JJ, Hamilton TA, et al. Sustained improvement with prolonged topical tretinoin (retinoic acid) for photoaged skin. *J Am Acad Dermatol.* 1990;23: 629-637.

7. Green LJ, McCormick A, Weinstein GD. Photoaging and the skin: the effects of tretinoin. *Dermatol Clin.* 1993;11:97-105.

8. Gilchrest BA. Treatment of photodamage with topical tretinoin: an overview. *J Am Acad Dermatol.* 1997;36:S27-36.

9. Olsen EA, Katz HI, Levine N, et al. Tretinoin emollient cream for photodamaged skin: results of 48-week, multicenter, double-blind studies. *J Am Acad Dermatol.* 1997;37:217-216.

10. Olsen EA, Katz HI, Levine N, et al. Sustained improvement in photodamaged skin with reduced tretinoin emollient cream treatment regimen: effect of once-weekly and three times-weekly applications. *J Am Acad Dermatol.* 1997;37:227–230.

11. Chew AL, Bashir SJ, Maibach HI. Topical retinoids. In: Elsner P, Maibach H., eds. *Cosmeceuticals: Drugs vs. Cosmetics.* New York: Marcel Decker; 2000:107-122.

12. Samuel M, Brooke RC, Hollis S, Griffiths CE. Interventions for photodamaged skin. *Cochrane Database Syst Rev.* 2005;CD001782.

13. Mukherjee S, Date A, Patravale V, et al. Retinoids in the treatment of skin aging: an overview of clinical efficacy and safety. *Clin Interv Aging.* 2006;1:327-348.

14. Sorg O, Antille C, Kaya G, Saurat JH. Retinoids in cosmeceuticals. *Dermatol Ther.* 2006;19:289-296.

15. Ting W. Tretinoin for the treatment of photodamaged skin. *Cutis.* 2010;86:47-52.

16. Griffiths CE, Kang S, Ellis CN, et al. Two concentrations of topical tretinoin (retinoic acid) cause similar improvement of photoaging but different degrees of irritation: a double-blind, vehicle-controlled comparison of 0.1% and 0.025% tretinoin creams. *Arch Dermatol.* 1995;131:1037-1044.

17. Bhawan J. Short- and long-term histologic effects of topical tretinoin on photodamaged skin. *Int J Dermatol.* 1998;37:286-292.

18. Fluhr JW, Vienne MP, Lauze C, et al. Tolerance profile of retinol, retinaldehyde and retinoic acid under maximized and long-term clinical conditions. *Dermatology.* 1999;199(Suppl 1):57-60.

19. Kligman AM, Grove GL, Hirose R, et al. Topical tretinoin for photoaged skin. *J Am Acad Dermatol.* 1986;15:836-859.

20. Kim BH, Lee YS, Kang KS. The mechanism of retinol-induced irritation and its application to anti-irritant development. *Toxicol Lett.* 2003;146:65-73.

21. Connor MJ, Smit MH. Terminal-group oxidation of retinol by mouse epidermis: inhibition *in vitro* and in vivo. *Biochem J.* 1987;244:489-492.

22. Duell EA, Derguini F, Kang S, et al. Extraction of human epidermis treated with retinol yields retro-retinoids in addition to free retinol and retinyl-esters. *J Invest Dermatol.* 1996;107:178-182.

23. Kang S, Duell EA, Fisher GJ, et al. Application of retinol to human skin *in vivo* induces epidermal hyperplasia and cellular retinoid binding proteins characteristic of retinoic acid but without measurable retinoic acid levels or irritation. *J Invest Dermatol.* 1995;105:549-556.

24. Kafi R, Kwak HSR, Schumacher WE, et al. Improvement of naturally aged skin with vitamin A (retinol). *Arch Dermatol.* 2007;143:606-612.

25. Fluhr JW, Vienne MP, Lauze C, et al. Tolerance profile of retinol, retinaldehyde and retinoic acid under maximized and long-term clinical conditions. *Dermatology.* 1999;199(Suppl 1):57-60.

26. Kurlandsky SB, Xiao JH, Duell EA, et al. Biological activity of all-trans retinol requires metabolic conversion to all-trans retinoic acid and is mediated through activation of nuclear retinoid receptors in human keratinocytes. *J Biol Chem.* 1994;269: 32821-32827.

27. Brisaert MG, Everaerts I, Plaizier-Vercammen JA. Chemical stability of tretinoin in dermatological preparations. *Pharmaceutica Acta Helvetiae.* 1995;70:16-166.

28. Ball Arefiev KL, Hantash BM. Advances in the treatment of melasma: a review of the recent literature. *Dermatol Surg.* 2012;38:971-984.

29. Rendon MI, Gaviria JI. Skin lightening agents. In: Draelos ZD, Dover JS, Alam M, eds. *Procedures in Cosmetic Dermatology: Cosmeceuticals.* Philadelphia: Saunders/ Elsevier; 2005:104.

30. Palumbo A, d'Ischia M, Misuraca G, et al. Mechanism of inhibition of melanogenesis by hydroquinone. *Biochim Biophys Acta.* 1991;1073:85-90.

31. Jimbow K, Obata H, Pathak MA, Fitzpatrick TB. Mechanism of depigmentation by hydroquinone. *J Invest Dermatol.* 1974;6:436-449.

32. Biewenga GP, Haenen GR, Bast A. The pharmacology of the antioxidant lipoic acid. *Gen Pharmacol.* 1997;29:315-331.

33. Burke KE: Nutritional antioxidants. In: Draelos ZD, Dover JS, Alam M, eds. *Procedures in Cosmetic Dermatology: Cosmeceuticals.* Philadelphia: Saunders/Elsevier; 2005:125-132.

34. Meister A, Anderson, ME. Glutathione. *Ann Rev Biochem.* 1983;52:711-760.

35. Linder J. Antioxidants: Essential preventative and corrective topicals. *Dermatologist.* 2011;19:28-33.

36. Chan AC. Partners in defense, vitamin E and vitamin C. Can *J Physiol Pharmacol.* 1993;71:725-731.

37. Montenegro L, Bonina F, Rigano L, et al. Protective effect evaluation of free radical scavengers on UVB induced human cutaneous erythema by skin reflectance spectrophotometry. *Int J Cosmet Sci.* 2007;17:91-103.

38. McDaniel DH, Neudecker BA, DiNardo JC, et al. Idebenone: a new antioxidant. Part I. Relative assessment of oxidative stress protection capacity compared to commonly known antioxidants. *J Cosmet Dermatol.* 2005;4:10-17.

39. Tournas JA, Lin FH, Burch JA, et al. Ubiquinone, idebenone, and kinetin provide ineffective photoprotection to skin when compared to a topical antioxidant combination of vitamins C and E with ferulic acid. *J Invest Dermatol.* 2006;126:1185-1187.

40. Huang C, Miller T. The truth about over-the-counter topical anti-aging products: a comprehensive review. *Aesthet Surg J.* 2007;27:402-412.

41. Farris PK. Topical vitamin C: a useful agent for treating photoaging and other dermatologic conditions. *Dermatol Surg.* 2005;31:814-818.

42. Heber GK, Markovic B, Hayes A. Anhydrous topical ascorbic acid on human skin. *J Cosmet Dermatol.* 2006;5:150-156.

43. Pinnell SR, Yang HS, Omar M, et al. Topical L-ascorbic acid: percutaneous absorption studies. *Dermatol Surg.* 2001;27:137-142.

44. Traikovich SS. Use of topical ascorbic acid and its effects on photodamaged skin topography. *Arch Otolaryngol Head Neck Surg.* 1999;125:1091-1098.

45. Lopez-Torres M, Thiele JJ, Shindo Y, et al. Topical application of alpha-tocopherol modulates the antioxidant network and diminishes ultraviolet-induced oxidative damage in murine skin. *Br J Dermatol.* 1998;138:207-215.

46. Thiele JJ, Traber MG, Packer L. Depletion of human stratum corneum vitamin E: an early and sensitive *in vivo* marker of UV induced photo-oxidation. *J Invest Dermatol.* 1998;110:756-761.

47. Shindo Y, Witt E, Han D, et al. Dose-response effects of acute ultraviolet irradiation on antioxidants and molecular markers of oxidation in murine epidermis and dermis. *J Invest Dermatol.* 1994;102:470-475.

48. Weber C, Podda M, Rallis M, et al. Efficacy of topically applied tocopherols and tocotrienols in protection of murine skin from oxidative damage induced by UV-irradiation. *Free Radic Biol Med.* 1997;22:761-769.

49. Weber SU, Thiele JJ, Cross CE, et al. Vitamin C, uric acid, and glutathione gradients in murine stratum corneum and their susceptibility to ozone exposure. *J Invest Dermatol.* 1999;113:1128-1132.

50. Thiele JJ, Traber MG, Podda M, et al. Ozone depletes tocopherols and tocotrienols topically applied to murine skin. *FEBS Lett.* 1997;401:167-170.

51. Valacchi G, Weber SU, Luu C, et al. Ozone potentiates vitamin E depletion by ultraviolet radiation in the murine stratum corneum. *FEBS Lett.* 2000;466:165-168.

52. Baumann L. Skin ageing and its treatment. *J Pathol.* 2007;211:241-251.

53. Thiele JJ, Ekanayake-Mudiyanselage S. Vitamin E in human skin: organ-specific physiology and considerations for its use in dermatology. *Mol Aspects Med.* 2007;28:646-667.

54. Bissett DL, Miyamoto K, Sun P, et al. Topical niacinamide reduces yellowing, wrinkling, red blotchiness, and hyperpigmented spots in aging facial skin. *Int J Cosmet Sci.* 2004;26:231-238.

55. Bissett DL, Oblong JE, Berge CA. Niacinamide: a B vitamin that improves aging facial skin appearance. *Dermatol Surg.* 2005;31:860-865.

56. Rivers JK. The role of cosmeceuticals in antiaging therapy. *Skin Therapy Lett.* 2008;13:5-9.

57. Dell'Acqua G, Schweikert K. A DNA repair complex to decrease erythema and UV-induced CPD formation. *Cosmetics Toiletries.* 2008;123:69-78.

58. Setlow RB. Cyclobutane-type pyrimidine dimers in polynucleotides. *Science.* 1966;153:379-386.

59. Sutherland BM, Delihas NC, Oliver RP, et al. Action spectra for ultraviolet light-induced transformation of human cells to anchorage-independent growth. *Cancer Res.* 1981;41:2211-2214.

60. Hart R, Setlow RB, Woodhead AD. Evidence that pyrimidine dimers in DNA can give rise to tumors. *Proc Natl Acad Sci U S A.* 1977;74:5574-5578.

61. Harm H. Repair of UV-irradiated biological systems: photoreactivation. In: Yang SY, ed. *Photochemistry and Photobiology of Nucleic Acids.* Vol. 2. New York: Academic Press; 1976:219-262.

62. Takahashi Y, Moriwaki S, Sugiyama Y, et al. Decreased gene expression responsible for post-ultraviolet DNA repair synthesis in aging: a possible mechanism of age-related reduction in DNA repair capacity. *J Invest Dermatol.* 2005;124:435-442.

63. Yamada M, Udono MU, Hori M, et al. Aged human skin removes UVB-induced pyrimidine dimers from the epidermis more slowly than younger adult skin in vivo. *Arch Dermatol.* 2006;297:294-302.

64. Yaar M, Gilchrest BA. Photoaging: mechanism, prevention and therapy. *Br J Dermatol.* 2007;157:874-887.

65. Sander CS, Chang H, Salzmann, S, et al. Photoaging is associated with protein oxidation in human skin in vivo. *J Invest Dermatol.* 2002;118:618-625.

66. Schweikert K, Gafner F, Dell'Acqua G. Uniprotect PT-3: bioactive complex for protection of skin proteins from UV-induced oxidation. *Int J Cosmet Sci.* 2010; 32:29-34.

67. Wulff BC, Schick JS, Thomas-Ahner JM, et al. Topical treatment with OGG1 enzyme affects UVB-induced skin carcinogenesis. *Photochem Photobiol.* 2008;84:317-321.

68. Ceccoli J, Rosales N, Tsimis J, et al. Encapsulation of the UV-DNA repair enzyme T4 endonuclease V in liposomes and delivery to human cells. *J Invest Dermatol.* 1989;93:190-194.

69. Berardesca E, Bertona M, Altabas K, et al. Reduced ultraviolet-induced DNA damage and apoptosis in human skin with topical application of a photolyase-containing DNA repair enzyme cream: clues to skin cancer prevention. *Mol Med Rep.* 2012;5:570-574.

70. Kiripolsky MG, Sundaram H, Bucay VW. A multi-center, open-label study to evaluate the effects of topically-applied DNA repair enzymes and substrates on photo-aged skin. 2012. White paper.

71. Schweikert K, McGregor W, Klein C, et al. Amino acids to increase DNA repair after UVB irradiation of reconstituted human skin. *SÖFW J.* 2006;132:22-26.

72. Milligan JR, Aguilera JA, Ly A, et al. Repair of oxidative DNA damage by amino acids. *Nucleic Acids Res.* 2003;31:6258-6263.

73. Bender K, Blattner C, Knebel A, et al. UV-induced signal transduction. *J Photochem Photobiol B.* 1997;37:1-17.

74. Petit-Frere C, Clingen PH, Grewe M, et al. Induction of interleukin-6 production by ultraviolet radiation in normal human epidermal keratinocytes and in a human keratinocyte cell line is mediated by DNA damage. *J Invest Dermatol.* 1998;111:354-359.

75. Wolf P, Maier H, Mullegger RR, et al. Topical treatment with liposomes containing T4 endonuclease V protects human skin *in vivo* from ultraviolet-induced upregulation of interleukin-10 and tumor necrosis factor. *J Invest Dermatol.* 2000;114:149-156.

76. Stege H, Roza L, Vink AA, et al. Enzyme plus light therapy to repair DNA damage in ultraviolet-B-irradiated human skin. *Proc Natl Acad Sci U S A.* 2000;97:1790-1795.

77. Schul W, Jans J, Rijksen YMA, et al. Enhanced repair of cyclobutane pyrimidine dimers and improved UV resistance in photolyase transgenic mice. *EMBO J.* 2002;21:4719-4729.

78. Berg RJW, Ruven HJT, Sands AT, et al. Defective global genome repair in XPC mice is associated to skin cancer susceptibility but not with sensitivity to UVB induced erythema and edema. *J Invest Dermatol.* 1998;110:405-409.

79. Dell'Acqua G, Schweikert K. A DNA repair complex to decrease erythema and UV-induced CPD formation. *Cosmetics Toiletries.* 2008;123:1-8.

80. Draelos ZD: Cosmeceutical botanicals: part 1. In: Draelos ZD, Dover JS, Alam M, eds. *Procedures in Cosmetic Dermatology: Cosmeceuticals.* Philadelphia: Saunders/Elsevier; 2005:75-77.

81. Katiyar SK, Elmets CA, Agarwal R, et al. Protection against ultraviolet-B radiation-induced local and systemic suppression of contact hypersensitivity and edema responses in C3H/HeN mice by green tea polyphenols. *Photochem Photobiol.* 1995;62:855-861.

82. Babu M, Wells A. Dermal-epidermal communication in wound healing. *Wounds.* 2001;13:183-189.

83. Bertaux B, Horneback W, Eisen AZ, et al. Growth stimulation of human keratinocytes by tissue inhibitor of metalloproteinases. *J Invest Dermatol.* 1991;97:679-85.

84. Finch PW, Rubin JS, Miki T, et al. Human KGF is FGF related with properties of a paracrine effector of epithelial cell growth. *Science.* 1989;245:752-55.

85. Eming SA, Krieg T, Davidson JM. Inflammation in wound repair: molecular and cellular mechanisms. *J Invest Dermatol.* 2001;127:514-525.

86. Schwartz E, Cruickshank FA, Christensen CC, et al. Collagen alterations in chronically sun-damaged human skin. *Photochem Photobiol.* 1993;58:841-844.

87. Bonin-Debs AL, Boche I, Gille H, et al. Development of secreted proteins as biotherapeutic agents. *Exp Opin Biol Ther.* 2004;4:551-558.

88. Mehta RC, Smith SR, Grove GL, et al. Reduction in facial photodamage by a topical growth factor product. *J Drugs Dermatol.* 2008;7:864-871.

89. Sundaram H, Mehta R, Norine J, et al. Role of physiologically balanced growth factors in skin rejuvenation. *J Drugs Dermatol.* 2009;8(5 Suppl):1-13.

90. Demidova-Rice TN, Hamblin MR, Herman IM. Acute and impaired wound healing: pathophysiology and current methods for drug delivery. Part 2. Role of growth factors in normal and pathological wound healing: therapeutic potential and methods of delivery. *Adv Skin Wound Care.* 2012;25:349-370.

91. Liu B, Earl HM, Baban D, et al. Melanoma cell lines express VEGF receptor KDR and respond to exogenously added VEGF. *Biochem Biophys Res Commun.* 1995;217:721-727.

92. Lazar-Molnar E, Hegyesi H, Toth S, et al. Autocrine and paracrine regulation by cytokines and growth factors in melanoma. *Cytokine.* 2000;12:547-554.

93. Draelos ZD. Exploring the pitfalls in clinical cosmeceutical research. *Cosmet Dermatol.* 2007;20:556-558.

94. Tribo-Boixareu MJ, Parrado-Romero C, Rais B, et al. Clinical and histological efficacy of a secretion of the mollusk *Cryptomphalus aspersa* in the treatment of cutaneous photoaging. *J Cosmet Dermatol.* 2009;22:247-252.

95. Wang X. A theory for the mechanism of action of the alpha hydroxy acids applied to the skin. *Med Hypothes.* 1999;53:380-382.

96. DiNardo JC, Grove GL, Moy LS. Clinical and histological effects of glycolic acid at different concentrations and pH levels. *Dermatol Surg.* 1996;22:421-424.

97. Draelos ZD. Dermatologic considerations of AHAs. *Cosmet Dermatol.* 1997;10:14-18.

98. Daniello NJ. Glycolic acid controversies. *Int J Aesthetic Restor Surg.* 1996;4:113-116.

99. Murad H, Shaman AT, Premo PS. The use of glycolic acid as a peeling agent. *Dermatol Clin.* 1995;13:285-307.

100. Moy LS, Murad H, Moy RL. Glycolic acid peels for the treatment of wrinkles and photoaging. *J Dermatol Surg Oncol.* 1993;19:243-246.

101. Piacquadio D, Dobry M, Hunt S, et al. Short contact glycolic acid peels as a treatment for photodamaged skin: a pilot study. *Dermatol Surg.* 1996;22:449-452.

102. Coleman WP, Futrell JM. The glycolic acid tricholoroacetic acid peel. *J Dermatol Surg Oncol.* 1994;20:76-80.

103. Newman NN, Newman A, Moy LS, et al. Clinical improvement of photoaged skin with 50% glycolic acid. *Dermatol Surg.* 1996;22:455-460.

104. Moy LS, Howe K, Moy RL. Glycolic acid modulation of collagen production in human skin fibroblast culture in vitro. *Dermatol Surg.* 1996;22:439-441.

105. Lim JT. Treatment of melasma using kojic acid in a gel containing hydroquinone and glycolic acid. *Dermatol Surg.* 1999;25:282-284.

106. Bontemps H, Mallaret M, Besson G, et al. Confusion after topical use of resorcinol. *Arch Dermatol.* 1995;131:112.

107. Baumbach JL, Sheth PB. Topical and intralesional antiviral agents. In: Wolverton SE, ed. *Comprehensive Dermatologic Drug Therapy.* Philadelphia: Saunders; 2001:532-533.

108. Stanley, MA. Imiquimod and the imidazoquinolones: mechanism of action and therapeutic potential. *Clin Exp Dermatol.* 2002;27(7):571-577.

109. Navi D, Huntley A. Imiquimod 5 percent cream and the treatment of cutaneous malignancy. *Dermatol Online J.* 2004;10:4.

110. Skinner RB Jr. Imiquimod. *Dermatol Clin.* 2003;21:291-300.

111. Cove JH, Holland KT. The effect of benzoyl peroxide on cutaneous micro-organisms in vitro. *J Applied Bacteriol.* 1983;54:379-382.

112. Oh CW, Myung KB. Retention hyperkeratosis of experimentally induced comedones in rabbits: the effects of three comedolytics. *J Dermatol.* 1996;23:169-180.

113. Hsu S, Quan LT. Topical antibacterial agents. In Wolverton SE, ed. *Comprehensive Dermatologic Drug Therapy.* Philadelphia: Saunders; 2001:480-481.

114. Mycek MJ, Gertner SB, Perper MM. *Lippincott's Illustrated Review: Pharmacology,* New York: JB Lippincott; 1992.

115. Puhvel SM. Effects of treatment with erythromycin 1.5 percent topical solution or clindamycin phosphate 1.0 percent topical solution on *P. acnes* counts and free fatty acid levels. *Cutis.* 1982;31:339-42.

116. Rappaport M, Puhvel SM, Reisner RM. Evaluation of topical erythromycin and oral tetracycline in acne vulgaris. *Cutis.* 1982;30:122-126, 130, 132-135.

117. Moreau D: *Physician's Drug Handbook.* Springhouse, PA: Springhouse Corporation; 1995.

118. Schmadel LK, McEvoy GK. Topical metronidazole: a new therapy for rosacea. *Clin Pharm.* 1990;9:94-101.

119. Gamborg Nielson P. Metronidazole treatment in rosacea with 1% metronidazole cream: a double-blind study. *Br J Dermatol.* 1983;108:327-332.

120. Eriksson G, Nord CE. Impact of topical metronidazole on the skin and colon microflora in patients with rosacea. *Infection.* 1987;15:8-10.

121. Gamborg Nielsen P. Metronidazole treatment in rosacea. *Int J Dermatol.* 1988;27:1-5.

122. Ward A, Campoli-Richards DM. Mupirocin: a review of its antibacterial activity, pharmacokinetic properties and therapeutic use. *Drugs.* 1986;32:425-444.

123. Parenti MA, Hatfield SM, Leyden JJ. Mupirocin: a topical antibiotic with a unique structure and mechanism of action. *Clin Pharm.* 1987;6:761-70.

124. Miller MA, Dascal A, Portnoy J, et al. Development of mupirocin resistance among methicillin-resistant *Staphylococcus aureus* after widespread use of nasal mupirocin ointment. *Infect Control Hosp Epidemiol.* 1996;17:811-813.

125. Lechevalier HA. The 25 years of neomycin. *CRC Crit Rev Microbiol.* 1975;3:359-97.

126. Winkelman W, Gratton D. Topical antibacterials. *Clin Dermatol.* 1989;7:156-162.

127. Marks JG Jr, DeLeo VA. *Contact and Occupational Dermatology.* St Louis: Mosby-Year Book; 1997.

128. Marone P, Monzillo V, Perversi L, et al. Comparative *in vitro* activity of silver sulfadiazine, alone and in combination with cerium nitrate, against staphylococci and gram-negative bacteria. *J Chemother.* 1998;10:17-21.

129. Phillips RM, Rosen T. Topical antifungal agents. In: Wolverton SE, ed. *Comprehensive Dermatologic Drug Therapy.* Philadelphia: Saunders; 2001:497-523.

130. Vanden Bossche H. Mode of action of pyridine, pyrimidine and azole antifungals. In: Berg G, Plempel M, eds. *Sterol Biosynthesis Inhibitors.* Chichester, UK: Ellis Horwood; 1988:9.

131. Vanden Bossche H, Marichal P. Mode of action of anti-Candida drugs: focus on terconazole and other ergosterol biosynthesis inhibitors. *Am J Obstet Gynecol.* 1991;165:1193-1199.

132. Vanden Bossche H. Cytochrome P450: target for itraconazole. *Drug Dev Res.* 1986;8:287-298.

133. Vanden Bossche H, Lauwers W, Willemsens G, et al. Molecular basis for the antimycotic and antibacterial activity of N-substituted imidazoles and triazoles: the inhibition of isoprenoid biosynthesis. *Pestic Sci.* 1984;15:188-198.

134. Vanden Bossche H. Biochemical targets for antifungal azole derivatives: hypothesis on the mode of action. In: Mcginnis MK, ed. *Current Topics in Medical Mycology.* Vol. 1. New York: Springer-Verlag; 1985.

135. Lester M. Ketoconazole 2% cream in the treatment of tinea pedis, tinea cruris, and tinea corporis. *Cutis.* 1995;55:181-183.

136. Taieb A, Legrain V, Palmier C, et al. Topical ketoconazole for infantile seborrhoeic dermatitis. *Dermatologica.* 1990;181:26-32.

137. Carr MM, Pryce DM, Ive FA. Treatment of seborrheic dermatitis with ketoconazole. I. Response of seborrheic dermatitis of the scalp to topical ketoconazole. *Br J Dermatol.* 1987;116:213-216.

138. Peter RU, Richarz-Barthauer U. Successful treatment and prophylaxis of scalp seborrhoeic dermatitis and dandruff with 2% ketoconazole shampoo: results of a multicenter, double-blind, placebo-controlled trial. *Br J Dermatol.* 1995;132:441-445.

139. Farr P, Shuster S. Treatment of seborrheic dermatitis with topical ketoconazole. *Lancet.* 1984;2:1271-1272.

140. McGrath J, Murphy GM. The control of seborrhoeic dermatitis and dandruff by antipityrosporal drugs. *Drugs.* 1991;41:178-184.

141. Stratigos JD, Antoniou C, Katsambas A, et al. Ketoconazole 2% cream versus hydrocortisone 1% cream in the treatment of seborrheic dermatitis: a double-blind comparative study. *J Am Acad Dermatol.* 1988;19:850-853.

142. Ive FA. An overview of experience with ketoconazole shampoo. *Br J Clin Pract.* 1991;45:279-284.

143. Green CA, Farr PM, Shuster S. Treatment of seborrhoeic dermatitis with ketoconazole. II. Response of seborrhoeic dermatitis of the face, scalp and trunk to topical ketoconazole. *Br J Dermatol.* 1987;116:217-221.

144. Katsambas A, Antoniou C, Frangouli E, et al. A double-blind trial of treatment of seborrhoeic dermatitis with 2% ketoconazole cream compared with 1% hydrocortisone cream. *Br J Dermatol.* 1989;121:353-357.

145. Cauwenbergh G, De Doncker P, Schrooten P, et al. Treatment of dandruff with a 2% ketoconazole scalp gel. A double-blind placebo-controlled study. *Int J Dermatol.* 1986;25:541.

146. Danby FW, Maddin WS, Margesson LJ, et al. A randomized, double-blind, placebo-controlled trial of ketoconazole 2% shampoo versus selenium sulfide 2.5% shampoo in the treatment of moderate to severe dandruff. *J Am Acad Dermatol.* 1993;29:1008-1012.

147. Rekacewicz I, Guillaume JC, Benkhraba F, et al. A double-blind placebo-controlled study of a 2 percent foaming lotion of ketoconazole in a single application in the treatment of pityriasis versicolor. *Ann Dermatol Venereol.* 1990;117:709-711.

148. el Euch D, Riahi I, Mokni M, et al. Ketoconazole 2% foaming gel in tinea versicolor: report of 60 cases. *Tunis Med.* 1999;77:38-40.

149. Caterall MD. Ketoconazole therapy for pityriasis versicolor (letter). *Clin Exp Dermatol.* 1982;7:679.

150. Savin RC, Horwitz SN. Double-blind comparison of 2% ketoconazole cream and placebo in the treatment of tinea versicolor. *J Am Acad Dermatol.* 1986;15:500-503.

151. Greer D, Jolly H. Topical ketoconazole treatment of cutaneous candidiasis. *J Am Acad Dermatol.* 1988;18:748-749.

152. Holt RJ, Newman RL. Laboratory assessment of the antimycotic drug clotrimazole. *J Clin Pathol.* 1972;25:1089-1097.

153. Gupta AK, Einarson TR, Summerbell RC, et al. An overview of topical antifungal therapy in dermatomycoses: a North American perspective. *Drugs.* 1998;55:645-674.

154. Clayton YM, Connor BL. Clinical trial of clotrimazole in the treatment of superficial fungal infections. *Postgrad Med J.* 1974;50(Suppl 1):66-69.

155. Gip L. The topical therapy of pityriasis versicolor with clotrimazole. *Postgrad Med J.* 1974;50(Suppl 1):59-60.

156. Oberste-Lehn H. Ideal properties of a modern antifungal agent: the therapy of mycoses with clotrimazole. *Postgrad Med J.* 1974;50(Suppl 1):51-53.

157. Fredriksson T. Topical treatment of superficial mycoses with clotrimazole. *Postgrad Med J.* 1974;50(Suppl 1):62-64.

158. Polemann G. Clinical experience in the local treatment of dermatomycoses with clotrimazole. *Postgrad Med J.* 1974;50(Suppl 1):54-56.

159. Zaias N, Battistini F. Superficial mycoses. Treatment with a new, broad-spectrum antifungal agent: 1% clotrimazole solution. *Arch Dermatol.* 1977;113:307-308.

160. Plempel M, Buchel KH, Bartmann K, et al. Antimycotic properties of clotrimazole. *Postgrad Med J.* 1974;50(Suppl 1):11-12.

161. Van Cutsem JM, Thienpont D. Miconazole, a broad-spectrum antimycotic agent with antibacterial activity. *Chemotherapy.* 1972;17:392-404.

162. Odds FC, Abbott AB, Pye G, et al. Improved method for estimation of azole antifungal inhibitory concentrations against *Candida* species, based on azole/antibiotic interactions. *J Med Vet Mycol.* 1986;24:305-311.

163. Botter AA. Topical treatment of nail and skin infections with miconazole, a new broad spectrum antimycotic. *Mykosen.* 1971;14:187-191.

164. Brugmans J, Van Cutsem J, Thienpont D. Treatment of long term tinea pedis with miconazole. *Arch Dermatol.* 1970;102:428-432.

165. Fulton JE Jr. Miconazole therapy for endemic fungal disease. *Arch Dermatol.* 1975;111:596-598.

166. Mandy SJ, Garrott TC. Miconazole treatment for severe dermatophytoses. *J Am Med Assoc.* 1974;230:72-75.

167. Ongley RC. Efficacy of topical miconazole treatment of tinea pedis. *Can Med Assoc J.* 1978;119:353-354.

168. Heel RC, Brogden RN, Speight TM, et al. Econazole: a review of its antifungal activity and therapeutic efficacy. *Drugs.* 1978;16:177-201.

169. Schaefer H, Stuttgen G. Absolute concentrations of an antimycotic agent, econazole, in the human skin after local application. *Arzneimittelforschung*. 1976;26:432-435.

170. Brenner M. Efficacy of twice-daily dosing of econazole nitrate 1% cream for tinea pedis. *J Am Podiatr Med Assoc*. 1990;80:583-587.

171. Cullen S, Millikan L, Mullen R. Treatment of tinea pedis with econazole nitrate cream. *Cutis*. 1986;7:388-389.

172. Cullen S, Rex I, Thorne E. A comparison of a new antifungal agent, 1% econazole nitrate (Spectazole) cream versus 1% clotrimazole cream in the treatment of intertriginous candidiasis. *Curr Ther Res*. 1984;35:606-609.

173. Vicik G, Mendiones M, Qinones C, et al. A new treatment for tinea versicolor using econazole nitrate 1.0 percent cream once a day. *Cutis*. 1984;33:570-571.

174. Fredriksson T. Treatment of dermatomycoses with topical econazole and clotrimazole. *Curr Ther Res*. 1979;25:590-594.

175. Daily A, Kramer S, Rex I, et al. Econazole nitrate (Spectazole) cream, 1 percent: a topical agent for the treatment of tinea pedis. *Cutis*. 1985;35:278-279.

176. Medoff G, Kobayashi G. The polyenes. In: Speller DCE, ed. *Antifungal chemotherapy*. London: John Wiley & Sons; 1980.

177. Hazen EL, Brown R. Nystatin. *Ann N Y Acad Sci*. 1960;89:258-266.

178. Fitzpatrick J. Topical antifungal agents. In: Freederg I, Eisen A, Wolff K, eds. *Dermatology in General Medicine*. New York: McGraw-Hill; 1999:2737-2741.

179. Bennett JE. Antimicrobial agents: antifungal agents. In: Gilman AG, Rall TW, Nies AS, eds. *The Pharmacological Basis of Therapeutics*. New York: McGraw-Hill; 1993:1165-1181.

180. Ryder N. Mode of action of allylamines. In: Berg D, Plempel M, eds. *Sterol Biosynthesis Inhibitors*. Chichester, UK: Ellis Horwood; 1988.

181. Ryder N, Dupont M. Inhibition of squalene epoxidase by allylamine antimycotic compounds: a comparative study of the fungal and mammalian enzymes. *Biochem J*. 1985;230:765-770.

182. Ryder N. The mechanism of action of terbinafine. *Clin Exp Dermatol*. 1989;14:98-100.

183. Georgopoulos A, Petranyi G, Mieth H, et al. *In vitro* activity of naftifine, a new antifungal agent. *Antimicrob Agents Chemother*. 1981;19:386-389.

184. Petranyi G, Georgopoulos A, Mieth H. *In vivo* antimycotic activity of naftifine. *Antimicrob Agents Chemother*. 1981;19:390-392.

185. Schuster I, Schaude M, Schatz F, et al. Preclinical characteristics of allylamines. In: Berg D, Plempel M, eds. *Sterol biosynthesis inhibitors*. Chichester, UK: Ellis Horwood; 1988:449-470.

186. Grassberger M, Mieth M, Petranyi G, et al. Aspects of antimycotic research exemplified by the allylamines. *Triangle*. 1986;25:711-784.

187. Jones TC. Treatment of dermatomycoses with topically applied allylamines: naftifine and terbinafine. *J Dermatol Treat*. 1990;1(Suppl 2):29-32.

188. Faruqi A, Khan K, Qazi A, et al. *In vitro* antifungal activity of naftifine (SN 105-843 GEL) against dermatophytes. *J Pakistani Med Assoc*. 1981;31:279-282.

189. Millikan LE, Galen WK, Gewirtzman GB, et al. Naftifine cream 1% versus econazole cream 1% in the treatment of tinea cruris and tinea corporis. *J Am Acad Dermatol*. 1988;18:52-56.

190. Kagawa S. Comparative clinical trial of naftifine and clotrimazole in tinea pedis, tinea cruris, and tinea corporis. *Mykosen*. 1987;30(Suppl 1):63-69.

191. Haas PJ, Tronnier H, Weidinger G. Naftifine in foot mycoses: double-blind therapeutic comparison with clotrimazole. *Mykosen*. 1985;28:33-40.

192. Smith EB, Wiss K, Hanifin JM, et al. Comparison of once- and twice-daily naftifine cream regimens with twice-daily clotrimazole in the treatment of tinea pedis. *J Am Acad Dermatol*. 1990;22:1116-1117.

193. Smith EB, Brenerman DL, Griffith RF, et al. Double-blind comparison of naftifine cream and clotrimazole/betamethasone dipropionate cream in the treatment of tinea pedis. *J Am Acad Dermatol.* 1992;26:125-127.

194. Zaun H, Luszpinski P. Multicenter double-blind contralateral comparison of naftifine and clotrimazole cream in patients with dermatophytosis and candidiasis. *Z Hautkr.* 1984;59:1209-1217.

195. Petranyi G, Meingassner JG, Mieth H. Antifungal activity of the allylamine derivative terbinafine in vitro. *Antimicrob Agents Chemother.* 1987;31:1365-1368.

196. Hill S, Thomas R, Smith SG, et al. An investigation of the pharmacokinetics of topical terbinafine (Lamisil) 1% cream. *Br J Dermatol.* 1992;127:396-400.

197. Stutz A. Allylamine derivatives: a new class of active substances in antifungal chemotherapy. *Angew Chemie* (International Edition: England). 1987;26:320-328.

198. Stutz A. Synthesis and structure-activity correlations within allylamine antimycotics. *Ann N Y Acad Sci.* 1988;544:46-62.

199. Clayton YM. *In vitro* activity of terbinafine. *Clin Exp Dermatol.* 1989;14:101-103.

200. Kagawa S. Clinical efficacy of terbinafine in 629 Japanese patients with dermatomycosis. *Clin Exp Dermatol.* 1989;14:116-119.

201. Villars V, Jones TC. Clinical efficacy and tolerability of terbinafine (Lamisil): a new topical and systemic fungicidal drug for treatment of dermatomycoses. *Clin Exp Dermatol.* 1989;14:124-127.

202. Nussenbaumer P, Dorfsatter G, Grassberger M, et al. Synthesis and structure-activity relationships of phenyl-substituted benzylamine antimycotics: a novel benzylamine antifungal agent for systemic treatment. *J Med Chem.* 1993;36:2115-2120.

203. Maeda T, Takase M, Ishibashi A, et al. Synthesis and antifungal activity of butenafine hydrochloride (KP-363), a new benzylamine antifungal agent. *Yakugaku Zasshi.* 1991;111:126-137.

204. Arika T, Hase T, Yokoo M. Anti-*Trichophyton mentagrophytes* activity and percutaneous permeation of butenafine in guinea pigs. *Antimicrob Agents Chemother.* 1993;37:363-365.

205. Arika T, Yokoo M, Hase T, et al. Effects of butenafine hydrochloride, a new benzylamine derivative, on experimental dermatophytosis in guinea pigs. *Antimicrob Agents Chemother.* 1990;34:2250-2253.

206. Tschen E, Elewski B, Gorsulowsky DC, et al. Treatment of interdigital tinea pedis with a 4-week once-daily regimen of butenafine hydrochloride 1% cream. *J Am Acad Dermatol.* 1997;36:S9-S14.

207. Greer D, Weiss J, Rodriguez D, et al. Treatment of tinea corporis with topical once-daily butenafine HCl 1%: a double-blind, placebo controlled trial. Presentation at 55th Annual American Academy of Dermatology Meeting, 1997.

208. Lesher J, Babel D, Stewart D, et al. Butenafine HCl 1% cream in the treatment of tinea cruris: A multicenter, vehicle controlled, double-blind trial. Presentation at 55th Annual American Academy of Dermatology Meeting, 1997.

209. Lesher JL Jr, Babel DE, Stewart DM, et al. Butenafine 1% cream in the treatment of tinea cruris: a multicenter, vehicle-controlled, double-blind trial. *J Am Acad Dermatol.* 1997;36:S20-S24.

210. Greer DL, Weiss J, Rodriguez DA, et al. A randomized trial to assess once-daily topical treatment of tinea corporis with butenafine, a new antifungal agent. *J Am Acad Dermatol.* 1997;37:231-225.

211. Savin R, De Villez RL, Elewski B, et al. One-week therapy with twice-daily butenafine 1% cream versus vehicle in the treatment of tinea pedis: a multicenter, double-blind trial. *J Am Acad Dermatol.* 1997;36:S15-S19.

212. Reyes BA, Beutner KR, Cukllen SI, et al. Butenafine, a fungicidal benzylamine derivative, used once daily for the treatment of interdigital tinea pedis. *Int J Dermatol.* 1998;37:450-453.

213. Savin R, Lucky A, Brennan B. One-week treatment of tinea pedis with butenafine HCl 1%: a multi-center, double-blind, randomized trial. Presentation at 55th Annual American Academy of Dermatology Meeting, 1997.

214. Biafine PDR drug information; as found on 1-8-12 on www.pdr.net/drugpages/ concisemonograph.

215. Coulomb B, Friteau L, Dubertret L. Biafine applied on human epidermal wounds is chemotactic for macrophages and increases the IL-1/IL-6 ratio. *Skin Pharmacol.* 1997;10:281-287.

216. Brown GL, Nanney LB, Griffen J, et al. Enhancement of wound healing by topical treatment with epidermal growth factor. *N Engl J Med.* 1989;321:76-79.

ZEIN OBAGI SYSTEM OF SKIN CLASSIFICATION

EXISTING SKIN CLASSIFICATION SYSTEMS

The best-known existing skin classification systems are the Fitzpatrick[1] system and the Glogau[2] system. The Fitzpatrick skin typing system was developed by Thomas B. Fitzpatrick in 1975, and, though subjective, it has had diagnostic and therapeutic value. This classification system denotes six different skin types, differentiated by skin color and typical reaction to sun exposure. The skin types are on a continuum and range from very fair (type I) to very dark (type VI), also depending on whether the patient burns or tans with sun exposure (Table 4.1). A major disadvantage of the Fitzpatrick system is that it fails to accurately predict a patient's response to topical treatments as well as the ideal depth for chemical peeling or other resurfacing procedures.

Another skin classification system, developed by Richard G. Glogau,[2] groups skin into four types, classifying patients according to their degree of photodamage, wrinkling, and scarring. This scale has limitations similar to those of the Fitzpatrick scale in that it does not help select the ideal procedure for each group or predict response or anticipated skin reactions to topical treatments.

DEVELOPMENT OF ZEIN OBAGI SKIN CLASSIFICATION SYSTEM

Recognizing the limitations of existing skin classification systems, Zein Obagi Skin Classification System more specifically addresses variables in skin types and their expected responses to various treatments. This new system came about after years of observing the factors that consistently influenced patient outcomes during treatment for a variety of skin problems. First, patients with the same skin condition or problem who were treated with the same treatment demonstrated a variable response to the treatment. To clarify, some patients improved greatly, some improved less, and others either did not improve at

TABLE 4.1 Fitzpatrick Skin Classification

Skin Type	Color	Reaction to Sun Exposure
I	Light, pale white	Always burns, never tans
II	White fair	Usually burns, only occasionally tans
III	Medium, white to light brown	Sometimes burns, gradually tans
IV	Olive, moderate brown	Rarely burns, tans easily
V	Brown, dark brown	Very rarely burns, tans very easily
VI	Black, very dark brown to black	Never burns, tans very easily

Box 4.1

Applications of the Zein Obagi Skin Classification System

- Select appropriate procedures for specific skin types.
- Determine the safe procedure depth for specific skin types.
- Determine the safety of repeating procedures.
- Determine the approach and duration of treatment to prepare skin before a procedure and to manage skin after the procedure.
- Control factors that influence procedure results, exacerbate certain skin conditions, and predispose certain skin types to developing complications. Select the appropriate topical agents.

all or actually appeared worse. Second, despite the same standards, a procedure sometimes led to a very good outcome in some patients but produced unwanted reactions or complications in others. Third, certain procedures were associated with undesirable effects in some patients but not in others. Specifically, patients with white skin often had good results, whereas patients with black or other darker skin types did not. Furthermore, some patients had poor outcomes following CO_2 fractional laser resurfacing yet had good results following a chemical peel that reached the same depth. Thus, the two existing skin classification systems described previously were of limited value because they address only a few variables and do not predict the skin's response to various treatments. Box 4.1 shows the applications of the Zein Obagi Skin Classification System, and Table 4.2 shows the attributes considered in the Zein Obagi Skin Classification System.

TABLE 4.2 Attributes Considered in Zein Obagi Skin Classification System

Attribute	Classification
Color	Original, deviated, complex
Thickness	Thick, medium, thin
Oiliness	Oily, normal, dry
Elasticity	Lax or firm
Fragility	Proper or improper healing

CLASSIFICATION OF SKIN TYPE ACCORDING TO COLOR

CONSIDERATION OF ETHNICITY IN SKIN CLASSIFICATION SYSTEMS

The Fitzpatrick system, although used widely, has major shortcomings. It describes colors (shades) of skin on a scale of I to VI, but does not take into account the ethnic purity or mixed nature of the skin color or how such color affects skin response to treatment or a procedure in terms of rate of healing, reactions, and ultimate outcome. If the Fitzpatrick skin classification considered ethnic purity of skin, it should include original white as types I or II, original black as type VI, and original Asian as types IV or V. In short, the Fitzpatrick system is inadequate in describing skin color, especially skin of patients of mixed ethnicity.

The color categories of original, deviated, and complex were developed to improve on the Fitzpatrick system and other systems of classifying skin color. Patients from India, Pakistan, Indonesia, Malaysia, and North and South America may have skin of mixed ethnicity (from several different or unknown origins) and are classified as having deviated skin. The skin of these patients can behave as black, Asian, or even white skin in unpredictable ways. Deviated skin types are more difficult to treat because they have a greater tendency to develop hypopigmentation, depigmentation, and severe postinflammatory hyperpigmentation (PIH). They are also more likely to have a prolonged recovery time after procedures.

Patients with the complex skin type have an uneven, variable skin color tone that is exacerbated by sun exposure. Examples include persons of indigenous (original) South American Indian and American Indian origin; those from India, Pakistan, and surrounding regions; and others of mixed racial origin. Complex skin could be considered as severely deviated. These patients also require a specific approach for safe and successful treatment. Recognizing whether the skin type is original, deviated, or complex facilitates individual treatment for each patient and assures the best outcome in Skin Health Restoration, procedure selection, and recommended procedure depth (Box 4.2).

SKIN COLOR STABILITY AND TIME TO NORMAL COLOR RECOVERY

Skin color stability refers to the skin's ability to quickly regain its natural color following various treatments or procedures. It is a major factor in

---

Box 4.2

The Role of Mixed Ethnicity

Mixed ethnicity plays a major role in skin response to disease treatment, procedures, and injury.

Box 4.3

Importance of Skin Color Stability

- Skin color stability refers to the skin's ability to regain its natural color quickly after a treatment or procedure.
- Stability of skin color is a major factor in classifying skin into the three Zein Obagi Skin Classification System color groups.

classifying skin into the three Zein Obagi color groups (Box 4.3). Skin in the original color category shows a fast and favorable response to Skin Health Restoration treatments that are aimed at correcting a pigmentation problem; this skin type also typically demonstrates a good outcome after a chemical peel or laser treatment that reaches the immediate reticular dermis (IRD) or the upper reticular dermis (URD). Conversely, skin in the deviated color category requires a longer preprocedure skin conditioning period and a more aggressive topical approach before and after a procedure. Also, those with deviated skin may show permanent changes in color tone after a procedure reaching the IRD or URD.

The most unstable skin type is the complex color category. Like skin in the deviated category, that in the complex category requires a more meticulous approach to treatment, a longer preprocedure conditioning period, and a longer post-procedure management period. The features of Zein Obagi skin color types are shown in Table 4.3.

TABLE 4.3   Features of Skin Color Types

Skin Color Category	Genetics	Features
Original	Not mixed racially or ethnically	Stable
		Color returns quickly after treatment
		PIH is rare and, when it occurs, is short lived
		Requires one KMC (6 weeks) of conditioning before and after procedures
		Deeper procedures (to the level of the URD) are typically safe
Deviated	Racially or ethnically mixed	Weakly stable
		PIH is darker, more pronounced, and lasts longer
		Requires one to three KMCs (12 weeks) of conditioning before and after procedures
		Deeper procedures (to the level of the URD) are possible but must be performed with caution
Complex	Racially or ethnically mixed	Extremely unstable
		PIH is stronger and responds slowly to treatment
		Requires two to three KMCs (12 to 18 weeks) of conditioning both before and after procedures
		Deeper procedures (to the level of the URD) are risky; results are unpredictable

KMC = keratinocyte maturation cycle; PIH = postinflammatory hyperpigmentation; URD = upper reticular dermis.

ORIGINAL SKIN COLOR TYPE

The original skin color type includes light white, dark black, and dark Asian (yellow) and is found in persons who are not racially or ethnically mixed (Figure 4.1, Figure 4.2, and Figure 4.3). This type is stable after most rejuvenation procedures, with the exception of certain deep procedures (discussed later). Melanocytes resume their normal function after healing has been completed, and skin returns to its original color. There may be short-lived PIH, but it responds rapidly to topical corrective treatment. However, skin of patients with black or dark Asian original color type undergoing deep procedures (below the level of the IRD, such as phenol peels, a ZO Controlled Depth Peel to the URD, CO_2 laser resurfacing, and dermabrasion) does not return to normal after such procedures. Instead, after these procedures, the skin of these patients can undergo variable degrees of melanocytic destruction with

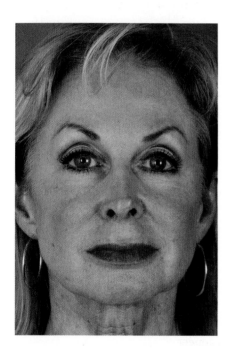

FIGURE 4.1 Patient with original white skin type (light).

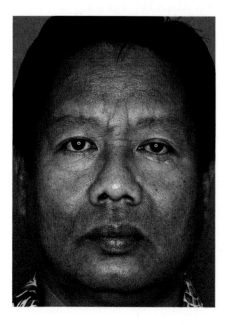

FIGURE 4.2 Patient with original Asian skin type (dark).

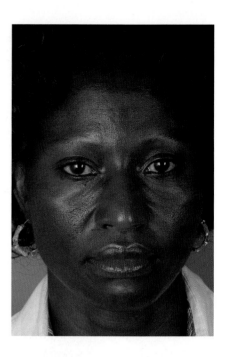

FIGURE 4.3 Patient with original black skin type (dark).

subsequent textural changes; together, these can result in a lighter color tone. It is important to warn patients with dark skin about these potential post-procedure color and textural changes because some may not welcome these changes. Table 4.4 shows the original color types and the corresponding Fitzpatrick types.

Regardless of a patient's color group classification, skin conditioning before and after a procedure must be performed in a specific manner that is appropriate for the skin's category. Specifically, the light white group needs one keratinocyte maturation cycle (KMC) of topical preprocedure skin conditioning (6 weeks), whereas the dark-skinned groups may need two to three cycles (12 to 18 weeks). After the procedure, all color groups need topical treatment for at least one KMC (6 weeks) to stabilize skin color; darker skin groups may need two to three cycles (12 to 18 weeks).

ZEIN OBAGI DEVIATED SKIN COLOR TYPE

The deviated skin type is found in persons who are racially or ethnically mixed. This skin color is unstable and more sensitive to the depth reached

TABLE 4.4 Zein Obagi Original Skin Color Types with Corresponding Fitzpatrick Skin Types		
Zein Obagi Original Color Type	*Fitzpatrick Type*	*Description*
Very light white, normal white	I, II, III	Light color; burns and does not tan; may have some light freckles. Chronically sun-exposed areas show telangiectasias, redness, actinic keratoses, and other forms of photodamage
Dark white	IV	Dark white (brunettes) same as above and higher tendency to pigmentation problems
Dark Asian	V	Brownish color; mildly darker in sun-exposed areas
Dark black	VI	Very dark; sun-exposed and nonexposed areas mostly similar in color

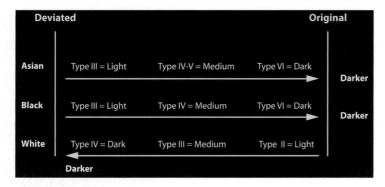

FIGURE 4.4 The spectrum of original to deviated Zein Obagi skin types in Asian, black, and white skin. In Asian skin, dark yellow is the original type, and the skin becomes more deviated as it becomes lighter. In black skin, dark black is the original type, and the skin becomes more deviated as it becomes lighter. In white skin, the original is light, and the skin becomes more deviated as it becomes darker.

by procedures and takes longer than skin in the original category to return to its natural color after a procedure. Although procedures that reach depths below the IRD (phenol peels, deep trichloroacetic acid [TCA] peels, deep CO_2 laser resurfacing, and dermabrasion) are likely to produce variable degrees of melanocyte reduction or destruction and a lighter color tone in all skin types, such deep procedures are even more likely to produce hypopigmentation in patients with deviated skin. Skin darkening in the form of PIH is also more likely, and it may persist longer and require more aggressive bleaching and blending. Figure 4.4 shows the spectrum of original to deviated skin types and the corresponding Fitzpatrick types.

Patients with skin in the deviated color category need more aggressive preprocedure topical skin conditioning and should have a procedure only after topical skin preparation for one to three KMCs (6 to 18 weeks) (Box 4.4). *The physician should not wait for the appearance of PIH before starting postprocedure treatment.* Bleaching and blending in moderately aggressive form should begin immediately after re-epithelialization. Table 4.5 shows the deviated color types and the corresponding Fitzpatrick types.

COMPLEX SKIN COLOR TYPES

Skin in the complex color category is variable, dark in some areas and lighter in others, and is extremely unstable and photosensitive (Figure 4.11). This kind

---

Box 4.4

Deviated Color Types

- Patients with skin in the deviated color categories need more aggressive topical preprocedure conditioning and should have a procedure only after color has been controlled and tolerance has been achieved.
- This is usually after one to three keratinocyte maturation cycles (6 to 18 weeks).

TABLE 4.5 Zein Obagi Deviated Color Types and Corresponding Fitzpatrick Types

Zein Obagi Deviated Color Type	Corresponding Fitzpatrick Type	Stability and Degree of PIH
Normal white	II, III	Unstable, mild PIH
Dark white	IV	
Light Asian	II, III	Unstable, strong PIH
Medium Asian	III, IV	Unstable, very strong PIH
Light and medium Black	III, IV	Unstable, very strong PIH

PIH = postinflammatory hyperpigmentation.

FIGURE 4.5 Patient with deviated white skin type (light white).

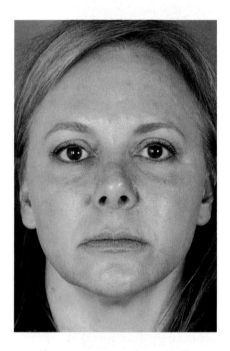

FIGURE 4.6 Patient with deviated white skin type (dark white).

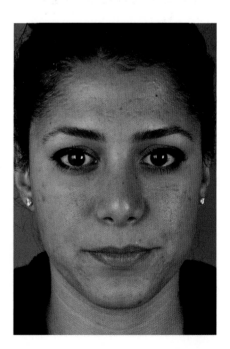

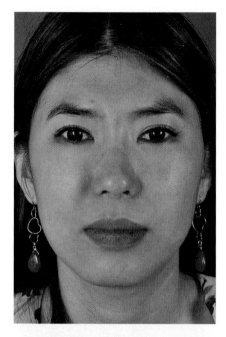

FIGURE 4.7 Patient with deviated Asian skin type (light).

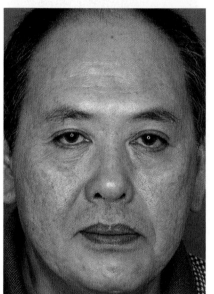

FIGURE 4.8 Patient with deviated Asian skin type (medium).

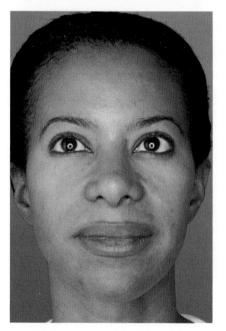

FIGURE 4.9 Patient with deviated black skin type (light).

FIGURE 4.10   Patient with deviated black skin
type (medium).

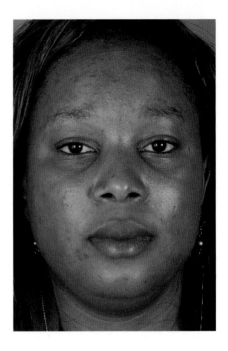

of skin naturally has an uneven, variable skin color tone that is exacerbated by sun exposure. Examples include persons of indigenous South American Indian and American Indian origin; those from India, Pakistan, and surrounding regions; and others of mixed racial origin. Most people in the complex category are considered to have Fitzpatrick skin type IV; however, occasionally they can also have Fitzpatrick skin type V or VI. Some patients have a combination of all three Fitzpatrick types.

Patients with skin in the complex category need two to three KMCs (12 to 18 weeks) of aggressive topical skin conditioning (see Chapter 2) to stabilize color before a procedure. Despite adhering to a post-procedure conditioning program, these patients typically have severe and long-lasting PIH following procedures. Hypopigmentation can also occur. Thus, procedures in patients with complex skin should not reach deeper than the level of the IRD. These

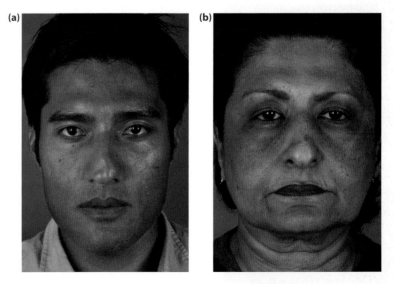

FIGURE 4.11   (a, b) Two patients with complex skin type (India).

TABLE 4.6 Number of Keratinocyte Maturation Cycles for Skin Health Restoration in Skin of Various Colors

Skin Color	Skin Conditioning	Number of KMCs (before and after the Procedure)*
Original	Aggressive	1
	Moderate	1-2
Deviated white	Aggressive	1-2
Deviated Asian, black	Aggressive	2
Complex	Aggressive	2-3

*Patients of all skin colors must have a minimum of one keratinocyte maturation cycle (KMC) before any procedure.

patients should also be told in advance that it will take some time for their skin to return to normal after a procedure. The complex skin type has no specific category in Fitzgerald classification.

The number of KMCs needed for Skin Health Restoration in skin of various colors is shown in Table 4.6.

SKIN TYPE CLASSIFICATION ACCORDING TO THICKNESS

Skin thickness is determined genetically and can be categorized into one of the following types: thin, medium, thick, and hamartomatous (Figure 4.12, Figure 4.13, Figure 4.14, and Figure 4.15). (Hamartomatous skin is described later in this chapter.) Distinctions between each type are not clear-cut and must be made by clinical examination of firmness, tightness, bulkiness, and

FIGURE 4.12 Patient with thin skin.

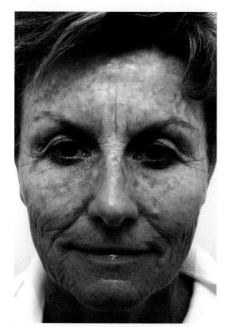

FIGURE 4.13 Patient with medium-thickness skin.

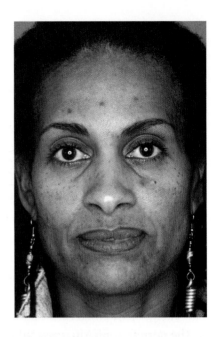

FIGURE 4.14 Patient with thick skin.

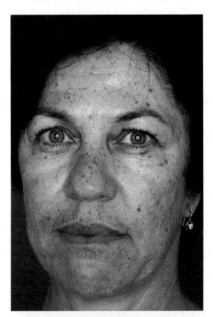

FIGURE 4.15 Patient with very thick skin (hamartomatous). Notice enlarged pores, dominant static lines.

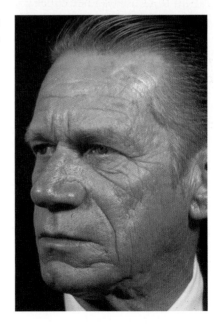

the ease with which the skin can be folded by the action of underlying muscles during facial expressions. Not only does overall skin thickness vary from person to person, but it also varies according to anatomical location. Specifically, the epidermis and papillary dermis (PD) are of approximately the same thickness in all anatomical locations; the stratum corneum is thickest in the palms and soles, and the dermis (papillary and reticular) is thickest on the back and thinnest on the eyelids. In general, in each skin thickness type, cheeks have thicker skin relative to the rest of the face, forehead skin thickness varies, and skin along the jawline is thinner than that on the cheeks. Efforts have been made to standardize the measurement of skin thickness through biopsies, ultrasound, and other methods, but results have been inconclusive, and standards are yet to be created.

There are also racial differences in skin thickness. Black patients generally have predominantly thick or medium-thick skin, whereas Asian patients typically are more likely to have medium-thick skin. The thickness of white skin can vary widely, with some patients having fairly thick skin and others, such as the very fair, having very thin skin. Sex also plays a role in skin thickness; men have thicker skin than women in all racial groups.

DETERMINATION OF SKIN THICKNESS BY PINCHING TECHNIQUE

In addition to using ultrasound devices and histological analysis, skin thickness can be determined easily by the cheek-pinching technique. By grabbing the cheek between the index finger and thumb, the size of the fold between the fingers reveals skin thickness. The skin is considered thin if the fold is 1 cm or less, medium-thick if the fold is 1½ cm, and thick if the fold is more than 2 cm (Table 4.7). Of note: the determination of skin thickness is not precise because it provides a range and a sufficient idea of thickness. Facial expression lines can also indicate skin thickness because skin appearance, aggregation, and extension of lines can be seen. Figure 4.16 shows a patient with original white skin color undergoing the pinching technique demonstrating variations in skin thickness on her cheeks, jawline, and eyelids.

EXPRESSION LINES AND FOLDS AND SKIN THICKNESS

Expression lines (dynamic lines) are folds in the skin seen when the underlying muscles contract while furrowing the eyebrows (Figure 4.17); during

TABLE 4.7 Identification of Skin Thickness by Pinching

Category	Thickness of Fold
Very thin	<½ cm
Thin	<1 cm to 1½ cm
Medium	1½ cm
Thick	>1½ to >2 cm

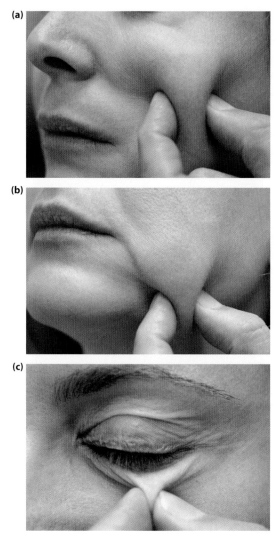

Figure 4.16 Patient with original white, medium-thickness, oily skin. (a) Each face has variable thickness based on anatomical areas. The thickest skin on a face is the cheek. (b) The skin on the jawline is of medium thickness for that particular skin. (c) The thinnest part of skin is on the eyelids.

elevation of the eyebrows (Figure 4.18); while smiling (Figure 4.19); or while pursing the lips (Figure 4.20). They are more numerous and prominent in persons with overall thin skin, as well as within thinner areas of skin in the same individual, such as the periorbital and perioral areas, forehead, and cheeks. Skin thickness can be determined by evaluating the extent of the

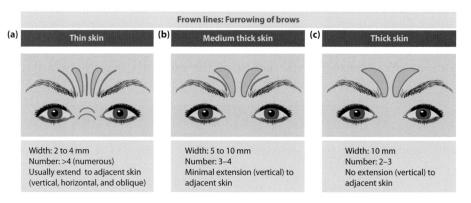

Figure 4.17 Effect of skin thickness on expression lines of patients while furrowing the brows: (a) thin; (b) medium; (c) thick.

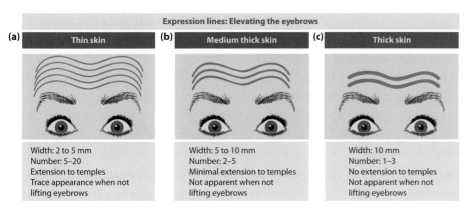

FIGURE 4.18 Effect of skin thickness on expression lines of patients while raising the eyebrows through contraction of the frontalis muscle (horizontal forehead lines): (a) thin skin; (b) medium-thickness skin; (c) thick skin.

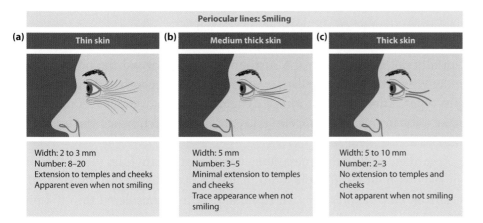

FIGURE 4.19 Effect of skin thickness on expression lines in the periocular areas of patients while smiling (crow's feet): (a) thin skin; (b) medium-thickness skin; (c) thick skin.

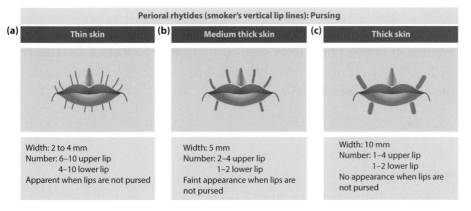

FIGURE 4.20 Effect of skin thickness on vertical perioral rhytides while pursing the lips, which is commonly seen in long-term cigarette smokers: (a) thin skin; (b) medium-thickness skin; (c) thick skin.

folds made with facial expressions. The physician should ask the patient to contract a muscle or muscle group to the extreme by frowning, smiling, lifting the eyebrows, pursing the lips as if whistling, and so forth. The physician should then observe the following three manifestations: the width of the "mountains," assessed by the depth of the "valleys," the degree of fold length extension, and the appearance of static rhytides in these same facial areas (which are present when the patient is not making any active facial expressions and the muscles are relaxed).

Expression folds (the mountains), otherwise known as dynamic rhytides, are a result of underlying muscle contraction. In thin skin, these folds are fine and numerous. The valleys, which are visible even when the patient is not contracting facial muscles to make an expression, are typically shallow. These folds extend to skin beyond the underlying anatomical demarcations of the individual muscles. They can be made to appear without extreme muscle contraction (i.e., with only mild expression) and are typically present to a lesser degree than when the muscles are relaxed.

In skin of medium thickness, expression folds are wider than in thin skin with deeper valleys. The folds typically extend just slightly beyond the underlying muscle demarcations to the surrounding skin. Some degree of facial expression (through muscular contraction) is necessary to make the folds appear; they are not apparent when the muscles are relaxed.

Thick skin has fewer folds, and they are wider than in thinner skin types, typically not extending to the surrounding skin beyond the borders of the underlying muscles. The valleys in thick skin are deeper than those in thinner skin types. Effort, in the form of dynamic facial movements, is required to make folds in thick skin appear; folds are not apparent when the underlying muscles are relaxed.

Regardless of skin thickness, long-standing static rhytides (those that present even without facial expression) may be a result of years of dynamic rhytides from facial expressions. In summary, skin is considered thin if a pinch test yields a fold less than or equal to 1 cm in thickness, medium if it is approximately 1½ cm in thickness, and thick if it is greater than 2 cm in thickness.

Skin thickness plays a significant role in Skin Health Restoration because it influences the necessary strength and duration of preprocedure and postprocedure skin conditioning, procedure selection (including target treatment depth), predictability of procedure results, potential for treatment-related complications, and suitability for repeating a specific procedure. Skin thickness also allows the practitioner to predict which wrinkles will disappear and which will only be minimized with specific procedures (chemical peels and laser treatments) (Box 4.5).

Box 4.5

Factors Influenced by Skin Thickness

- Strength and duration of skin conditioning
- Selection of a procedure and its depth of penetration
- Predictability of post-procedure outcome
- Wrinkle minimization versus eradication
- Suitability for a repeat procedure
- Propensity for periprocedural complications (permanent color changes and scarring)

TABLE 4.8 Characteristics of Thin Skin

Characteristic	Features
Firmness	Minimal; the dermis is thin because of a lower collagen content
Translucence	Translucent; underlying blood vessels are easily visible
Adnexal structures	Few
Aging	Wrinkles appear early; jowling and laxity appear later and can be quite prominent
Dynamic rhytides	Numerous on forehead and periocular areas; periocular areas and perioral areas develop numerous shallow folds
Dryness/oiliness	Tendency toward dryness
Procedural safety margin	Narrow for all invasive resurfacing procedures (because of fewer adnexal structures)
Post-procedure complications	Higher rate of complications (hypopigmentation, depigmentation, hypertrophic reactions, keloids) than with thicker skin types
Rate of healing	Slow after procedures below the IRD
Bruising	Easily bruised after injectables (fillers, neurotoxins)
Response to nonsurgical tightening procedures	Optimal; one procedure may be sufficient (e.g., a ZO Controlled Depth Peel reaching the PD or IRD)
Maximum procedure depth	PD to the IRD

IRD = immediate reticular dermis; PD = papillary dermis.

Defining characteristics of thin, medium, and thick skin are further delineated in Table 4.8, Table 4.9, and Table 4.10.

Atrophic skin, a subtype of thin skin, results from certain diseases, chronic application of topical corticosteroids, radiation treatment, and malnutrition (including in those patients with anorexia nervosa). This skin type shows minimal firmness and a very thin dermis (like cigarette paper) due to a sparse content

TABLE 4.9 Characteristics of Medium-Thickness Skin

Characteristic	Features
Firmness	Good; sufficiently thick (more collagen within the dermis than thin skin has)
Translucence	None
Adnexal structures	Adequate or average number
Aging	Wrinkles in areas of thin skin (e.g., periorbital sites); laxity and moderately deep folds in areas of thicker skin (e.g., the forehead)
Dynamic rhytides	Less numerous; appear as thicker and deeper folds
Dryness/oiliness	Tendency toward oiliness
Procedural safety margin	Good safety margin for invasive or ablative resurfacing
Post-procedure complications	Less frequent (hypopigmentation, depigmentation, hypertrophic reactions, keloids)
Rate of healing	Good even after procedures below the level of the IRD
Bruising	Less bruising after injectables (fillers, neurotoxins) than in patients with thin skin
Response to nonsurgical tightening procedures	Good; optimal after a ZO Controlled Depth Peel down to the level of the PD or IRD
Safe procedure depth	PD to IRD; focal URD in the designed peel

IRD = immediate reticular dermis; PD = papillary dermis; URD = upper reticular dermis.

TABLE 4.10 Characteristics of Thick Skin

Characteristic	Features
Firmness	Strong; thick dermis because of abundant amount of collagen
Translucence	None
Adnexal structures	Rich, numerous
Aging	Mainly laxity (jowling and deeper folds); wrinkles appear later and are less deep
Dynamic rhytides	Few, but with thicker folds and deeper valleys
Dryness/oiliness	Tendency toward oiliness
Procedural safety margin	Excellent safety margin for resurfacing or ablative procedures
Post-procedure complications	Infrequent (hypopigmentation, depigmentation, hypertrophic reactions, keloids)
Rate of healing	Good even after procedures that penetrate below the IRD
Bruising	Rare after injectables (fillers, neurotoxins)
Response to nonsurgical tightening procedures	Weak response to nonsurgical tightening procedures (e.g., ZO Controlled Depth Peel) reaching the level of the IRD
Safe procedure depth	PD, IRD, URD

IRD = immediate reticular dermis; PD = papillary dermis; URD = upper reticular dermis.

of collagen fibers. It is translucent with visible underlying blood vessels, has minimal adnexal structures, and is highly sensitive and dry. Aging changes in thin skin are mainly skin mummification, with no wrinkles or laxity. This skin type is not suitable for any procedures other than a mild exfoliation because post-procedural complications, including severe atrophic and hypertrophic scarring and permanent dyschromia, can follow more invasive procedures.

Hamartomatous (bulldog or lion face) skin is abnormally thick with many deep folds, greatly enlarged pores, and lumps and bumps from sebaceous gland hyperplasia and adenomas. Certain areas may be so thick that they cannot be folded, and thickness cannot be assessed. Aging changes are mostly seen as skin sagging, jowling, and deep folds. Rhytides may not be present. Because of the great degree of firmness and the low degree of elasticity in hamartomatous skin, nonsurgical tightening procedures are not suitable. However, procedures that improve texture, such as fully ablative or CO_2 fractional laser resurfacing and dermabrasion, are ideal treatment options. Additionally, depending on the severity of the hamartomatous skin texture, photodynamic therapy, a course of systemic isotretinoin, or both, may be necessary to shrink the sebaceous glands to produce an optimal cosmetic result.

Table 4.11 shows the significant effect of skin thickness on Skin Health Restoration objectives and their outcomes. Box 4.6 shows factors to consider in selecting a procedure.

A COMBINED PROCEDURE APPROACH TO SKIN THICKNESS

Skin can be rejuvenated by a variety of distinct procedures performed concurrently to reduce injury and yield synergistic beneficial effects. For example, the ultimate result after the combination of relaxing dynamic rhytides with neurotoxin injections, restoring volume deficits through filler injections, and

TABLE 4.11   Skin Health Restoration Objectives in Relation to Skin Thickness

Objectives	Thin Skin	Medium and Thick Skin
Restore a strong barrier function	Eliminate sensitivity	Same as in thin skin
	Improve natural or inherent hydration	
Control sebum production	Only if skin is oily	When skin is normal or oily
Stimulate	Increase epidermal cell turnover	Improve epidermal cell turnover and increase dermal elasticity
	Increase dermal collagen production	
Optimal treatment strength	As tolerated	Moderate to aggressive approach
	Increase to build tolerance	

Box 4.6

Skin Thickness and Procedure Selection

THIN SKIN

- Use caution with any resurfacing procedures; avoid penetrating deeper than the papillary dermis or immediate reticular dermis (IRD).
- Avoid ablative laser resurfacing.
- Tightening procedures, such as the ZO Controlled Depth Peel, are ideal.

MEDIUM TO THICK SKIN

- Tightening procedures, such as the ZO Controlled Depth Peel, can be safely performed down to the IRD.
- One to two procedures may be needed for optimal tightening (ZO Controlled Depth Peel).
- CO_2 fractional laser resurfacing is the gold standard for improving texture.

---

tightening skin and evening out texture and tone using a chemical peel produce much more comprehensive and aesthetically pleasing results than any of those treatment modalities alone. As noted previously, the selection of a proper procedure approach (whether singular or combined) must be guided by the nature of the skin problem and by the patient's skin thickness. Table 4.12 shows specific skin treatment goals and the appropriate procedures.

Selection of a Procedure for Thin Skin

Skin thickness is the most important variable in selection of a rejuvenation procedure. Thin skin is ideal for a tightening procedure that does not extend beyond the IRD in depth. This depth will provide sufficient tightening and mild leveling and will not make the skin thinner or change its color. The procedure can be repeated at intervals of 6 to 8 weeks or longer for gradual

TABLE 4.12 Skin Treatment Goals and the Appropriate Procedures	
Goal	*Procedure*
Increase dermal collagen	Stimulate with topical retinoids
Exfoliate the epidermis	Alpha-hydroxy acid peels, microabrasion, ZO 3-Step Peel composed of a cocktail of TCA, salicylic acid, and lactic acid
Tightening	ZO Controlled Depth Peel (20% to 28% TCA) to the level of the PD or IRD
Leveling	CO_2 fractional laser resurfacing, ZO Controlled Depth Peel (20% to 28%) to varying depths
Volume restoration	Fillers, biostimulatory molecule injections
Softening of dynamic rhytides	Neurotoxin injections to immobilize underlying facial muscles

IRD = immediate reticular dermis; PD = papillary dermis; TCA = trichloroacetic acid.

improvement. Leveling procedures, such as a ZO Controlled Depth Peel, laser resurfacing, or a phenol peel, are risky in thin skin because they may make skin even thinner and accelerate long-term aging changes. In patients with thin skin, prolonged stimulation with topical agents to increase dermal thickness is essential. Scarring, such as keloids, and permanent hypopigmentation are more common in patients with thin skin following procedures that reach below the IRD. Thin skin has a narrow safety margin for deep procedures.

Combination Procedures in Thin Skin

Patients with thin skin can benefit from the combination of a focal leveling procedure and a tightening procedure, both of which can be done at the same time. Focal leveling limited to deep unstretchable wrinkles or scars can be obtained with the CO_2 fractional laser, which is safer than deeper chemical peels. The IRD-level peel is performed first, followed by leveling that is limited to the affected areas and extends no deeper than the URD. Leveling of the entire face should be avoided. However, even with this approach, expression lines are only minimally improved, and a long-term neurotoxin treatment to soften dynamic rhytides may be necessary to maintain optimal cosmesis.

Medium and Thick Skin

Medium and thick skin is ideal for leveling and tightening procedures. Expression lines can be significantly minimized, and some can be eliminated entirely for a prolonged period of time. However, as in thin skin, expression lines will not be minimized, and additional treatment with a neurotoxin may be necessary to weaken the underlying muscles responsible for dynamic rhytides.

SKIN TYPE ACCORDING TO OILINESS

Skin can be classified as *oily,* secreting excessive sebum; *normal,* secreting a moderate amount of sebum; or *dry,* secreting a below-average amount of sebum (Box 4.7). Oily skin is seen predominantly in persons with thick and medium-thickness skin and is only occasionally seen in patients with thin skin. Figure 4.21 shows a patient with thick, oily skin, and Figure 4.22

Box 4.7

In terms of oiliness and dryness, skin should be grouped into two categories: dry (for genetic reasons) and oily. The terms *normal skin* and
combination skin should be avoided.

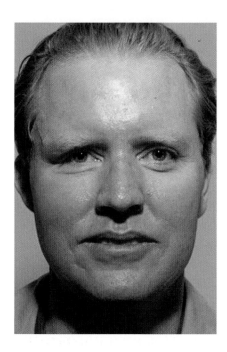

FIGURE 4.21 Patient with thick, oily skin.

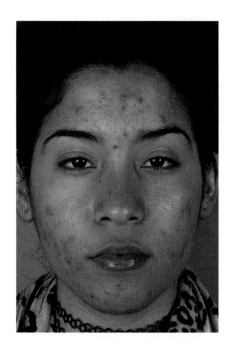

FIGURE 4.22 Patient with medium-thickness, oily skin.

FIGURE 4.23   Patient with thin, dry skin.

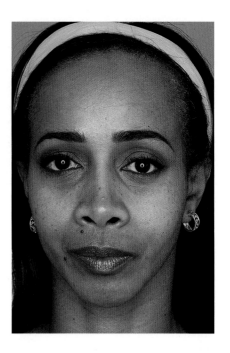

shows a patient with medium-thickness, oily skin. Oily skin is associated with large or hyperactive sebaceous glands. It is also frequently associated with enlarged pores. Despite a common misconception, oily skin does not age more slowly than dry skin; aging changes in skin are directly proportional to the amount and quality of collagen and elastin within the dermis. Also, a relative lack of sebum is not the cause of skin dryness. For example, an infant's skin has no surface sebum (the sebaceous glands are small and inactive), yet it does not appear dry. Dryness is actually related to dermal and epidermal hydration, as well as effective barrier function, which regulates transepidermal water loss. Figure 4.23 shows a patient with thin, dry skin. The amount of glycosoaminoglycans and natural moisturizing factors that attract and retain water within the dermis influences the skin's ultimate hydration status. Table 4.13 shows commonly held misconceptions related to skin dryness.

Sebum provides antibacterial activity and yields a natural smoothness and glow to skin. Excess sebum, on the other hand, is detrimental. Hypersecretion of sebum leads to clogged pores, comedone formation (as in acne and rosacea), and seborrheic dermatitis. Although naturally produced by one's own skin, sebum is a highly inflammatory substance that induces a significant immune response; this resultant inflammation is manifested as acne, rosacea, seborrheic dermatitis, PIH, and scarring. Patients with oily skin pose more

TABLE 4.13 Misconceptions Regarding Skin Dryness	
Misconception	Fact
Those with oily skin appear to age more slowly	Skin aging is not related to the amount of sebum; instead, it is proportional to the amount and quality of collagen and elastin within the dermis.
Sebum prevents skin dryness	Dryness is due to a relative decreased amount of dermal glycosaminoglycans and natural moisturizing factors as well as to an impaired barrier function (increased transepidermal water loss).

challenging treatment approaches (regardless of the treatment type) because sebum reduces the efficacy and penetration of many topical agents. It also reduces the ultimate efficacy of chemical peels and laser treatments and may even cause treatment failure, especially when treating stubborn hyperpigmentation. Extreme caution is advised when treating skin with excess sebum using resurfacing procedures because they can result in an uneven penetration and skin response and in post-procedure acne or rosacea flares. Additionally, premature treatment of skin with chemical peels or lasers (before first controlling excess sebum production) can increase the potential for PIH that is resistant to topical treatment.

SKIN TYPE ACCORDING TO ELASTICITY AND LAXITY

Skin laxity is manifested as wrinkles, eyebrow dropping, redundancy of upper and lower eyelid skin, deepened nasolabial folds, redundant skin on the cheeks and jawline, and jowling. These changes begin at approximately the age of 30 years with the appearance of fine lines and the loss of skin tightness and are accelerated by the degenerative effects of chronic photodamage on elastin within the dermis. Histologically, lax skin is characterized by a thinner epidermis and dermis. Specific dermal changes include solar elastosis (degenerating elastin fibers) and disorganization and a reduced amount of collagen fibers. Although often seen together in advanced skin aging, muscle laxity is not synonymous with skin laxity for treatment purposes. Examples of muscle laxity include platysmal banding and redundancy (which can lead to jowl formation) and orbicularis oculi and frontalis muscle drooping, which can ultimately lead to eyelid and eyebrow ptosis. Loss of elasticity in the face can be categorized as early versus late skin laxity. Features of facial laxity are delineated in Box 4.8. Figure 4.24 shows a patient with skin laxity, and Figure 4.25 shows a patient with skin and muscle laxity.

ATYPICAL HEALING EFFECTS IN RELATION TO SKIN TYPE

Although skin displaying atypical healing is not a distinct skin classification, its presence can be the cause of many complications following procedures (e.g., chemical peels and laser treatments). Complications from atypical or impaired healing include hypertrophic scars and keloids. The potential for atypical healing should be assessed in every patient before performing any procedure; this is especially important in more invasive procedures such as resurfacing below the level of the IRD.

Evaluation of skin thickness by measuring the fold created when applying pressure simultaneously with the practitioner's thumb and index finger reveals that skin in certain patients does not offer resistance to firm squeezing

Box 4.8

Features of Early and Late Facial Laxity

EARLY LAXITY

■ Appearance of wrinkles

■ Lack of resistance to pulling of the skin (decreased elasticity)

■ Deepening of nasolabial folds and exaggeration of expression lines (dynamic rhytides)

■ Improvement with gentle skin stretching in one direction (the Dr. Zein Obagi Stretch Test)

■ Minimal textural changes

■ Can be reversed at a very early stage with topical retinoic acid or retinol and with a trichloroacetic acid chemical peel reaching the immediate reticular dermis

■ Not significantly improved by a surgical procedure (such as a facelift)

LATE LAXITY

■ Muscle laxity and skin laxity

■ Dermatochalasis

■ Eyebrow ptosis

■ Jowl formation

■ Redundancy of neck muscles

■ Fat pad migration (downward and inward/medially)

■ Minimal to no improvement with the Dr. Zein Obagi Stretch Test

■ Ideal for the combination of surgical and non-surgical skin tightening

FIGURE 4.24 Patient with skin laxity.

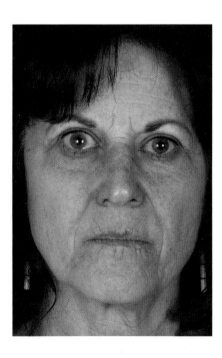

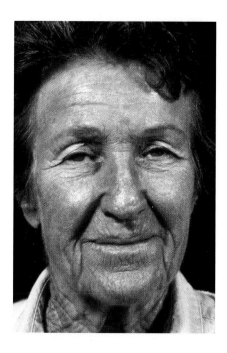

FIGURE 4.25 Patient with skin and muscle laxity.

Box 4.9

Skin Types Showing Lack of Resistance

Lack of resistance to the fold-pinch test can be seen in all skin types but appears most often in Asian and black patients.

---

or pinching. This lack of resistance can be compared with what one feels when attempting to pinch a sponge: the thumb and index finger can touch, and the created fold bulges wide above the squeezed area. In other patients, such squeezing indicates strong resistance, similar to what one would encounter with a firm substance such as leather. In addition, skin resistance in patients with a propensity for keloid formation after surgery or deep resurfacing procedures, as well as in those who developed keloids after resolution of individual inflammatory acne lesions, reveals little or no resistance to the fold-pinch test. Lack of resistance can be seen in all skin types but appears most often in Asian and black patients (Box 4.9). After identifying skin with a propensity toward atypical healing, the practitioner should avoid penetrating deeper than the papillary dermis when performing resurfacing procedures.

REFERENCES

1. Fitzpatrick scale. Wikipedia. Available from: http://en.wikipedia.org/wiki/Fitzpatrick_scale. Retrieved June 23, 2014.
2. Fitzpatrick TB. The validity and practicality of sun-reactive skin types I through VI. *Arch Dermatol.* 1988;124:869-871.
3. Glogau RG. Chemical peeling and aging skin. *J Geriatr Dermatol.* 1994;2:30-35.

4. Roberts WE. Skin type classification systems: old and new. *Dermatol Clin.* 2009;27:529-533.

5. Holck DE, Ng JD. Facial skin rejuvenation. *Curr Opin Ophthalmol.* 2003;14:246-252.

6. Sachdeva S. Fitzpatrick skin typing: applications in dermatology. *Indian J Dermatol Venereol Leprol.* 2009;75:93-96.

7. Kim MM, Byrne PJ. Facial skin rejuvenation in the Asian patient. *Facial Plast Surg Clin North Am.* 2007;15:381-386.

8. Sehgal VN, Verma P, Srivastava G, et al. Melasma: treatment strategy. *J Cosmet Laser Ther.* 2011;13:265-279.

SKIN REJUVENATION
The Art, the Science, and the Procedures

SKIN REJUVENATION DEFINED

The popularity of skin rejuvenation procedures has increased exponentially over the past decade as a result of increased patient interest and technological advancements. Patients are becoming better educated and more aware of different treatment options for skin rejuvenation through the Internet. However, the seemingly endless variety of claims in advertisements sponsored by product and device companies can confuse patients. This most likely arises from the different perceptions among professionals of the meaning of "skin rejuvenation." To many physicians, skin rejuvenation indicates performance of a procedure. To cosmeceutical companies, it implies use of their anti-aging topical products, and to laser and device manufacturers, it implies treatment with one of their own devices.

Skin rejuvenation, however, is not a cream used to improve the skin's surface; it is not a procedure, such as use of a laser or other energy-emitting device, a chemical peel, or filler or neurotoxin injections; and it is not invasive surgery, such as a facelift. Skin rejuvenation is a *comprehensive treatment plan* with a combined approach, as defined in Box 5.1.

This definition makes the concept of skin rejuvenation simple, straightforward, and suitable for all patients. Restoring and maintaining skin in its optimal original state is the main objective of skin rejuvenation (Box 5.2). This is accomplished by designing an appropriate topical protocol and overall treatment plan that is appropriate for each patient's needs. Such a plan is based on the following:

- Topical agents that restore general skin health and treat any concurrent skin disease
- When indicated, an additional appropriate procedure, based on its mechanism of action and the desired result
- When choosing a procedure, identification of the safe depth of penetration for a particular skin type (see Chapter 4) to ensure maintenance of skin integrity and natural appearance

---

Box 5.1

Skin Rejuvenation Defined

Skin rejuvenation is the art of transforming skin to its original state through combined use of the following:

- Topical agents that restore general skin health
- Topical agents to treat existing disease (e.g., acne, rosacea, actinic keratoses) when they are present.
- Procedures (e.g., lasers and other energy-emitting devices, chemical peels, and injections of fillers or neurotoxins) when topical agents alone do not completely restore skin to its original state.

Box 5.2

Restoring and maintaining skin in its original state is the main objective of skin rejuvenation.

PATIENT SELECTION

In all aesthetic procedures, proper patient selection is a crucial component of a successful outcome. Prospective patients seeking skin rejuvenation often come to the physician with a "consumer" attitude. They want to look younger and better and are interested in finding out the specific out-of-pocket expenses for such improvement. As consumers, however, patients often "doctor shop," seeking the lowest price for a given procedure, yet also expect an excellent outcome, a predictable post-procedure course, and minimal downtime during recovery. Because of the considerable variation in individual expectations, demands, and levels of understanding of preprocedure skin conditioning and procedures, the physician must make every effort to ensure that each patient has realistic expectations and is fully informed about alternative treatment options, the expected duration of post-procedure healing time, and potential adverse events associated with each procedure.

Patients seeking better skin may ask for one treatment from the physician, without knowing that another treatment would better achieve the specific desired results. For example, patients often point to static rhytides around the mouth and ask for administration of a neurotoxin. However, in this scenario, volume restoration using filler injection, not the use of neurotoxin, which relaxes muscles and softens the appearance of dynamic rhytides, is the most appropriate method of achieving the desired improvement. Furthermore, a patient's expectations may seem realistic before a specific procedure, yet after the procedure has been performed, the same patient may reveal his or her actual, but unrealistic, expectations. The physician must make every attempt to screen for these problem patients during the initial consultation to avoid

Box 5.3

Patients to Exclude from Treatment

- Pregnant women and, occasionally, lactating women (depending on the treatment type)
- Those who fail to keep appointments
- Those demonstrating poor compliance with the topical skin conditioning regimen
- Those who have unreasonable expectations
- Those who mention a myriad of "complications" they have had with other physicians
- Those who believe that their appearance is responsible for a failed marriage or other relationship
- Those who are unable to allow enough time for necessary post-procedural healing
- Those who are depressed, undergoing emotional crises, or taking several psychotropic medications

time-consuming post-procedure complaints and lawsuits. Finding a tactful way to exclude patients who appear to have unrealistic expectations, as well as those displaying traits suggesting they may not be compliant with preprocedure and post-procedure instructions, will ultimately provide invaluable peace of mind.

The physician must also consider the patient's motivation for the rejuvenation procedure. Patients seeking aesthetic treatments may suffer from emotional dysfunction and a lack of self-confidence. On the severe end of the spectrum, patients may have a serious mental health disorder, such as body dysmorphic disorder. These and other patients are often not prepared psychologically or financially for a lengthy treatment program and are more likely to be dissatisfied with their results, regardless of the treatment type. The physician should avoid accepting patients with psychological and emotional problems for cosmetic and rejuvenation procedures. Box 5.3 lists patients who should be excluded from cosmetic treatments.

DIAGNOSTIC CONSIDERATIONS

A patient's diagnosis has a significant effect on the time needed to complete the rejuvenation program. For example, scars and rhytides can be corrected relatively quickly (by intralesional steroid injections and/or laser treatments and injections of neurotoxins and fillers, respectively). In contrast, the correction of melasma or other forms of dermal melanosis typically takes much longer, often involving a combination approach with multiple distinct treatment modalities.

Any concurrent skin conditions must be corrected before performing a rejuvenation procedure. Specifically, inflammatory skin conditions such as acne vulgaris, rosacea, seborrheic dermatitis, and folliculitis must be controlled because they can impair or prevent optimal post-procedure healing. Similarly, other skin conditions, such as melasma, excessive skin oiliness, or sensitivity, should also be treated before a rejuvenation procedure. For example, before treating melasma with a chemical peel, the physician must ensure that the patient has adequately preconditioned his or her skin, which includes daily application of a product containing a retinoid to stabilize melanocytes, as well as a product containing hydroquinone (HQ) to control melanocytes. These creams should be used for at least 6 weeks before the rejuvenation procedure to optimize results and minimize the risk for potential complications. Furthermore, patients with these conditions should be counseled regarding their required participation in prepeel and postpeel care; the potential need for multiple treatments, such as chemical peels for melasma; and long-term topical treatment to reduce excess sebum and restore and maintain the skin's barrier function to prevent skin sensitivity and other complications. Occasionally, low-dose (20 mg/day) isotretinoin is started *after* a rejuvenation procedure and used for approximately 3 to 5 months to minimize oiliness that leads to post-procedure hyperpigmentation and acne flares. Textural skin changes, such as solar elastosis, diffuse acne scarring, disseminated sebaceous gland hyperplasia, and rhinophyma, may require different types of procedures (e.g., hyfrecation, subscission, wire loop surgery) or combined or multiple procedures for optimal cosmesis.

The depth of the problem should guide the choice of corrective procedure (Figure 5.1). Conditions limited to the epidermis respond well to any exfoliative procedure, whereas conditions located within the dermis can be improved

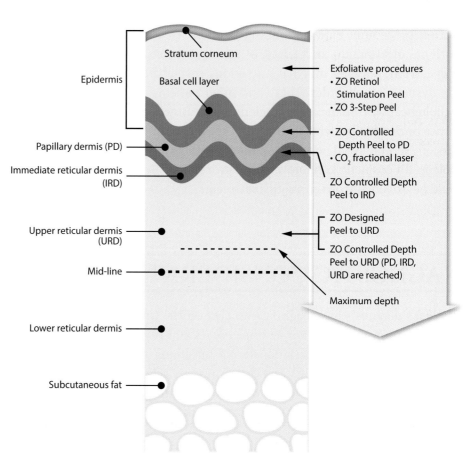

FIGURE 5.1 Skin layers and corrective procedures.

with tightening or leveling (deep chemical peels and/or CO_2 fractional laser treatment). Subcutaneous volume loss responds best to injections of fillers, biostimulatory molecules, and/or autologous fat. Surgical removal of excess lax skin is also appropriate in certain circumstances. Neurotoxin injections can add further benefit on the muscular level by "softening" the appearance of dynamic rhytides.

TREATMENT PLANNING

After classifying the patient's skin and making the diagnosis, the physician should formulate a comprehensive treatment plan that includes both short- and long-term goals. The plan must clearly inform the patient of the reason for each part of the overall plan, the importance of patient compliance, and the complexity of the plan. Monitoring patient compliance with short-term treatment recommendations—for example, assessing the patient's daily use of a comprehensive topical regimen—allows the physician maximal control over the entire process. A patient's inability or unwillingness to follow the recommended, pre-procedure daily skin care regimen should be a "red flag," signaling the physician to avoid any subsequent invasive rejuvenation procedures. These noncompliant patients are much more likely to experience suboptimal overall results and adverse events. See Box 5.4 for an overview of skin rejuvenation treatment planning, which has been broken down into seven parts for the sake of simplicity.

Regardless of specifics related to each patient's individualized rejuvenation treatment plan, certain physician guidelines should always be followed. One must always maintain the clear objective of restoring overall skin health while also treating concomitant skin disorders. As such, before *any* rejuvenation

---

Box 5.4

Overview of Skin Rejuvenation Treatment Planning

1. Classify the patient's skin (according to color/ethnicity and thickness).
2. Diagnose conditions to be treated.
3. Treat any active disease.
4. Maintain the objective of restoring skin health while initiating a plan for skin conditioning (through the use of daily topical products) before any upcoming planned procedures.
5. If one or more rejuvenation procedures are indicated, choose them based on the match of the procedure's mechanism of action to the depth of the condition being treated.
6. Have a clear plan for expediting recovery, minimizing potential for post-procedural complications, and treating complications if they do occur.
7. Establish a comprehensive, effective post-procedure maintenance regimen.

Box 5.5

Before *any* rejuvenation procedure, the skin must be conditioned for at least 6 weeks by at-home daily application of a comprehensive topical regimen.

Box 5.6

Essential Physician-to-Patient Communication before a Procedure

- Explain the overall treatment plan or program.
- Inform of the possibility of adverse events or complications.
- Explain the possible need for a repeated procedure.
- Communicate the expected "downtime" following the procedure.
- Explain the need for a maintenance program.
- Answer the patient's questions.

---

procedure, the skin must be prepared and conditioned adequately for at least 6 weeks by at-home daily application of a comprehensive topical regimen (Box 5.5). The patient should know that the doctor may terminate the overall treatment plan if he or she fails to comply with individual recommendations.

Effective, two-way communication between the physician and the patient is essential. The physician should explain the overall treatment plan or program, answer all of the patient's questions, and clearly inform the patient that, despite best intentions and one's overall experience, the treatment program may not succeed and could result in unintentional, adverse events or complications. The physician should also clearly explain that a procedure might need to be performed more than once (e.g., more than one treatment with the CO_2 fractional laser may be necessary to optimally correct severe facial acne scarring). The expected "downtime" should also be made clear so that patients can schedule their work and social commitments accordingly. It is always best to underpromise and overdeliver when treating any patient. Furthermore, a thorough discussion of alternative treatment options should be included when proposing a treatment plan to a patient. And, the patient should know that a post-procedure, daily topical maintenance program will be essential for overall treatment success. The essential physician-to-patient communication is shown in Box 5.6.

PROCEDURE SELECTION

Physicians currently choose light, medium, or deep procedures for their patients without understanding the meaning of these terms. They also tend to focus mainly on skin color (such as the Fitzpatrick skin type) when choosing a procedure, while overlooking other important factors, such as skin thickness, laxity, and tendency to form hypertrophic scars or keloids. In choosing the best procedure for a patient, physicians need to take a broader post-treatment perspective that evaluates and optimizes the skin's overall quality, health, and function.

There are currently no adequate, standardized guidelines for choosing a procedure or procedures for correction of a given condition involved in skin rejuvenation. Physicians tend to select procedures based on their personal experience, mostly acquired during training in residency and fellowship. The popularity (from media and advertising influences) and profitability of procedures seem also to guide a physician's choice. This is a clear danger in that profitability and popularity do not necessarily correlate with effectiveness or appropriateness of that procedure. For example, exfoliative chemical peels are being performed to correct wrinkles and scars, which actually necessitate chemical peels or laser treatments that penetrate deeper. On the other hand, there are many cases in which physicians are choosing to perform rejuvenative procedures that are more invasive than necessary for the specific patient.

Selecting procedures should be based on multiple factors:

1. Skin type (color, thickness, oiliness, laxity, and healing properties)
2. The nature of the patient's skin problems
3. The skin's response to Dr. Zein Obagi Skin Stretch Test
4. Thermal versus chemical procedures
5. Proper procedure depth

PROCEDURE SELECTION ACCORDING TO SKIN TYPE

Skin type is a broad term encompassing skin color, thickness, oiliness, laxity, and healing properties.

Skin Color

Skin color that is light white and original white (Zein Obagi Skin Classification System; see Chapter 4) is suitable for thermal (i.e., lasers and other energy-emitting devices that employ radiofrequency and ultrasound) and chemical procedures. Darker skinned patients, of African or Asian descent, are best treated with nonthermal procedures such as chemical peels. This avoids potential complications such as postinflammatory hyperpigmentation (PIH), which can occasionally occur after excessive heating of melanocytes with certain laser procedures. Furthermore, to avoid complications and maximize cosmetic improvement in darker skin types, the penetration depth for chemical peels should not exceed the immediate reticular dermis (IRD). For patients with more severe or persistent conditions (e.g., certain cases of melasma), the physician should consider performing a second procedure—again, limited in depth to the IRD—at a future visit. For skin in the deviated category, nonthermal procedures are preferred. Thermal procedures can be performed in these patients, but recovery time will be longer because PIH is more likely to occur and responds more slowly to post-procedure topical corrective treatments, although it does ultimately respond well in the long run.

Skin Thickness

Keeping in mind the previous recommendations on optimal treatments for specific skin color types (assuming all else is equal), thick skin is better equipped to tolerate invasive and ablative procedures and is thus ideal for thermal as well as nonthermal procedures. For patients with thick skin (for lighter skin types, see earlier discussion), chemical peels can safely be performed down to the level of the upper reticular dermis (URD), when appropriate. For thin skin, nonthermal procedures, such as chemical peels, are preferred, and penetration depth should be limited to the IRD to avoid complications. Figure 5.2 shows a patient with thin to medium-thickness skin treated with a ZO Controlled Depth Peel to the IRD.

Skin Oiliness

Preceding all procedures, sebum must be reduced during skin conditioning. In oily skin, including skin prone to acne or rosacea, a course of low-dose (20 mg) daily isotretinoin should be considered. However, this oral medication should only be started *after* any deep chemical peel or laser procedure because there have been reports in the literature that isotretinoin used immediately before or during ablative or invasive procedures can impair the skin's ability to heal optimally. If the decision is made to control severe cases of acne or rosacea with a 5-month course of isotretinoin before an ablative or invasive procedure, a "washout period" of at least 6 months (during which the patient is completely off the isotretinoin) is recommended. After the patient's skin has completely re-epithelialized following the rejuvenation procedure, a course of daily low-dose isotretinoin should be started or restarted and topical skin conditioning resumed. Adherence to these recommendations accelerates the return of skin to normal and minimizes potential post-procedure

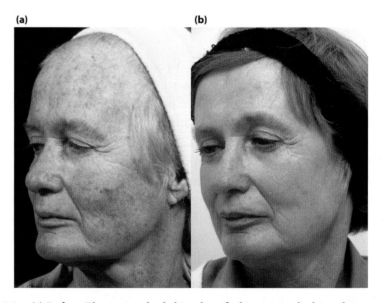

(a) **(b)**

FIGURE 5.2   (a) Before. The patient had skin classified as original white, thin to medium thickness, and nonoily. She was diagnosed as having skin laxity and photodamage. (b) After. The patient was treated with 6 weeks of Skin Health Restoration followed by a ZO Controlled Depth Peel to the immediate reticular dermis.

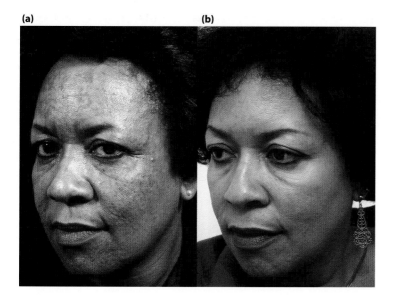

FIGURE 5.3 (a) Before. The patient had skin classified as deviated black, thick, and oily. She was diagnosed as having rosacea and dermal melasma. (b) One year later. The patient was treated with 6 weeks of HQ-based Skin Health Restoration followed by a medium-depth ZO Designed Controlled Depth Peel. This was followed by HQ-based Skin Health Restoration and use of isotretinoin, 20 mg/day for 5 months.

complications, such as PIH. Taking into consideration the degree of oiliness in a patient's skin is also important because excessive sebum, as seen in oily skin, decreases the efficacy of the preprocedure and post-procedure topical conditioning programs. This, in turn, increases the potential for periprocedural complications. Figure 5.3 shows a patient with thick, oily skin, diagnosed with rosacea and melasma, who was treated with Skin Health Restoration to condition skin and reduce sebum, followed by a medium-depth ZO Designed Controlled Depth Peel.

Skin Laxity

When there is skin laxity, which is different from muscle laxity, a nonthermal, nonablative procedure that tightens is best. Specifically, a chemical peel penetrating to the level of the papillary dermis (PD) or IRD is optimal for correcting skin laxity because this restores the production of healthy elastin. Skin laxity is best corrected by a procedure that penetrates to the depth of the IRD, such as a tightening procedure (Figure 5.4). This is in contrast to the temporary tightening effect seen following treatment with thermal devices, including many lasers, because these cause collagen denaturation and shrinkage, yet do not induce elastin production. Furthermore, skin with concomitant, underlying muscle laxity—for example, in patients with loose skin of the neck due to platysmal muscle laxity—usually requires a surgical approach to correction (platysmaplasty), in addition to a tightening procedure that treats lax skin for optimal cosmesis.

Skin with Suboptimal Healing

Nonthermal, nonablative procedures, such as chemical peels penetrating to the depth of the PD, are the ideal choice for patients with a history of suboptimal or atypical healing (e.g., those with a propensity to form hypertrophic scars and keloids). These procedures should not exceed depths beyond

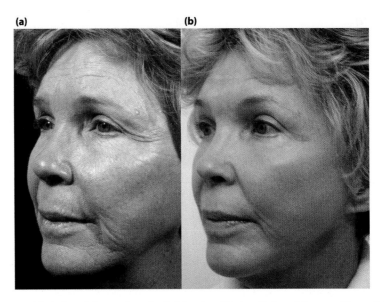

FIGURE 5.4 (a) Before. The patient had skin classified as light white, medium thickness, and nonoily. She was diagnosed as having photodamage, laxity, and stretchable rhytides. (b) One year later. The patient was treated for 10 weeks with non-HQ-based Skin Health Restoration, followed by a ZO Controlled Depth Peel to the immediate reticular dermis. This was followed by 12 weeks of non-HQ-based Skin Health Restoration.

the level of the PD in all patients in this category. Furthermore, to avoid the potential for hypopigmentation in patients with dark skin (original type), the procedures should not penetrate to depths below the level of the IRD.

The recommended procedures for Zein Obagi Skin Classification System are shown in Table 5.1.

PROCEDURE SELECTION ACCORDING TO THE NATURE OF THE SKIN PROBLEM

Presence of Active Disease

Patients with an underlying active disease, such as acne, rosacea, psoriasis, or irritant or allergic contact dermatitis, should not undergo a tightening or leveling procedure (thermal or nonthermal, ablative or nonablative) until *after* the disease has been adequately treated and controlled. In contrast, more superficial, exfoliative procedures, such as mechanical exfoliation (microdermabrasion), as well as light chemical peels (glycolic and salicylic acid), can in fact be very beneficial

TABLE 5.1 Skin Type and Recommended Procedures

Zein Obagi Skin Type	Recommended Procedures
Light white and original white skin	Thermal and nonthermal procedures, such as chemical peels
Darker skin patients of African or Asian descent	Nonthermal procedures, such as chemical peels
Deviated skin	Nonthermal procedures, such as chemical peels
Thick skin	Thermal and nonthermal procedures (such as chemical peels, possibly down to the level of the upper reticular dermis)
Thin skin	Chemical peels
Skin with laxity	Chemical peels to the papillary dermis or immediate reticular dermis
Skin with suboptimal healing	Chemical peels to the papillary dermis

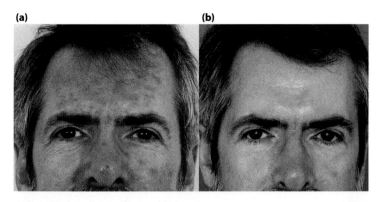

(a) **(b)**

FIGURE 5.5 (a) Before. The patient had skin classified as deviated normal white, medium thickness, and oily. He was diagnosed as having active severe rosacea and seborrheic dermatitis. (b) One year later. The patient was treated with 3 months of non-HQ-based Skin Health Restoration, metronidazole in the morning, and isotretinoin, 20 mg/day. Two treatments with the ZO 3-Step Peel were performed after 6 and 10 weeks of starting Skin Health Restoration. Note that no procedure should be performed on a patient until rosacea has been cleared.

in correcting skin with active disease and are best used in combination with a comprehensive daily topical treatment regimen. Figure 5.5 shows a patient with active disease—severe rosacea and seborrheic dermatitis—who was treated with a program of Skin Health Restoration first and then a ZO Controlled Depth Peel.

Patients with epidermal and dermal melasma usually respond well to chemical peels. Because melanocytes are heat sensitive, thermal procedures are best avoided because they have the potential to worsen the post-procedural dyschromia. In contrast, those with hyperpigmented patches due to an underlying disorder referred to as a nevus of Ota or a nevus of Ito respond best to thermal procedures (e.g., sequential treatments with the 1064-nm QS-Nd:YAG laser) because they are due to an excessive proliferation of melanocytes and their presence in the dermis and subcutaneous tissue (as opposed to melasma, which is due to an overproduction of melanin from a relatively normal number of individual melanocytes). As such, thermal and laser treatments in these patients are beneficial because they induce selective destruction of excessive melanocytes.

A lentigo is a discrete hyperpigmented macule or patch due to an increased number of melanocytes located within the epidermis in the cell layer directly above the basement membrane. Lentigines are distinguished from ephelides (freckles) based on the etiology of the outwardly observed hyperpigmented macules. Specifically, ephelides have a relatively normal total number of individual melanocytes, but these melanocytes are producing an increased *amount* of melanin. Again, lentigines, in contrast, are histologically distinct in that they have an increased *number* of melanocytes. Both lentigines and ephelides are easily treated by intense pulse light (IPL), certain lasers (QS-alexandrite and QS-ruby), and chemical peels. As with all skin treatments, proper preprocedure and post-procedure topical skin conditioning is essential for patients with active underlying pigmentary disorders.

Presence of Photodamage

Chronic photodamage is most commonly manifested as numerous, scattered, diffuse, poorly demarcated actinic keratoses, lentigines, ephelides, telangiectasias, atrophic patches, and skin with textural irregularities. Regardless of a patient's skin color, the optimal rejuvenation approach to correcting chronic

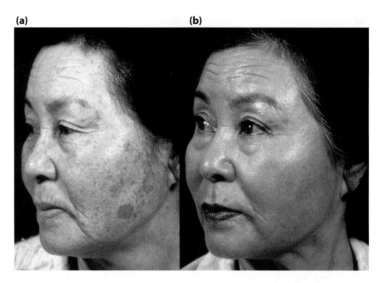

(a) **(b)**

FIGURE 5.6   (a) Before. The patient had skin classified as Asian (light) and thick. She was diagnosed as having photodamage and lentigines on her cheeks. (b) One year later. The patient underwent 6 weeks of aggressive HQ-based Skin Health Restoration followed by a ZO Controlled Depth Peel to the papillary dermis. Aggressive HQ-based Skin Health Restoration was continued for 12 weeks following the peel. Maintenance involved a non-HQ-based skin health program.

actinic damage is one or more chemical peels to the level of the IRD. Figure 5.6, Figure 5.7, and Figure 5.8 show patients with photodamage and/or lentigines who were treated with a program of Skin Health Restoration and a ZO Controlled Depth Peel. Of note, photodamaged skin is atrophic, fragile, and thus susceptible to scarring following ablative procedures. Finally, IPL treatments, when administered by experienced providers using optimal devices, can correct the overall poikilodermatous appearance of photodamaged skin. Box 5.7 lists the common manifestations of chronic photodamage. Box 5.8 summarizes the procedures that can be used for rejuvenation of skin in patients with certain conditions.

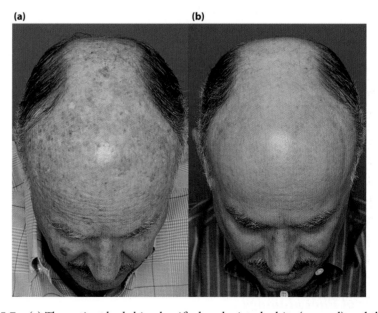

(a) **(b)**

FIGURE 5.7   (a) The patient had skin classified as deviated white (normal) and thick. He was diagnosed as having severe photodamage, lentigines, actinic keratoses, and a basal cell carcinoma on his right cheek. (b) One year later. The patient underwent 6 weeks of HQ-based Skin Health Restoration and DNA repair, epidermal stabilization, and stimulation, followed by a ZO Controlled Depth Peel to the papillary dermis.

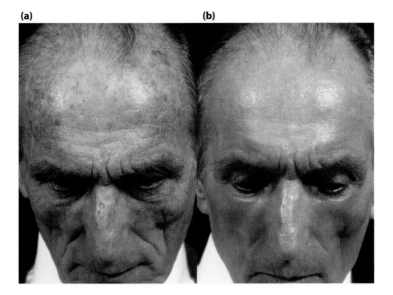

(a) **(b)**

FIGURE 5.8 (a) Before. The patient had skin classified as original white, medium thickness, and nonoily. He was diagnosed as having photodamage, lentigines, and actinic keratoses. (b) One year later. The patient was treated with 5 months of HQ-based Skin Health Restoration, followed by a ZO Controlled Depth Peel to the immediate reticular dermis on his face and scalp. This was followed by 6 weeks of HQ-based Skin Health Restoration.

Box 5.7

Manifestations of Chronic Skin Photodamage

Chronic skin photodamage is commonly manifested as actinic keratoses, lentigines, ephelides, telangiectasias, atrophic patches, and textural irregularities.

Box 5.8

Procedures for Patients with Certain Conditions

- Patients with an underlying active disease, such as acne, rosacea, psoriasis, or irritant or allergic contact dermatitis, should not undergo a tightening or leveling procedure until *after* the disease has been adequately treated and controlled.
- Exfoliative procedures, however, are beneficial for patients with these conditions.
- Patients with epidermal and dermal melasma usually respond well to chemical peels.
- Patients with nevus of Ota or nevus of Ito respond best to thermal procedures.
- Patients with chronic actinic damage are best treated with one or more chemical peels to the level of the IRD.

Box 5.9

Dr. Zein Obagi Skin Stretch Test

When an area of skin with hyperpigmentation is stretched:

- Epidermal melasma will appear lighter, and dermal melasma will appear darker.

When an area of skin with wrinkles is stretched:

- Rigid wrinkles and scars will not improve or fade. This reveals severe textural damage and indicates a leveling procedure for correction.
- Wrinkles and scars that improve or disappear indicate minimal textural damage, and less invasive procedures (tightening) are needed.

Dr. Zein Obagi Skin Stretch Test

Dr. Zein Obagi Skin Stretch Test is a simple way to identify the nature and depth of certain problems. The test is performed by gently stretching, with both hands, the affected areas of the patient's skin and observing subsequent specific changes on the skin surface (Box 5.9).

The importance of Dr. Zein Obagi Skin Stretch Test is two-fold. First, it allows the physician to determine the depth of skin involved with hyperpigmentation. With this information, an appropriate procedure and depth of procedure penetration can be determined. Second, this test allows the physician to choose the correct rejuvenation procedure based on evaluation of how the wrinkles and scars responded to the test. Specifically, rigid wrinkles and scars are best treated by a leveling procedure reaching the URD (e.g., CO_2 fractional laser treatment or a medium-depth ZO Designed Controlled Depth Peel). In contrast, soft wrinkles and scars are best treated by a tightening procedure (e.g., a ZO Controlled Depth Peel to the IRD).

THERMAL VERSUS NONTHERMAL PROCEDURES

All lasers, as well as other energy-emitting devices, such as IPL, radiofrequency, and ultrasound, are considered thermal devices. They are very useful for treating a wide variety of skin problems and play an important role in Skin Health Restoration and rejuvenation. The physician must carefully determine safe and effective parameters for each individual patient based on skin type, skin thickness, the target for correction, and the depth of treatment required to reach the target, among other factors. The most important laser parameters that must be adjusted specifically for each patient include the wavelength, pulse width, spot size, and amount of energy emitted. The CO_2 fractional laser and the erbium lasers are optimal treatment choices for skin resurfacing, particularly for treating rigid wrinkles and scars. Figure 5.9 and Figure 5.10 show patients treated with CO_2 fractional laser treatment.

Chemical peels are considered nonthermal procedures. The most important parameters to be considered when choosing a specific chemical peel include

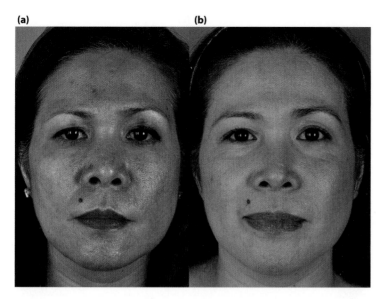

Figure 5.9 (a) Before. The patient had skin classified as deviated Asian (medium), medium thickness, and oily. She was diagnosed as having acne, rosacea, sebaceous gland hyperplasia, and severe textural irregularities due to acne scarring. (b) After. The patient was treated with 6 weeks of aggressive HQ-based Skin Health Restoration, followed by CO_2 fractional laser treatment. This was followed by a 5-month course of low-dose isotretinoin (20 mg/day) and aggressive, HQ-based Skin Health Restoration for another 6 weeks.

the type of acid used (TCA, salicylic acid, glycolic acid, lactic acid, and phenol, among others), the concentration of the acid, and the total amount of acid applied to the treatment area. For those chemical peels that do not self-neutralize, the amount of time that the chemical solution is in contact with the skin is also a consideration.

Regardless of whether a thermal or a nonthermal procedure is chosen, the depth of skin penetration is proportional to the extent of rejuvenation, as well as to the possibility of adverse events or complications (including treatment failure). The physician should consider the safety of a chosen depth for a particular skin type and whether the treatment can be safely permitted to penetrate deeper in certain focal areas within the full treatment site when these

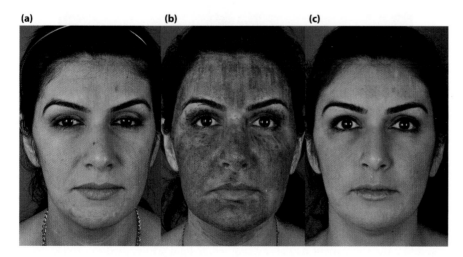

Figure 5.10 (a) Before. The patient had skin classified as deviated white (dark) and medium thickness. She was diagnosed as having cystic acne and variable acne scars. (b) Six days after a CO_2 fractional laser procedure. Following the laser procedure, she had 18 weeks of aggressive Skin Health Restoration and used isotretinoin, 20 g/day. (c) Six months later.

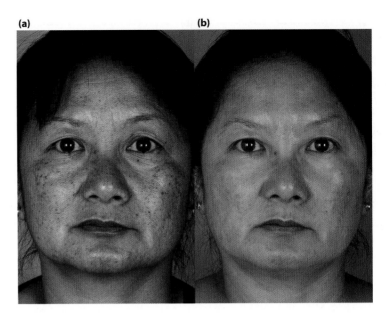

FIGURE 5.11 (a) The patient had skin classified as original Asian and medium thickness. She was diagnosed as having photodamage, lentigines, and dermatosis papulosa nigra. (b) One year later. The patient underwent HQ-based Skin Health Restoration for 6 weeks, followed by hyfrecation and a ZO Controlled Depth Peel to the immediate reticular dermis. The patient continued for 12 weeks following the peel.

focal areas could benefit from deeper or stronger correction. Figure 5.11 and Figure 5.12 show patients who underwent Skin Health Restoration followed by a chemical peel (ZO Controlled Depth Peel) to the level of the IRD.

Peel Terminology

Current terminology used to describe the depth of a chemical peel tends to be confusing, unscientific, and easily subject to misinterpretation. For example, a "light" peel to one physician may be a "medium-depth" peel to another. Thus,

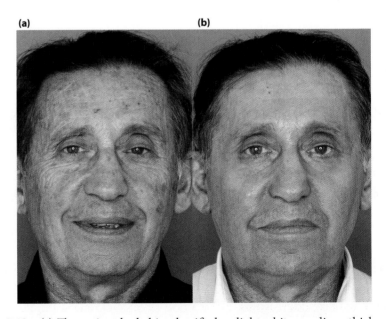

FIGURE 5.12 (a) The patient had skin classified as light white, medium thickness, and oily. He was diagnosed as having photodamage and actinic keratoses. He had a history of basal cell carcinomas. (b) One year later. The patient underwent aggressive HQ-based Skin Health Restoration for 5 months. A ZO Controlled Depth Peel to the immediate reticular dermis level was performed after 6 weeks of Skin Health Restoration (skin conditioning).

Box 5.10

Describing Chemical Peel Depth

- Terms such as "light," "medium," and "deep" are inadequate descriptors for chemical peels. (See the classification of peel depth and terminology shown in Table 5.2.)
- The concentration of an acid does not directly correlate to its depth of penetration.
- With continuous application, any concentration of acid can reach any depth in the skin.

when describing chemical peels, the terms "light," "medium," and "deep" are relatively meaningless and are best avoided to prevent confusion. Regardless of the term used to describe the intensity of the chemical peel, it is important to remember that one should never administer a peel that penetrates deeper than the URD.

The concentration of an acid is another incorrect indicator for describing the depth of a peel. As discussed in Chapter 8, with continuous application, any concentration of acid can reach deep into the URD (and beyond, when used incorrectly) (Box 5.10). Of note, this concept applies not just to trichloroacetic acid (TCA) but also to all types of chemical peel acids that are applied to the skin. Classification of peel depth and terminology is shown in Table 5.2.

PROCEDURE SELECTION ACCORDING TO MECHANISM OF ACTION

Rejuvenation procedures differ in their mechanism of action. These include 1) exfoliation, 2) tightening, 3) leveling, 4) extracellular matrix stimulation and thickening, 5) volume restoration, and 6) immobilization of muscular contraction. The ideal skin rejuvenation approach consists of 1) improving the appearance and function of skin (restoring skin health) by using proper

TABLE 5.2 Classification of Rejuvenation Procedures Based on Depth	
Depth of Penetration	**Appropriate Procedure to Reach Desired Depth**
Epidermis	Exfoliative or "false" peels
Papillary dermis (PD)	Tightening procedure, such as the ZO Controlled Depth Peel to the PD
Immediate reticular dermis (IRD)	Tightening procedure, such as the ZO Controlled Depth Peel to the IRD
PD, IRD, or upper reticular dermis (URD)	Combined tightening and leveling procedures, such as:
The ZO Designed Controlled Depth Peel when the URD is reached in small areas	The ZO Controlled Depth Peel to the PD, IRD, and the URD, or
The medium-depth ZO Designed Controlled Depth Peel when the URD is reached in large areas	The combination of the ZO Controlled Depth Peel to the IRD followed by the CO_2 fractional procedure to the URD

TABLE 5.3   Rejuvenation Procedures: Penetration and Mechanism of Action

Procedure	Depth of Penetration	Propensity for Leveling	Propensity for Tightening
CO_2 Fractional Laser	URD	Strong	Weak
ZO Controlled Depth Peel (trichloroacetic acid)	IRD	Weak	Strong
	URDs	Strong	Strong
Phenol peel	Mid-dermis	Strong	Weak
Dermabrasion	URD	Strong	Weak
Neurotoxin injections	Muscles	None	None
Microabrasion, intense pulse light, "false" or superficial peels	Epidermal exfoliation	None	None

topical agents and 2) performing select procedures to correct problems that cannot be corrected by topical agents alone (Table 5.3).

When a physician's main goal is to correct mild skin textural irregularities such as tactile roughness, minimize comedone formation, or normalize dyschromia limited to the epidermis, a procedure that achieves only superficial exfoliation is best. Microdermabrasion, a retinol home peel (see Chapter 9), an alpha-hydroxy acid (AHA) chemical peel, or a chemical peel that combines relatively low concentrations of salicylic acid, TCA, lactic acid, and retinol (the ZO 3-Step Peel) can be chosen for simple exfoliation. Fine to medium stretchable wrinkles, stretchable scars, and lax skin are optimally improved through a tightening procedure, such as the ZO Controlled Depth Peel to the PD. Of note, the CO_2 fractional laser is best suited for leveling because it does not provide sufficient tightening.

Deep, nonstretchable wrinkles and scars are optimally improved through leveling procedures, which include the CO_2 fractional laser, a chemical peel that penetrates to the URD (by TCA in the ZO Controlled Depth Peel), or dermabrasion. For optimal improvement, in certain patients with more severe, extensive, or numerous wrinkles, skin laxity, photodamage, and textural irregularities or scarring, a combination approach, using both a chemical peel and a laser procedure, may offer optimal results while allowing the physician to avoid individual procedures penetrating to unnecessarily deep levels over all of the face.

EXFOLIATION AND EXFOLIATIVE PROCEDURES

Current exfoliative procedures remove parts of the epidermis above the basal layer. They are beneficial for *temporary* correction of epidermal problems but have no beneficial effect on dermal problems, such as wrinkles or scars, *regardless of how many times they are repeated*. Healing is rapid (3 to 6 days) after an exfoliating procedure.

In general, exfoliation can be classified as "natural," "induced," or "false." Natural exfoliation is innate and involves daily shedding of mature, nonviable cells from the upper stratum corneum. Natural exfoliation is the body's natural method of continually renewing the epidermis and maintaining its barrier function. It is impaired or slowed down with advanced age, overuse of moisturizers, and the use of oil-based cosmetics; it can be accelerated by manual friction or rubbing. The rate of natural exfoliation is increased in those with psoriasis (within the areas of the psoriatic papules or plaques), seborrheic dermatitis, or hypertrophic actinic keratoses, as well as by several other, more rare dermatologic disorders.

As bonds between corneocytes break and individual corneocytes become partially separated (which occurs in both intrinsic and extrinsic aging), skin develops a rough texture, which patients typically interpret as dryness and subsequently begin habitual application of moisturizers. Although this produces temporary relief of the perceived dryness, chronic use of moisturizers actually reduces the rate of epidermal mitosis and leads to reduced natural exfoliation, a weakened barrier function, and a thinner epidermis. Together, these lead to skin that is more sensitive or reactive to external insults.

Figure 5.13 and Figure 5.14 show patients who used exfoliative procedures as part of their Skin Health Restoration programs. In Figure 5.13, the patient used the ZO Retinol Stimulation Peel, and in Figure 5.14, the patient used the ZO 3-Step Peel for effective exfoliation.

Induced exfoliation results from various concentrations of topical AHAs, beta-hydroxy acids (BHAs), and kojic acid. These substances disrupt the hemidesmosomal bonds between corneocytes and, to some extent, between keratinocytes. More specifically, the topical application of AHAs (glycolic, lactic, citric, and malic acids), which are water soluble, leads to exfoliation of individual corneocytes and keratinocytes, whereas the application of BHAs (e.g., salicylic acid), which are lipid soluble, "melts" cells through keratolysis.

False exfoliation refers to stratum corneum *dehydration* leading to subsequent exfoliation induced by topically applied tretinoin, benzoyl peroxide, or several other agents. With these specific agents, groups of cells are shed (coarse exfoliation). However, in most patients, this exfoliation phenomenon subsides

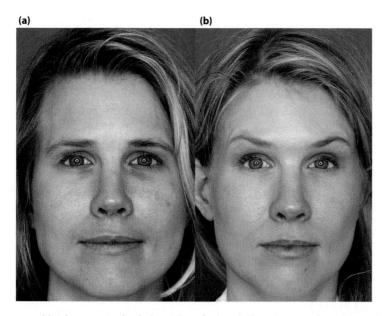

(a) (b)

FIGURE 5.13 (a) The patient had skin classified as light white and medium thickness. She was diagnosed as having photodamage, discoloration, and dullness. (b) One year later. The patient was treated for 5 months with a non-HQ-based program of Skin Health Restoration and had two ZO Retinol Stimulation Peels and an injection of Botox.

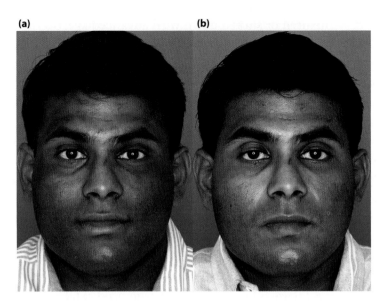

FIGURE 5.14 (a) Before. The patient had skin classified as complex (Indian) thick and oily. He was diagnosed as having postinflammatory hyperpigmentation. (b) Six months later. The patient was treated with 3 months of HQ-based Skin Health Restoration and isotretinoin, 20 mg/day. This was followed by 3 months of non-HQ-based Skin Health Restoration and one ZO 3-Step Peel.

after a few weeks of steady, daily use. Thus, they are considered "false" exfoliators. False exfoliation can also be mechanically induced through microdermabrasion, vigorous scrubbing with a porous material like sandpaper, scraping with a blade (dermaplaning), and stripping with adhesive tape.

TIGHTENING PROCEDURES

Skin tightness is related to the amount and quality of elastin in the dermis and, to a lesser extent, to the amount and quality of collagen. The opposite of skin tightness is skin laxity, as is seen in both intrinsic and extrinsic aging. Inherent skin laxity (with advancing age) is accelerated with chronic photodamage. Laxity can be reversed and tightness restored through the regeneration of new elastin and collagen, which is induced by certain tightening procedures. Referring to certain procedures as "tightening" procedures originated from the observation that patients who underwent a ZO Controlled Depth Peel with TCA, which was allowed to penetrate to at least the level of the PD, had reduced skin laxity and increased skin tightness. Specifically, skin tightening occurs from procedures that penetrate to the level of the PD, the IRD, or occasionally even the URD. These procedures are ideal for epidermal and dermal stretchable wrinkles, scars, large pores, sun damage, and dermal melasma.

CHARACTERISTICS OF TIGHTENING PROCEDURES

Tightening procedures are minimally invasive procedures that heal quickly (7 to 10 days) with almost no potential for hypopigmentation or scarring, assuming they are performed by well-trained individuals who follow patients closely during the healing process. After tightening procedures, most of the adnexal structures in the treatment field remain intact, and deep irregularities in skin texture (areas of rolling and boxcar acne scarring) are not significantly affected. These procedures can be performed on all skin types and on facial as well as nonfacial skin. Of note, in areas of nonfacial skin with a lower concentration of adnexal structures, such as the neck and upper chest, special care should be taken to avoid penetration below the level of the PD because these areas are more prone to scarring if they are treated too aggressively.

In general, the ideal candidate for a tightening procedure, such as the ZO Controlled Depth Peel, is someone with fine to medium stretchable wrinkles or scars with or without concurrent signs of photodamage (telangiectasias and/or diffuse poikiloderma). For a greater tightening effect, more than one peel can be performed, ideally spaced at least 6 to 8 weeks apart for peels penetrating to the PD and 8 to 12 weeks apart for peels penetrating to the level of the IRD. More than one ZO Controlled Depth Peel procedure (usually two to three treatments) is often necessary to achieve optimal tightening and cosmesis in thick skin. Figure 5.15 shows a patient who had Skin Health Restoration followed by a ZO Controlled Depth Peel for tightening.

Combining Procedures

Immediately following application of the ZO Controlled Depth Peel to the PD or IRD, a CO_2 fractional laser procedure can be performed to the level of the URD in areas of unstretchable wrinkles or scars during the same procedural

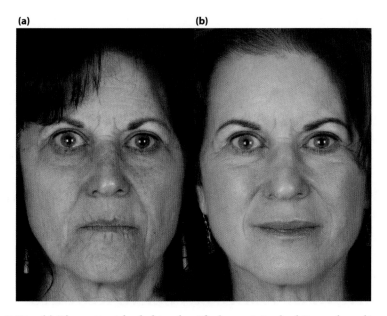

FIGURE 5.15   (a) The patient had skin classified as original white and medium thickness. She was diagnosed as having photodamage, early solar elastosis, wrinkles, and discoloration. (b) One year later. The patient underwent aggressive HQ-based Skin Health Restoration for 6 weeks, followed by a ZO Designed Controlled Depth Peel to the papillary dermis and immediate reticular dermis, as well as to the upper reticular dermis periorally. Skin Health Restoration was continued for 12 weeks following the peel.

visit. However, combined procedures should only be considered by those highly trained in chemical peels and lasers because they are more invasive and have more potential for complications.

LEVELING PROCEDURES

Leveling procedures are intended to smooth out skin surface textural irregularities, as is seen in patients with deep static rhytides who respond negatively to Dr. Zein Obagi Skin Stretch Test. Chemical peels that penetrate to the level of the IRD can produce mild leveling (smoothing out or correction of the texture), but optimal results are achieved following procedures that penetrate deeper, to the level of the URD (e.g., CO_2 fractional laser treatment). However, because no reliable depth signs (see Chapter 10) are available for monitoring the safety and efficacy of leveling procedures that penetrate below the depth of the IRD, a safe and effective outcome depends on the skill and experience of the physician. The deeper the leveling, the more injury is inflicted on the skin, including destruction of adnexal structures, which house the stem cells that allow re-epithelialization during the healing process.

PENETRATION ISSUES

Allowing a leveling procedure to penetrate too deeply can result in permanent skin thinning, dyschromia (including areas of depigmentation), demarcation lines, and scarring (atrophic, hypertrophic, and keloidal). Furthermore, *even greater caution* should be used when treating patients with skin that is dark or of the deviated color type because these patients have an increased chance of developing *permanent* post-procedural dyschromia.

If a scar or wrinkle does not improve during Dr. Zein Obagi Skin Stretch Test, it most likely extends to below the level of the IRD. Thus, as opposed to conditions that do improve with this stretch test and are best treated with tightening procedures, those that do not improve are best treated with procedures that are capable of penetrating to the depth of the URD, and thus provide effective leveling. These include CO_2 fractional laser procedures and certain chemical peels (e.g., the ZO Controlled Depth Peel). Figure 5.16 and Figure 5.17 show patients who had a ZO Designed Controlled Depth Peel for leveling.

OBTAINING OPTIMAL LEVELING RESULTS

Factors associated with leveling procedures, including selection of the most suitable, specific leveling procedure, as well as the determination of the optimal depth of penetration (taking into account skin color, thickness, propensity toward abnormal healing and scarring, and other characteristics), make it difficult to formulate a cookie-cutter approach to routinely

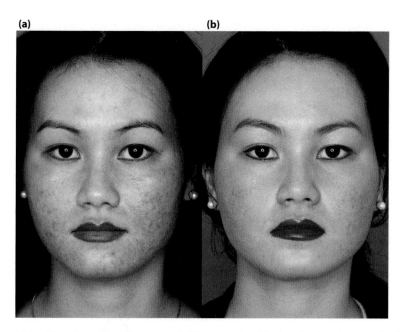

FIGURE 5.16 (a) Before. The patient had skin type classified as deviated Asian (light) and thick. She was diagnosed as having stretchable and unstretchable acne scars. (b) One year later. The patient had 6 weeks of aggressive HQ-based Skin Health Restoration and then underwent a ZO Designed Controlled Depth Peel to the papillary dermis and immediate reticular dermis, as well as to the upper reticular dermis in areas with unstretchable scars on the cheeks. She was then treated for 3 months with a Skin Health Restoration program and used isotretinoin, 20 mg/day.

obtain optimal results. First and foremost, physicians should attempt to master a leveling procedure that they can best control. As noted elsewhere in this chapter, for patients with thin skin, the maximum safe penetration depth is the IRD. However, for patients with very thin skin, the procedure should not extend deeper than the PD. Furthermore, patients with a history

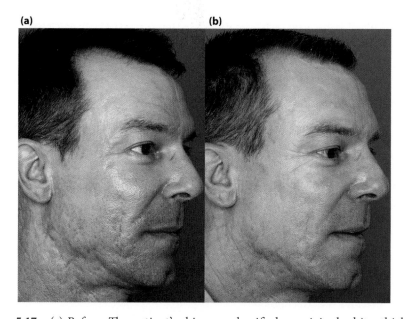

FIGURE 5.17 (a) Before. The patient's skin was classified as original white, thick, and oily. He was diagnosed as having acne scars (severe atrophic, fibrotic, and rolling). (b) One year later. The scars on the patient's cheeks and jaw line were treated with subscissions using a 21-gauge needle, 1 month apart, while he was being treated with HQ-based Skin Health Restoration. Six weeks later, he underwent a medium-depth ZO Designed Controlled Depth Peel, followed by HQ-based Skin Health Restoration for 3 months.

of keloid formation or other signs of poor or impaired healing, as can be revealed by the presence of hypertrophic or keloidal scars, as well as atrophic scars elsewhere on their body, should not undergo procedures that exceed the level of the PD.

Leveling procedures that reach the URD or the mid-dermis (phenol peels and dermabrasion) alter skin texture permanently and are associated with a higher rate of complications. They cannot be repeated safely in every skin type. In general, as a leveling modality, the CO_2 fractional laser is an easily learned and controlled procedure that is ideal for this purpose. It is too risky, however, on thin skin, and the ZO Controlled Depth Peel to the PD or IRD is the preferred modality for treating patients with thin skin.

In general, tightening procedures are ideal for patients with all skin types. Patients with concurrent muscle and skin laxity may be best suited for a treatment plan that includes surgical correction, such as a facelift, combined with a tightening procedure to address skin laxity. As mentioned previously, these can be performed at the same time. Leveling procedures are best for thick and medium-thick skin and should be limited to areas that require depth to the URD. Of note, compared with tightening procedures, which typically have a healing time of 8 to 10 days, leveling procedures are associated with a longer healing time (typically 10 to 12 days). Furthermore, recovery time (resolution of diffuse erythema and blotchiness) is approximately 4 to 6 weeks longer after leveling procedures compared with

TABLE 5.4   Tightening or Leveling Procedures: Summary

Procedure Type	Comment
Tightening	Ideal for thin skin, epidermal and dermal stretchable rhytides, scars, large pores, sun damage, dermal melasma
	Can be achieved by procedures that penetrate to the level of the papillary dermis (PD) or immediate reticular dermis (IRD), such as the ZO Controlled Depth Peel
	Nonablative lasers or other energy-emitting devices (e.g., radiofrequency or ultrasound) can be used, but results are generally suboptimal and inconsistent
	Does not correct deep irregularities in skin texture
	Can be performed on nonfacial skin (only to the PD level)
	More than one procedure can be performed
	Can be combined with a CO_2 fractional laser procedure for nonstretchable scars
	Healing time of 8 to 10 days
Leveling	Ideal for patients with deep static rhytides and nonstretchable scars
	Can be achieved by procedures that penetrate to the upper reticular dermis (URD) by means of the ZO Controlled Depth Peel
	Can be achieved with CO_2 fractional laser treatment
	Can be achieved by a combination of the ZO Controlled Depth Peel and the CO_2 fractional laser procedure
	Cannot be repeated safely (with a few exceptions)
	Alter skin texture permanently and are associated with a higher rate of complications
	Healing time of 10 to 12 days
	Leveling procedures should be attempted only after the physician has mastered the technique

TABLE 5.5 Complications Correlated with Procedure Action and Depth

Mechanism of Action	Depth of Penetration	Likelihood of PIH	Likelihood of Scarring	Likelihood of Persistent Erythema, Sensitivity, Disease Flare-Ups
Exfoliation	Epidermis	Very rare	None	None
Tightening	PD or IRD	Common	Possible	Rare
Leveling	URD	Common	Possible	Common

tightening procedures. A summary of tightening and leveling procedures is shown in Table 5.4.

Leveling Procedures and Procedure Depth

Selecting a procedure based on its mechanism of action—for example, leveling versus tightening—ensures that the procedure penetrates to the depth necessary to improve the patient's specific conditions, while avoiding unnecessary depths that can reduce adnexal structures, melanocytes, and fibroblasts and possibly cause postoperative complications. As mentioned elsewhere, the patient's skin type (see Chapter 4) is also important in determining the optimal depth of penetration for a specific procedure because certain skin types necessitate depth limitations. Examples include thinner versus thicker skin, original color versus deviated color, and so forth. Reactions and complications as correlated to procedural depth are shown in Table 5.5.

COMBINATION APPROACHES TO SKIN REJUVENATION

Combining two or more procedures with different mechanisms of action can maximize ultimate results, minimize invasiveness, and optimize safety. A combination of procedures is recommended to avoid unnecessary depth in areas where there might be higher risk for textural changes or other complications. Using multiple procedures can also maximize results as each procedure approaches the problems in a different way. To further clarify, following a leveling procedure, the skin has fewer adnexal structures and melanocytes and is typically permanently thinner. These changes make it more difficult for a physician to perform a second leveling procedure safely, especially in patients with initially thinner skin. For that reason, a combined tightening and leveling procedure is the safest approach and allows these procedures to be repeated, if necessary.

Possible combinations of procedures for optimal skin rejuvenation are shown in Table 5.6. Figure 5.18 and Figure 5.19 show patients who underwent a ZO Controlled Depth Peel followed by CO_2 fractional laser treatment. Figure 5.20 shows a patient who underwent hyfrecation of the dermatosis

TABLE 5.6 Combination Procedures for Skin Rejuvenation

Procedures	Example	Comment
A tightening procedure to the papillary dermis (PD) to tighten skin and correct stretchable scars and wrinkles combined with a leveling procedure to the URD in areas where such depth is needed	A ZO Controlled Depth Peel to the PD and immediate reticular dermis (IRD) on the entire face, followed immediately by the CO_2 fractional laser to the URD in certain areas	This combination provides better results than either procedure alone. It increases safety because it avoids penetrating to unnecessarily deep levels (e.g., the upper reticular dermis [URD]) to achieve the desired tightness while limiting the depth only to areas where leveling is desired
A surgical procedure to remove excessive skin and/or muscle combined with a nonsurgical skin tightening procedure to the entire face	A facelift followed by a ZO Controlled Depth Peel to the PD or IRD on the entire face	The tightening from the facelift is heightened by additional tightening from the peel.
A tightening procedure combined with neurotoxin injections	A ZO Controlled Depth Peel performed *after* Botox/Dysport/Xeomin	This combination maximizes the tightening results from a peel.
		Neurotoxin immobilizes the muscles of expression and allows maximal tightening of skin in the forehead, glabella, and around the eyes.
		For optimal results, injection of the neurotoxin should be performed at least 1 week before the tightening procedure to achieve maximal muscle relaxation and optimize skin surface area treated with the tightening procedure (e.g., ZO Controlled Depth Peel).
A vascular or pigment laser treatment combined with a ZO Controlled Depth Peel to the PD	Pulse dye laser (FLPD), KTP, or other laser that selectively targets vasculature *or* QS-alexandrite, QS-ruby, or other laser that selectively targets excessive brown pigment—to individual lesions—followed by a ZO Controlled Depth Peel to the entire face or other full treatment area	This combination simultaneously improves skin texture, restores even color tone (e.g., in those with dermal melanosis, nevi of Ito/Ota/Huri, or tattoos), and corrects stretchable wrinkles and scars.
		This combination is performed in two steps: first the vascular or pigment laser is used to treat vascular or pigmentary lesions, respectively. An endpoint of bruising of nonstretchable scars is typically used when the FLPD is chosen as the vascular laser treatment modality. This is followed by a ZO Controlled Depth Peel to the PD or IRD.
Electrodessication and gentle hyfrecation combined with a ZO Controlled Depth Peel to the PD or IRD		Dermatosis papulosa nigra, condyloma accuminata, syringomas, and actinic keratoses are first treated by electrodessication and immediately followed by a ZO Controlled Depth Peel to the PD or IRD.

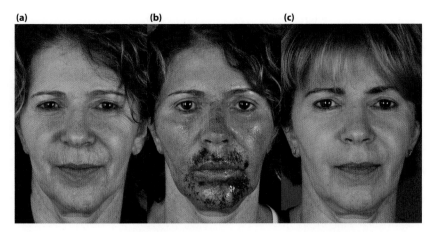

Figure 5.18 (a) Before. The patient had skin classified as original white (normal), medium thick, and not oily. She was diagnosed as having skin laxity and stretchable and unstretchable rhytides around the mouth. (b) The patient was treated for 6 weeks with HQ-based ZOMD treatment, followed by a ZO Controlled Depth Peel to the immediate reticular dermis. This was immediately followed by perioral CO_2 fractional laser during the same treatment session (a combined approach). The patient then continued the ZOMD HQ-based program for 3 months. (c) Six months later.

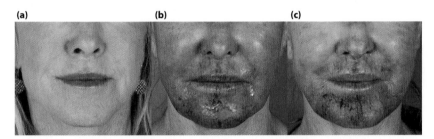

Figure 5.19 (a) Before. The patient had skin classified as white (light), medium thick, and nonoily. She was diagnosed as having laxity and rhytides (stretchable on cheeks, nonstretchable in the perioral area). (b) After 6 weeks of non-HQ-based Skin Health Restoration treatment, she underwent a ZO Controlled Depth Peel to the immediate reticular dermis followed by CO_2 fractional laser treatment in the perioral area. (c) Six days after the combined procedures.

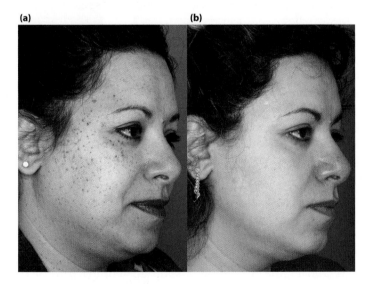

Figure 5.20 (a) Before. The patient had skin classified as deviated white (medium), thick, and oily. She was diagnosed as having dermatosis papulosa nigra (DPN). (b) One year later. After 6 weeks of treatment with HQ-based Skin Health Restoration, she underwent hyfrecation of the DPN and had a ZO Controlled Depth Peel to the papillary dermis at the same surgical session. This was followed by 3 months of HQ-based Skin Health Restoration.

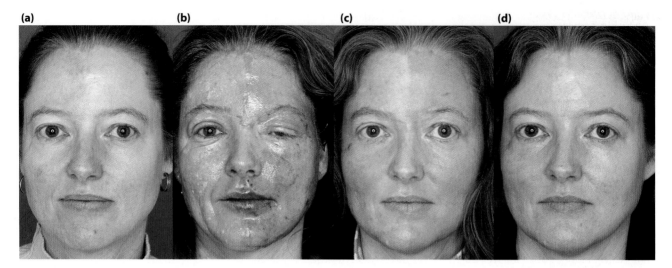

FIGURE 5.21   (a) Before. The patient had skin classified as light white, medium thick, and oily. She was diagnosed as having laxity and wrinkles. (b) The right side of the patient's face was treated with a ZO Controlled Depth Peel and the left side with CO_2 fractional laser. (c) One month after the procedures. Notice greater tightness and less erythema on the peel side compared with the laser-treat left side. (d) Three months later. The patient is being treated with non-HQ-based Skin Health Restoration.

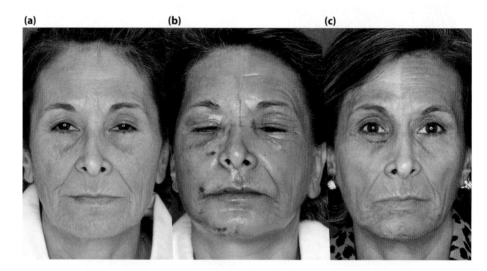

FIGURE 5.22   (a) Before. The patient had skin classified as deviated white, medium thick, and normal oiliness. She was diagnosed as having rhytides and laxity. (b) Immediately postoperatively. The patient was treated with 6 weeks of HQ-based Skin Health Restoration, followed by CO_2 fractional laser treatment on the right side of her face and a ZO Controlled Depth Peel to the immediate reticular dermis on the left side of her face. The purpose was to compare the tightening effects produced individually by the two different procedures. (c) Four months after the procedure. Notice that a greater tightening effect was achieved on the patient's left side (the ZO Controlled Depth Peel side).

papulosa nigra followed by a ZO Controlled Depth Peel during the same treatment session.

Figure 5.21 and Figure 5.22 show a split-face comparison of the tightening effects obtained with CO_2 fractional laser resurfacing and with a ZO Controlled Depth Peel. Figure 5.23 shows the steps of a combination of a ZO Controlled Depth Peel and an ablative CO_2 fractional laser treatment.

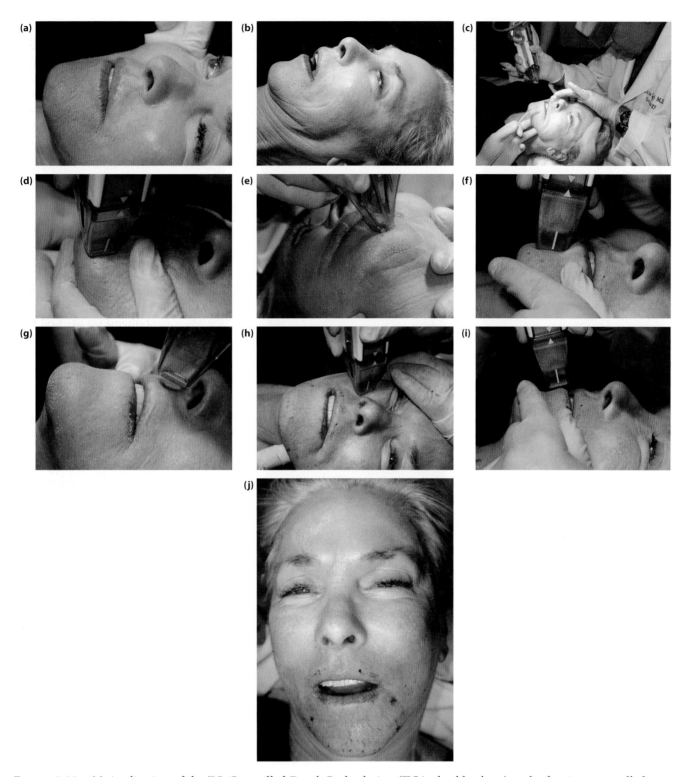

Figure 5.23 (a) Application of the ZO Controlled Depth Peel solution (TCA plus blue base) to the face in a controlled, even fashion. (b) Characteristic endpoints specific to a successfully completed ZO Controlled Depth Peel to the immediate reticular dermis on the face (with the exception of the eyelids, which were treated to the papillary dermis). Notice the confluent, white, sheet-like frost without an underlying pink background on the face (with the exception of the upper and lower eyelids). (c, d) Immediately following completion of the ZO Controlled Depth Peel, the patient is treated with the CO_2 fractional laser. In this patient, the perioral areas are being treated with this combined method to target the unstretchable wrinkles, which are due to long-standing solar elastosis. (e, f, g) Notice the irregular texture of the damaged skin on the chin (a combination of sebaceous gland hyperplasia and solar elastosis). (h, i) The endpoints of this combined treatment approach: pinpoint bleeding to total effacement of surface wrinkles/textural irregularities. Feathering of the surrounding areas, including the border of the mandibular line and the upper neck, is performed through lower laser energy and density. (j) The appearance of the face, immediately following the combined approach (both procedures).

135

REFERENCES

1. Moran ML. Office-based periorbital rejuvenation. *Facial Plast Surg.* 2013;29:58-63.

2. Mangat DS, Tansavatdi K, Garlich P. Current chemical peels and other resurfacing techniques. *Facial Plast Surg.* 2011;27:3-49.

3. Goldman A, Wollina U. Facial rejuvenation for middle-aged women: a combined approach with minimally invasive procedures. *Clin Interv Aging.* 2010;23;5:293-299.

4. Kumari R, Thappa DM. Comparative study of trichloroacetic acid versus glycolic acid chemical peels in the treatment of melasma. *Indian J Dermatol Venereol Leprol.* 2010;76:447.

5. Wollina U, Payne CR. Aging well—the role of minimally invasive aesthetic dermatological procedures in women over 65. *J Cosmet Dermatol.* 2010;9:50-58.

6. Rullan P, Karam AM. Chemical peels for darker skin types. *Facial Plast Surg Clin North Am.* 2010;18:111-131.

7. Fabbrocini G, De Padova MP, Tosti A. Chemical peels: what's new and what isn't new but still works well. *Facial Plast Surg.* 2009;25:329-336.

8. Berson DS, Cohen JL, Rendon MI, et al. Clinical role and application of superficial chemical peels in today's practice. *J Drugs Dermatol.* 2009;8:803-811.

9. Hirsch R, Stier M. Complications and their management in cosmetic dermatology. *Dermatol Clin.* 2009;27:505-520.

10. Ho SG, Chan HH. The Asian dermatologic patient: review of common pigmentary disorders and cutaneous diseases. *Am J Clin Dermatol.* 2009;10:153-168.

11. Fitzgerald R, Graivier MH, Kane M, et al. Appropriate selection and application of nonsurgical facial rejuvenation agents and procedures: panel consensus recommendations. *Aesthet Surg J.* 2010;30(Suppl):36S-45S.

SEBUM-INDUCED INFLAMMATORY DISORDERS AND TREATMENTS

This chapter will address a variety of skin problems without systemic involvement that are seen daily in our clinics. These conditions are grouped into categories, based on the causative factors, their depth of involvement (epidermal or dermal), and their clinical manifestations (Box 6.1). Treatment approaches for each of the various conditions within a specific category are similar. Throughout this chapter, these topics will be addressed in a way that serves dermatologists, plastic surgeons, and other professionals interested in treating specific skin disorders, while also maintaining focus on Skin Health Restoration.

ACNE AND ITS CAUSES

Acne is a common skin disorder that arises from pilosebaceous unit dysfunction, which consists of a hair follicle and its associated sebaceous gland. Acne affects approximately 85% of individuals between the ages of 12 to 24 years. Typically, it first manifests at puberty, when increasing androgen levels activate the sebaceous glands, which begin producing sebum. As androgen levels continue to rise, sebaceous glands become hypertrophic, and the amount of sebum greatly increases. Sebum is a powerful inflammatory agent that leads to the more severe forms of acne and scarring when produced in excess. Sebum also disturbs the maturation of keratinocytes (dyskeratosis) by inducing epidermal inflammation. These two factors—increased sebum production and the dyskeratotic keratinocytes—cause occlusion of pores and the subsequent appearance of whiteheads. When the trapped material in the pores oxidizes and turns dark, whiteheads appear as blackheads. Blackheads are commonly seen in areas with enlarged pores, such as the nose. The immune system's response to the excessive sebum on the skin surface, together with the trapped sebum in the hair follicle and the bacterial flora (*Propionibacterium acnes*), leads to the appearance of inflammatory cystic lesions that involve the dermis

---

Box 6.1

Etiologic Categories of Skin Problems Addressed

- Sebum-induced pilosebaceous unit abnormalities
- Melanocytic dysfunction (pigmentary disorders)
- Textural (photodamage, extrinsic aging, and scars)

---

and lead to acne scars. The severity of inflammation leads to the spread of acne lesions and the formation of pustules, inflammatory nodules, and more cysts.

Inflammation induced by the presence of increased sebum and *P. acnes* leads to variable degrees of scarring and postinflammatory hyperpigmentation (PIH) in certain patients. Over time, the chronic inflammation with its destructive effects damages skin texture, producing rolling, boxcar, and ice-pick scarring. Occasionally, hypertrophic scars and keloids can appear in predisposed individuals with severe acne. Factors contributing to acne development and severity are shown in Box 6.2. The chronological changes in acne are shown in Table 6.1.

Box 6.2

Factors Contributing to Acne Development and Severity

- Heredity: the size, number or density, sensitivity, and activity level of sebaceous glands
- Disorders of keratinization, in which corneocytes are not shed at an adequate rate. This can cause occlusion of pores and microcomedone formation.
- Lifestyle, including exposure to:
  - Practices that increase sebum production (e.g., hot showers or baths, saunas or steam rooms, and sweating from physical exertion or warm climates)
  - Dietary factors (nonorganic dairy products from cows that have been given hormones, a diet with a high glycemic index [which induces inflammation], and stimulants, such as caffeine)
  - Inappropriate skin care products (moisturizers, which weaken skin, and oil-based makeup)
- Hormonal factors: systemic hormonal abnormalities (e.g., polycystic ovarian syndrome and other conditions associated with excessive androgens). Additionally, hormonal changes before and during a woman's monthly menses, as well as those that occur during pregnancy, may cause acne to develop or flare.
- Patient manipulation of acne lesions: attempts to squeeze or extract whiteheads or cysts can increase lesion depth, inflammation, and the immune response, creating more aggravated acne flare and increasing the potential for postinflammatory hyperpigmentation.

TABLE 6.1   Chronological Changes in Acne

Features	Stage of Life		
	Adolescence	*Adulthood*	*Elderly*
Sebaceous glands			
Size	Normal or large	Larger (rosacea)	Smaller
Activity	Active	Active or very active	Less active
Skin oiliness	Normal or oily	Normal or oily	Normal or dry
Acne	None or all types may be present	None or all types and rosacea	None or mild
Inflammation	None to strong	Strong or very strong	Little to none
Acne course	Continuous*	Continuous	Diminished

*Acne that persists into adulthood converts to rosacea.

APPROACH TO TREATING ACNE

The range of topical and oral acne treatment options currently on the market is so broad that it may seem limitless. Similarly, recommendations on how to use specific products (alone or in combination) are numerous. The approach presented here is based on several fundamental beliefs that may contradict what many physicians accept as standard in acne treatment. One such belief, which lays the foundation for the treatment protocols in this chapter, is that acne is preventable. Patients with various types of acne and their treatment are shown in Figures 6.1 to 6.7.

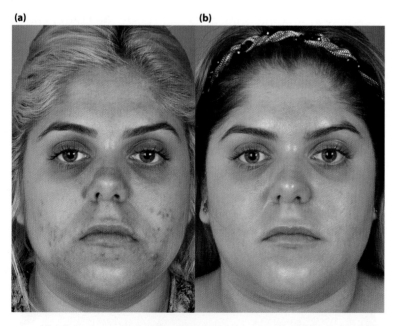

FIGURE 6.1   (a) The patient had skin classified as original white, thick, and oily. She was diagnosed as having cystic acne and postinflammatory hyperpigmentation. (b) Six months later. The patient had aggressive HQ-based Skin Health Restoration and applied benzoyl peroxide and used isotretinoin, 20 mg/day, simultaneously with topical treatment for 5 months. She also underwent two ZO 3-Step Peel treatments (an exfoliation and stimulation procedure).

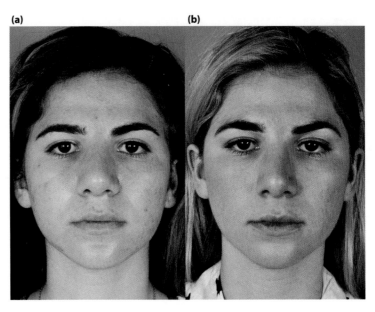

FIGURE 6.2 (a) The patient had skin classified as deviated white (light), oily, with large pores. She was diagnosed as having cystic acne. (b) Six months later. The patient underwent 5 months of HQ-based Skin Health Restoration (to provide exfoliation, stimulation blending, and epidermal melanocyte stabilization) and acne treatment (with benzoyl peroxide). She used isotretinoin, 20 mg/day, simultaneously with topical treatments. After 5 months of treatment, she began a maintenance program.

ACNE PREVENTION

Acne is preventable only if addressed at the initial stages, when whiteheads and blackheads begin to appear, but before sebum-induced inflammation can trigger the immune response. Every effort should be made to eliminate whiteheads and blackheads in the early, noninflammatory acne lesions stage. They can be extracted with a comedone extractor, which applies equal pressure circumferentially around the comedone and causes the sebum and follicular

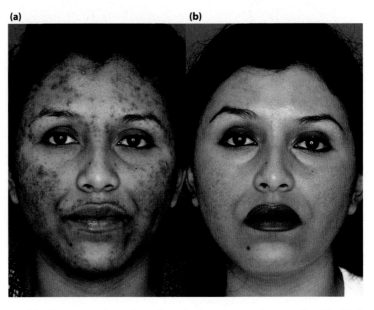

FIGURE 6.3 (a) The patient had skin classified as deviated white (dark), thick, and oily. She was diagnosed as having cystic acne, postinflammatory hyperpigmentation, and acne scars. Before her visit, she had been treated by another physician with isotretinoin, 60 mg/day, for 5 months but was not prescribed any topical treatment.

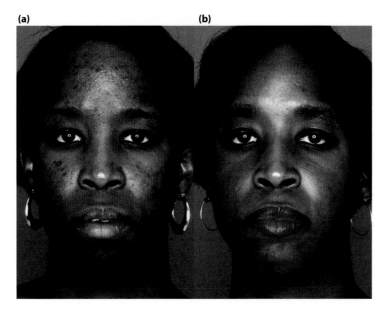

FIGURE 6.4 (a) The patient had skin classified as black (medium), medium thickness, and oily. She was diagnosed as having cystic acne, postinflammatory hyperpigmentation, and acne scars. She had been treated only with isotretinoin and moisturizers at another clinic. (b) Six months later. The patient was treated with HQ-based Skin Health Restoration to provide correction, stabilization, and stimulation.

debris to be expelled outward. Manual picking should be avoided because it can push the sebum and follicular debris deeper and induce inflammation and cyst formation. Use of a good acne preventive program, consisting of cleanser, scrub, and a sebum-reducing agent, can help eliminate whiteheads and blackheads in an early stage (Table 6.2). If, however, some inflammatory acneiform cysts appear, intralesional steroid injections (triamcinolone acetonide, diluted

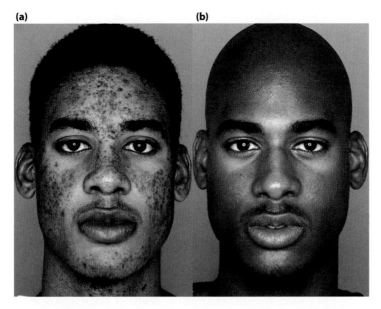

FIGURE 6.5 (a) The patient had skin classified as deviated black (light), medium thick, and oily. He was diagnosed as having cystic acne, postinflammatory hyperpigmentation, and acne scars. (b) Six months later. The patient was treated with non-HQ-based Skin Health Restoration for melanocyte stabilization and stimulation. He was also treated with isotretinoin, 20 mg/day, and underwent one ZO Controlled Depth Peel to the papillary dermis. Notice the restoration of natural skin color tone.

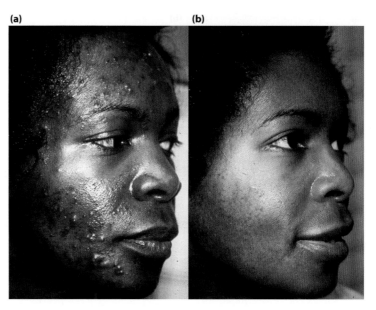

FIGURE 6.6   (a) The patient had skin classified as medium black, thick, and oily. She was diagnosed as having active cystic acne and postinflammatory hyperpigmentation. (b) Five months later. The patient followed an aggressive HQ-based Skin Health Restoration program. On week 6, she had a ZO Controlled Depth Peel to the papillary dermis. After healing, she restarted the same Skin Health Restoration regimen as before and began using isotretinoin, 20 mg/day, for 5 months.

to a concentration of 2.5 mg/mL) should be used to prevent or arrest the focal inflammation early.

Moreover, *P. acnes* does not directly cause acne. Rather, these bacteria play a secondary role in the condition. The complete pathophysiology of acne has not yet been elucidated, and the etiology appears to be multifactorial. Focusing on

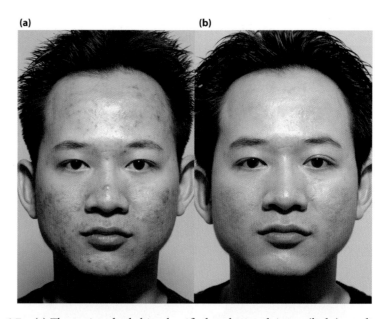

FIGURE 6.7   (a) The patient had skin classified as deviated Asian (light), medium thickness, and very oily. He was diagnosed as having cystic acne, acne scars, and postinflammatory hyperpigmentation. Treatment with antibiotics and acne topical treatments by other physicians had failed to improve his condition. (b) Five months later. The patient had HQ-based Skin Health Restoration to provide exfoliation, stimulation and blending (tretinoin plus HQ), and epidermal melanocyte stabilization. He also used topical benzoyl peroxide and isotretinoin, 20 mg/day.

TABLE 6.2   Acne Prevention Steps and Products

Steps	Products
Skin Preparation	
Cleansing	Oily skin cleanser, AM and PM
Scrub	Nonirritating Ossential Exfoliating Polish once daily
Sebum reduction	Offects TE-Pads (sebum-reducing agent), AM and PM
Stabilization and correction	
Alpha-hydroxy acids (AHAs) for exfoliation	Glycogent (topical exfoliator), AM
Acne-specific topical agents	Alternate AHAs with acne-specific topical agents, such as Aknetrol (benzoyl peroxide), every 4-5 months to prevent bacterial resistance
Barrier repair and stabilizing agents	Ossential Daily Power Defense (combination of retinol, antioxidants, and anti-inflammatory agents)
Lifestyle Changes	
Modify lifestyle factors to prevent increased sebum production	Never use moisturizers, even the noncomedogenic variety, or heavy foundation. Both can alter skin barrier function and increase skin irritability, which can lead to inflammation and cystic acne

bacteria does not address the pathogenesis of the condition and, in practice, leads to high rates of reoccurrence and treatment failure. In actuality, sebum and the resulting inflammation are the main problems in acne, and the control of sebum may be the key to acne prevention and treatment.

ACNE TREATMENT STRATEGY

Acne treatment should represent only a portion of the broader approach that aims to restore general skin health. Healthy skin is less susceptible to acne. Accordingly, the treatment objective should be not only to temporarily slow down sebaceous gland activity and dry up the pimples but also to restore skin health while correcting all of the contributing factors responsible for causing acne at the same time.

The patient's first consultation is especially important. It should provide the patient (and physician) with an idea of what's going on medically and what treatment options are available. This sets the stage for the formulation of both a long- and short-term treatment strategy. As such, the first consultation should include a thorough patient history and a physical examination. If an underlying systemic hormonal abnormality is suspected as contributing to the patient's acne, the patient should have appropriate blood tests ordered during the visit; a consult with an endocrinologist may also be appropriate in this setting. In female teenagers, it appears that certain birth control pills can help tremendously to regulate hormonal factors that play a major role in their acne condition. Such pills include drosperinone (Yaz), which counteracts the androgens that drive sebum production. Additionally, other agents such as spironolactone or insulin resistance agents (e.g., metformin) can be used. The physician must also determine whether a systemic antibiotic or isotretinoin is indicated. In short, the physician must determine the acne type (comedogenic [cystic and nonscarring] or severe [cystic and scarring]) and, based on the type, inform the patient (Box 6.3) and discuss treatment options. Patient

> **Box 6.3**
>
> **Patient Education**
>
> Necessary discussion points with the acne patient include the following:
>
> - Causative factors (etiology)
> - Treatment course and expected duration, including the products "essential" for treatment
> - Anticipated reactions, which usually include initial irritation, dryness, and flaking or peeling of skin caused by topical medications
> - Patient responsibilities during treatment, which include strict adherence to the treatment program and ability to return for regular follow-up visits

compliance with a daily treatment regimen is essential, and drawing pictures for patients while explaining their condition is helpful.

The topical approach to treating acne, while at the same time improving overall skin health, includes the following: skin preparation, addition of disease-specific agents (if indicated), exfoliation and stimulation of epidermal renewal, barrier repair, stimulation of the dermis (for deep repair), hydration and calming (only if needed for skin dryness), and sun protection (Box 6.4).

Treatment should begin with appropriate topical agents; systemic agents can be added when needed. Procedures such as exfoliative peels and photodynamic

> **Box 6.4**
>
> **Skin Health Restoration and Treatment in Acne Patients**
>
> 1. Skin preparation:
>   - Washing face twice daily with a cleanser specifically formulated for oily skin
>   - Mechanical exfoliation
>   - Application of a sebum-reducing astringent
> 2. Addition of disease-specific agents
>   - Examples include topical benzoyl peroxide, antibiotics, dapsone, adapalene, tazarotene
> 3. Epidermal renewal—alternate daily with the disease-specific agents
>   - Exfoliation: all patients should use topical alpha-hydroxy acids
>   - Postinflammatory hyperpigmentation, if present: hydroquinone (HQ) or non-HQ agents can be added
> 4. Barrier repair agents (for epidermal stabilization), AM
> 5. Stimulation of the skin (for deep repair), PM
>   - Tretinoin (retinoic acid) or tretinoin plus HQ (blending)
> 6. Hydration and calming of the skin (as needed, to reduce reactions and improve compliance) (optional)
> 7. Protection of the skin—sunscreen daily, nonoily makeup

therapy (PDT), with blue or red light, can be used to assist treatment, but never as the first line of treatment. For example, if PDT is going to be used, one should start with all essential and supportive topical agents (see Chapter 3). When the acne is somewhat controlled and the skin is more tolerant (e.g., after at least 6 weeks on a topical regimen containing essential topical agents), PDT sessions can be added to the overall treatment plan to accelerate and improve results. The topical photosensitizing agent applied before PDT treatment collects preferentially in sebaceous glands, and the subsequent exposure to light of the appropriate wavelength destroys those glands.

Immediate Interventions during Initial Visits

Along with the discussion and planning that occurs at a patient's first visit, the physician can take certain steps to resolve some of the patient's most pressing acne issues during that same visit. These include extraction of comedones, intralesional steroid injection into inflammatory acneiform nodules, and initiation of a short course of oral steroids (Box 6.5). Furthermore, to help unclog pores and dry cystic lesions faster, physicians can use exfoliative procedures or products, including alpha-hydroxy acids (AHAs), beta-hydroxy acids (BHAs), or exfoliative chemical peels (Invisapeel, Non-irritating Ossential Exfoliating Polish once daily, Ossential Advanced Radical Night Repair, ZO 3-Step Peel) after the first maturation cycle of treatment (6 weeks) has been completed.

The Skin Health Restoration program for the acne patient is shown in Box 6.6, and the treatment duration and phases are shown in Box 6.7.

Dr. Zein Obagi's Revised Acne Classification

Current acne classifications (mild, recalcitrant, severe; comedogenic, cystic adult acne—conglobata, necrotica, keloidae) are merely descriptive terms that

---

Box 6.5

Early Acne Interventions (during Initial Visits)

- Extraction of individual comedones
- Injection of active inflammatory acneiform nodules and cysts (to stop inflammation and prevent scarring)
- Initiation of a 1-week course of oral systemic steroids (if not contraindicated) in patients with severe cystic acne that involves the face, back, or chest
- Methylprednisolone in tapered doses (60-50-40-30-20-10-5 mg/day), which can be helpful in severe cases
- If needed to arrest inflammation (while the patient is also starting on oral isotretinoin): repeated additional courses of oral systemic steroids (1 week per month for two to three courses) until isotretinoin benefits become apparent
- If systemic steroids are contraindicated, an alternate anti-inflammatory agent, such as 200 mg ibuprofen daily for 10 days, repeated once a month during the first three keratin maturation cycles (18 weeks) of treatment

---

Box 6.6

Skin Health Restoration Program for the Acne Patient

- Preparation of the skin with oily skin cleanser, mechanical exfoliation, and a sebum-reducing astringent
- Addition of a disease-specific agent or agents, such as topical benzoyl peroxide, antibiotic, dapsone, adapalene, or tazarotene, AM
- Epidermal renewal: alternated daily with the disease-specific agents
  - Exfoliation: topical alpha-hydroxy acids in all patients
  - Postinflammatory hyperpigmentation (if present): addition of hydroquinone (HQ) or non-HQ agents
- Barrier repair agents, AM
- Stimulation of the skin (for deep repair), PM
- Tretinoin (retinoic acid) or tretinoin + HQ (blending)
- Hydration and calming of the skin (as needed, to reduce reactions and improve compliance) (optional)
- Protection of the skin: sunscreen daily, nonoily makeup (optional)

---

do little more than confuse physicians and patients. Instead, the following suggested classification (Table 6.3) provides more clear objectives and frees physicians from the restrictions that conventional wisdom imposes on proper treatment choice.

SYSTEMIC TREATMENTS FOR ACNE

At the first visit, when discussing and formulating the treatment plan, physicians should inform patients that more severe cases of acne and those cases that are not responding to topical treatment may require concomitant

---

Box 6.7

Treatment Duration and Phases in Acne Treatment

Treatment duration: three keratinocyte maturation cycles (KMCs), which are 6 weeks each (18 weeks total), in which each cycle represents a treatment phase. These include the following:

1. Repair phase: *expected* skin reaction to topical medications
2. Tolerance phase: reactions begin to subside; skin improvement starts to become noticeable
3. Completion phase: minimal to no skin reactions persist, and maximal improvements are seen

Every patient should follow a maintenance program after completion of active treatment to prevent recurrence.

TABLE 6.3   Acne Classification

Type of Acne	Comment
Comedogenic	Comedones without cysts or scars: Prevention is possible and recommended.
Cystic, no scars	Acne with cysts but no visible scars
Cystic with scars	Cystic acne with visible scars

systemic treatment. Similarly, patients presenting with cystic acne and subsequent active scarring may require concurrent systemic treatments such as oral antibiotics, isotretinoin, spironolactone, or other agents.

If acne improvement after one keratin maturation cycle (KMC) (6 weeks) is minimal and new lesions continue to appear despite patient compliance with a thorough topical regimen, the physician has two options:

- Add antibiotics for 1 to 2 months (if acne scars are not present), with the plan to wean the patient off the antibiotics as soon as improvement is achieved.
- Add isotretinoin (especially if acne scarring is actively occurring).

Role of Antibiotics

Many physicians prescribe topical and/or oral antibiotics for acne, using the rationale that these agents will kill *P. acnes* and other potential strains of bacteria and reduce inflammation. However, such an approach introduces concerns that likely outweigh these treatments' merits. In particular, research shows that patients using topical or systemic antibiotics for acne should use them in pulsed fashion to reduce the potential for the development of antibiotic resistance. Specifically, after a patient has used one antibiotic agent for 2 or 3 months, he or she should be switched to another agent.

Additionally, oral antibiotics have the potential for many side effects. These include, but are not limited to, bacterial resistance, gastrointestinal upset, photosensitivity, allergic reactions (including anaphylaxis), and, rarely, severe cutaneous immune system reactions, such as Stevens-Johnson syndrome. For these reasons, the physician should limit acne treatment with systemic antibiotics to 2- to 3-month intervals and repeat only when necessary (Box 6.8). Overall, the benefits of systemic antibiotics in acne are likely overstated.

Box 6.8

Antibiotic Treatment of Acne

- Systemic antibiotics are not essential in acne treatment.
- If systemic antibiotics are used, they should be administered in 2- to 3-month "pulses," followed by rest and subsequent treatment with a different antibiotic, if necessary.
- This applies only in cases in which the acne is responding well to the systemic antibiotics and no postinflammatory scarring is appearing.

Role of Oral Isotretinoin

Isotretinoin is extremely effective in the treatment of acne because it addresses the role of sebum. Namely, isotretinoin reduces sebum production that then decreases inflammation, lowers *P. acnes* counts, and inhibits microcomedone formation. According to the U.S. Food and Drug Administration (FDA), it is indicated for patients who have severe, inflammatory, recalcitrant nodular or cystic acne.

In 2006, the FDA implemented the iPLEDGE Program, which manages potential risks of isotretinoin use by educating patients in an attempt to eliminate fetal exposures to this highly teratogenic drug. Accordingly, it cannot be given to women who are breastfeeding, pregnant, or planning a pregnancy in the upcoming 6 months or so (assuming a 5-month treatment course with isotretinoin).

Isotretinoin also has been associated with increased risk for developing or worsening depression (including suicidal ideation). The association between isotretinoin use and an increased risk for inflammatory bowel disease has not been completely elucidated, but evidence for an association does not appear to be strong. Other potential contraindications include hepatic dysfunction (isotretinoin is metabolized in the liver), severe hyperlipidemia (isotretinoin can lead to a slight elevation in cholesterol), anorexia nervosa, and osteoporosis. If isotretinoin is contraindicated or the patient declines the drug after a thorough discussion of its risks and benefits, the physician may prescribe a series of treatments with photodynamic therapy.

Guidelines Regarding Isotretinoin

During the past decade, the reputation of isotretinoin has been tarnished, particularly in the popular press, as lawsuits over potential and purported side effects have garnered headlines by targeting prescribers and manufacturers of isotretinoin. These developments have created a fear of isotretinoin that the public and many physicians now share. Many patients, even those with severe, recalcitrant, scarring acne, refuse to consider the drug because they have researched it online and have come across various sources claiming harmful effects from the medication. Also, many physicians, afraid of lawsuits and averse to the additional work required to initiate and maintain patients on isotretinoin through the FDA iPLEDGE Program, hesitate to prescribe isotretinoin.

Many of these concerns appear to be exaggerated. To date, isotretinoin has usually been prescribed for patients with severe nodulocystic acne that resists traditional treatments such as topical agents, as well as systemic antibiotics and hormonal therapies. The dosage recommended by the FDA and isotretinoin manufacturers is 0.5 to 1 mg/kg of body weight/day, taken for an average of 5 months. Our clinic has had great success using oral isotretinoin in much lower doses (i.e., 10 to 20 mg/day) for a similar total treatment duration of 5 months, while concomitantly treating the acne in an aggressive topical fashion. In contrast to our method (low-dose daily isotretinoin in combination with aggressive daily topical treatment), many doctors tell patients not to use any topical acne treatments, while treating patients with much higher doses (i.e., 60 to 80 mg/day) of isotretinoin. Instead, these patients are instructed to use moisturizers to reduce the skin dryness that invariably accompanies high-dose isotretinoin use. The latter approach suffers from the following three fundamental flaws:

1. The recommendation that physicians prescribe isotretinoin only for patients with severe acne unresponsive to traditional treatments is ambiguous and unfair to many patients who otherwise could benefit from the drug. Rather, a more flexible indication considers the following factors:
   - Acne severity
   - Presence of early acne scarring
   - Patient's psychological condition and social requirements
   - Presence of other skin diseases or abnormalities

   Following these guidelines will provide patients with a more effective, compassionate treatment plan, which prevents unnecessary long-term suffering, scarring, and complications.

2. The current recommended daily dose (0.5 to 1 mg/kg/day) is too high. Our clinic has found that the dose of isotretinoin is relatively proportional to the severity and the incidence of certain side effects, such as skin dryness, that patients experience. The FDA selected this dose to maximize the benefits of isotretinoin (shrinking sebaceous glands and reducing sebum) within 5 months. However, side effects of all systemic retinoids are similar, and most of them are dose related. Being prescribed a dose of isotretinoin that is all but guaranteed to cause severe skin and mucosal dryness and irritation has turned away many patients who could benefit from isotretinoin.

3. The trend of not prescribing topical acne therapies to patients while they are taking isotretinoin is also highly counterproductive. Using a lower daily dose allows patients to incorporate topical treatments that can restore the skin's barrier function and the integrity of the pilosebaceous units, while also addressing pigmentary changes and eliminating comedones. In our experience, lower dose systemic isotretinoin treatment in combination with more aggressive, concomitant topical acne treatment leads to longer remissions and better overall results.

Isotretinoin is a potent drug with a high potential for serious complications when used on improperly screened patients and warrants strict prescribing guidelines. However, after spending several years evaluating varying doses and monitoring recurrence rates achieved with isotretinoin monotherapy versus concomitant use of topical agents at our clinic, we now recommend the following for prescribing isotretinoin therapy:

- Use a fixed dose of 10 to 40 mg daily (most commonly 20 mg/day) taken twice a week. This is enough to reduce sebum production, arrest sebum-induced inflammation, and prevent the immune response that creates tissue destruction and scarring. In fact, the remission lengths and recurrence rates achieved by our patients are exactly the same as those achieved with high daily isotretinoin doses. Yet the lower dose creates less dryness and other systemic side effects, while also allowing patients to incorporate beneficial topical treatments. Specifically, we recommend that physicians never prescribe more than 40 mg daily and that they use topical acne treatments simultaneously.
- In teenagers, start at 10 to 20 mg of isotretinoin daily, or even every other day, along with a daily topical Skin Health Restoration regimen (correction, stimulation, and acne-specific agents).
- Continue daily systemic acne treatment with isotretinoin, in combination with topical treatments, for 5 months.

> **Box 6.9**
>
> ## Conditions Indicating Discontinuation of Isotretinoin
>
> ■ Significant elevation of cholesterol or liver enzymes
> ■ Development of colitis, depression, or any other systemic complaint

- After 5 months of treatment, do not discontinue isotretinoin abruptly. Rather, reduce dosing from daily to twice a week for 2 months after the 5-month course of daily treatment.
- After patients fully complete isotretinoin treatment (including the taper), begin a 3-month observation period. If acne flares during this time, restart isotretinoin for an additional 1 to 2 months.
- Be flexible. Monitor patients for depression (work with the patient's therapist in this regard) and evaluate for severe dryness or other side effects. If any of these side effects occur, allow the patient to reduce dosing to twice weekly, or even to temporarily stop isotretinoin and restart, as appropriate.

Isotretinoin Caveats

Whichever regimen one selects, because isotretinoin is a potent drug with the potential to cause serious side effects, physicians should follow all precautions suggested by the iPLEDGE Program. Accordingly, prescribers must administer monthly pregnancy tests for females of childbearing potential (and ensure they remain negative throughout the course of treatment), monitor patients' blood levels at baseline and during treatment if indicated, and stop isotretinoin whenever any of the conditions shown in Box 6.9 occur.

Addressing Teratogenicity

Because of public misconceptions and fears about isotretinoin, many women incorrectly believe that they should wait 1 year after stopping isotretinoin to become pregnant. However, we now know that the body does not store isotretinoin, as it does vitamin A, and that isotretinoin is not detectable in the blood within 5 to 7 days of discontinuing use. Therefore, we can tell women of childbearing potential that they can become pregnant 1 month after stopping isotretinoin. Also, because isotretinoin does not affect sperm quality in any way, males taking isotretinoin need no such restrictions.

ROSACEA

Rosacea, a subtype of acne, is a disorder of the pilosebaceous units, which affects both the skin's appearance and texture. In acne, sebaceous glands can be large and/or hyperactive, whereas in rosacea, the glands enlarge gradually as the person ages. Dermatologic and popular literature frequently characterizes rosacea as red or pink skin; however, this is inaccurate because some patients may not show redness. In general, hallmarks of rosacea include transient redness (flushing), which can sometimes be persistent, plus an increased number of visible telangiectasias and, in many cases, papules and pustules. These symptoms typically appear on the central face in a symmetrical distribution, although other body sites, including the upper trunk and neck, can also be affected. Figures 6.8 to 6.12 show that rosacea can present in a wide spectrum

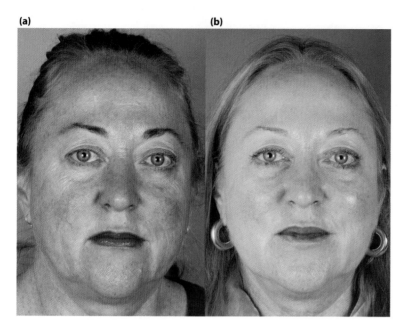

FIGURE 6.8 (a) The patient had skin classified as light white and oily. She was diagnosed as having large pores, rosacea, and erythema. (b) Six months later. The patient followed non-HQ-based Skin Health Restoration to provide correction, stabilization, and stimulation for five months, during which time she received two FLDP laser treatments for erythema.

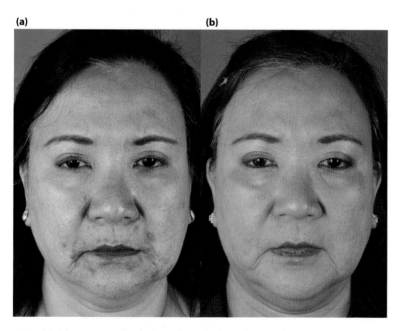

FIGURE 6.9 (a) The patient had skin classified as deviated Asian, medium thick, and very oily. She was diagnosed as having rosacea, enlarged pores, sebaceous gland hyperplasia, and postinflammatory hyperpigmentation. Topical treatments and antibiotics had failed to improve her condition. (b) Five months later. The patient had HQ-based Skin Health Restoration with exfoliation, correction, blending (tretinoin and HQ), and epidermal melanocyte stabilization. She was treated with isotretinoin, 20 mg/day, simultaneously with the topical medication. During the treatment, she underwent two ZO Retinol Stimulation Peel treatments.

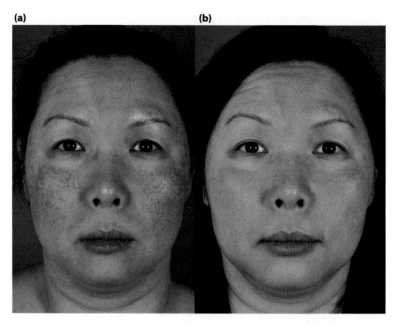

Figure 6.10 (a) The patient had skin classified as deviated Asian (medium), thick, and oily. She was diagnosed as having rosacea, manifested by general erythema, telangiectasias, and skin sensitivity. Her history revealed many years of treatment with fluorinated corticosteroids (which caused steroid atrophy) and moisturizers. (b) Eight months later. The patient had non-HQ-based Skin Health Restoration with emphasis on barrier function repair, epidermal stabilization, and mild stimulation initially. Stimulation strength was gradually increased, and her skin became tolerant after 4 months. She underwent four FLDP laser treatments for the erythema. On her third month of treatment, she began isotretinoin, 20 mg/day, twice weekly to suppress sebum and sebum-induced inflammation.

of clinical situations and with many variations. With an overall prevalence of up to 10% in the general population, rosacea strikes women more often than men. However, affected men are more likely to progress to advanced stages (including prominent rhinophyma). Rosacea is typically diagnosed in the third or fourth decade of life and in those with a history of adolescent acne. The chronological changes characteristic of rosacea are shown in Table 6.4.

Experts disagree about the precise etiology of rosacea; it is likely multifactorial with hereditary and environmental influences. In many patients, acne first appears in the teenage years and over time can gradually evolve into rosacea, often without being recognized by the patient or physician until significant skin texture damage has occurred. Rosacea usually progresses through the following stages:

- Erythema
- Flushing (with or without generalized facial edema and/or ocular symptoms; namely, blepharitis and conjunctivitis)
- Papules and pustules
- Rhinophyma (hypertrophic sebaceous glands leading to an enlarged nose)

The range of clinical manifestations makes rosacea a great imitator of many other dermatologic conditions (Box 6.10). Because of this, rosacea is frequently misdiagnosed by physicians. The cyclical (recurring and remitting) nature of rosacea further contributes to physicians' propensity to misdiagnose the condition as adult acne or one of several types of dermatitis. Misdiagnosis results in the prescription of inappropriate treatment.

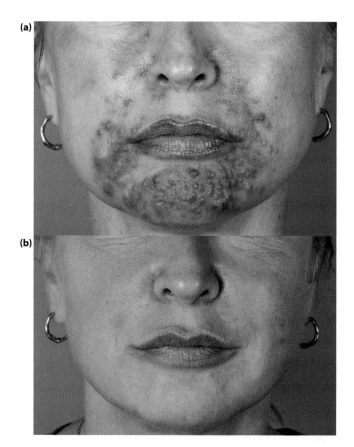

FIGURE 6.11 (a) The patient had skin classified as light white, medium thickness, and oily. She was diagnosed as having granulomatous rosacea, resistant to traditional treatment. Notice the deformity of the chin. (b) One year later. The patient had aggressive non-HQ-based Skin Health Restoration along with metronidazole, intralesional steroid injections, and isotretinoin, 20 mg/day. She had FLPD laser treatment to decrease erythema and break up the granulomas. Five months after discontinuing isotretinoin, a ZO Controlled Depth Peel to the immediate reticular dermis was performed.

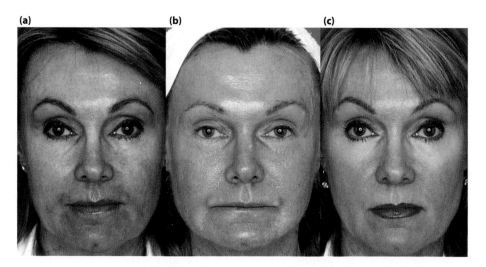

FIGURE 6.12 (a) The patient had skin classified as normal white, medium, and oily. She was diagnosed as having enlarged pores, rosacea, seborrheic dermatitis, stretchable acne scars, and mild laxity. (b) The patient immediately after a ZO Controlled Depth Peel to the immediate reticular dermis, performed after 6 weeks of non-HQ-based Skin Health Restoration. Notice the even blue frost with no pink background. (c) Five months later. The patient had Skin Health Restoration (correction, epidermal stabilization, and stimulation) and also used metronidazole in the morning. Isotretinoin, 20 mg/day, was added to the Skin Health Restoration program after complete healing from the peel and continued for 4 months.

TABLE 6.4 Chronological Changes in Sebaceous Glands

		Period of Life	
Features	Adolescence	Adulthood	Advanced Years
Sebaceous gland size*	Large or hyperactive, resulting in acne and oily skin	Large or enlarging, resulting in hyperplasia, adenomas, and rosacea	Hypertrophy, adenomas, rhinophyma
Skin oiliness	Oily	Excessively oily	Variable
Acne	Present	Texture changes, acne-like cysts, granulomas	Severe textural damage
Inflammation	Strong	Increasing	Variable

*Increased size of the sebaceous glands implies increased activity (sebum production).

Box 6.10

Conditions that May Be Mistaken for Rosacea

- Adult acne
- Seborrheic dermatitis
- Allergic contact or irritant dermatitis
- Folliculitis
- Infections
- Photosensitizing conditions

DIAGNOSING ROSACEA

To counter the misconceptions and uncertainties about rosacea, consider that a diagnosis of rosacea generally requires the presence of sebaceous gland abnormalities plus two or more of the manifestations shown in Box 6.11. The only exception is that, rarely, rosacea may initially present as a perioral dermatitis-like rash or edema alone, without any other symptoms.

With these symptoms in mind, diagnosing rosacea requires inspecting skin carefully, looking for sebaceous gland hyperplasia and adenomas, as well as signs

---

Box 6.11

Rosacea Signs and Symptoms

- Erythema, telangiectasias
- Oily skin and history of acne
- Changes in skin texture (hypertrophy, rhinophyma)
- Thick, glabrous skin with enlarged pores
- Skin sensitivity, irritability
- Involvement of the mucosal surfaces of the eyes and eyelids (blepharitis, conjunctivitis) and scalp (pustules, dandruff)
- Pustules, acne-like cysts, granulomas
- Postinflammatory hyperpigmentation

of inflammation and hypertrophic changes (in the nose, cheeks, and chin). About 15% to 20% of patients with cutaneous rosacea have concurrent ocular involvement (ocular rosacea). In about one out of five of these cases, the ocular manifestations appear first. These can include irritation, redness, dry eyes, itching, burning, a foreign body sensation, photosensitivity, and recurrent styes and eye infections.

No single histological, serological, or other diagnostic test can specifically confirm the presence or absence of rosacea. However, physicians can perform various diagnostic tests, such as bacterial cultures, skin scrapings (with KOH evaluation to look for fungi and spores), patch tests, and biopsies to rule out conditions with a similar appearance.

POTENTIAL CAUSES OF ROSACEA

Though there's a dearth of definitive research regarding the causes of rosacea, experts have identified several factors that appear to play major roles in its development and severity (Box 6.12).

Although some of the conflicting opinions regarding the cause or causes of rosacea have merit, as in acne, sebaceous gland size and activity are the main culprits (Box 6.13). Therefore, to better understand the skin signs of rosacea and how best to treat them, one must understand the activities of sebaceous

Box 6.12

Possible Causes of Rosacea

- Genetic tendency: rosacea occurs in families, in fair-skinned people of Celtic or northern European descent, and in individuals with oily skin.
- Hormonal fluctuations: rosacea typically begins appearing from the age of 30 years and older; it also commonly strikes women during menopause.
- Lifestyle triggers: for some sufferers, avoiding a wide range of the most common potential triggers (e.g., alcohol, spicy foods, hot temperatures, ultraviolet exposure, and physical exertion) appears to minimize rosacea flares.
- Parasitic mites (*Demodex folliculorum*, *Demodex brevis*): some studies have shown that the skin of patients with rosacea harbors above-normal amounts of these mites.
- Bacterial: treatment of *Helicobacter pylori*, for example, often improves rosacea symptoms.

Box 6.13

Main Causes of Rosacea

Sebaceous gland size and activity are the main causes of rosacea.

glands over a normal lifespan and the various skin changes that this activity can induce.

At puberty, rising androgen levels increase sebaceous gland activity, leading to increased sebum production. Increased sebum induces a severe level of inflammation, which is the source of most rosacea symptoms. Focal and generalized skin hypertrophy due to the enlargement of sebaceous glands also occurs. In some patients, acne lesions and nodules, as well as granulomas, continue to appear, whereas in others, erythema, telangiectasias, hyperpigmentation, and textural damage are the dominant forms of presentation.

ROSACEA TREATMENT

As reflected in the current lack of consensus regarding how best to define rosacea and establish its cause, physicians typically focus mainly on relieving its symptoms instead of addressing its cause. To that end, physicians commonly prescribe topical metronidazole, steroids, moisturizers, sulfa-based products, retinoids (occasionally), and oral antibiotics. Also, doctors frequently use laser and intense pulsed light (IPL) treatments to treat the erythema of rosacea and photodynamic therapy (PDT) to suppress sebaceous gland activity. These regimens deliver short-lived improvements at best because they fail to address the underlying sebaceous gland hyperactivity and the damage to the skin's barrier function. Following a comprehensive treatment plan, with attention paid to concurrent Skin Health Restoration measures, maximizes each patient's chance for successful treatment and long-term management of rosacea. This treatment plan rests on the following fundamental principles: 1) rosacea cannot be prevented or cured; however, it can be treated and controlled, and its manifestations can be reversed; and 2) for treatment to succeed, well-defined targets and objectives must be addressed.

Rosacea can aggravate and contribute to the failure of treatment of other skin conditions. For example, melasma will not respond to treatment if the patient's rosacea is not simultaneously treated. And trying to treat erythema or telangiectasias using IPL devices or vascular lasers before controlling rosacea can aggravate the condition. Attempting to perform any procedures while rosacea is still active can lead to a flare-up and a high risk for complications

Rosacea Treatment Steps

Early, mild rosacea (with minor textural changes and acne activity) generally responds to topical agents and PDT. Advanced rosacea (with severe textural changes and acne), however, requires a more aggressive approach with topical agents and systemic isotretinoin. If isotretinoin is contraindicated, a series of PDT treatments, in addition to the daily topical treatment regimen, is recommended. Also, certain other procedures such as chemical peels, focal electrodessication, the CO_2 fractional laser, and certain other laser treatments, can be of additional use.

Step A. **Treat sebaceous gland enlargement and hyperactivity** to reduce sebum production, which helps in suppressing skin inflammation, arresting breakouts (papules and pustules, cysts, and nodules)

and preventing further textural damage. To that end, use one or more of the following therapies:

- PDT (for milder cases)
- Oral isotretinoin (for more effective treatment and more advanced cases)
- CO_2 fractional laser: in patients desiring improvement in skin texture, we perform the CO_2 fractional laser treatment first, then, immediately after the laser procedure, start that patient on a 5-month course of daily oral, low-dose isotretinoin.

Step B: Improve skin tolerance. Restoring a strong skin barrier function requires using Skin Health Restoration principles (correction and stabilization).

Step C: Treat rosacea-induced PIH and discoloration. This can be accomplished by using HQ (bleaching and blending) or by non-HQ melanocyte stabilization in a Skin Health Restoration program.

Step D: Calm acne-like eruptions and shrink enlarged pores. As discussed with acne treatment, targeting whiteheads and blackheads, cysts, nodules, and granulomas requires using the following measures:

- To prepare the skin, patients should use a cleanser designed for oily skin, followed by mechanical exfoliation with an exfoliating scrub once daily to stimulate epidermal renewal and provide deep pore cleansing, and then application of a topical astringent to eliminate surface sebum twice daily.
- The physician may add one or more of the following disease-specific agents, as needed:
  - Benzoyl peroxide has antibacterial properties that reduce rosacea-related inflammation. This agent may initially cause stinging and erythema in patients with barrier dysfunction. However, reactions are generally short lived, and improvement is quickly realized by patients with acneiform eruptions and granulomatous rosacea.
  - Retinoids: vitamin A–derived topical agents promote tissue remodeling and help in combatting skin inflammation. Their use is associated with an initial phase of anticipated reactions (see Chapter 2).
  - AHAs are essential for epidermal exfoliation and renewal.
  - Metronidazole: an antibiotic of the nitroimidazole class, metronidazole (which can be used topically or orally) kills bacteria and protozoa.
  - Sodium sulfacetamide: this topical antibiotic is available, often combined with sulfur, in a variety of vehicles (foams, washes, lotions), for use in acne, rosacea, and seborrhea.

Step E: Improving skin, texture, and color. To address skin texture (enlarged pores and sebaceous gland hyperplasia and adenomas), use strong stimulation (tretinoin) and certain procedures, such as chemical peels, PDT, or laser fractionation. But to eliminate skin redness that does not respond well to laser treatment, it is necessary to arrest skin inflammation (see Step A). Telangiectasias, which represent proliferation and permanent dilation of small blood vessels, respond only to vascular laser treatment.

Step F: Use of systemic antibiotics. Oral antibiotics (tetracycline and its derivatives) are of limited value in the treatment of rosacea. Because bacteria play only a minor role in the etiology of rosacea, reduction of

TABLE 6.5 Choice and Timing of Treatment Based on Signs and Symptoms of Rosacea

Signs and Symptoms	Treatment Choice	Timing of Treatment
Erythema, telangiectasias	Intense pulsed light or vascular-specific lasers	At any time after 6 weeks of skin conditioning*
Postinflammatory hyperpigmentation, discoloration	Topical agents alone or in conjunction with exfoliative peels	At any time after 6 weeks of skin conditioning*
Sebaceous gland hyperplasia	Photodynamic therapy	Once a month while patient is treated with topical agents
	Isotretinoin	Once or twice yearly during maintenance
	CO_2 fractional laser	20 mg/day for 5 months, along with topical agents
		20 mg/2 weeks during maintenance in patients with no risk for pregnancy

*Treatment of the skin with at least 6 weeks of a topical regimen to strengthen and stabilize the skin's barrier function and its melanocytes is recommended before any energy- or light-based treatment (including intense pulsed light and laser treatments) to optimize overall results. This preconditioning topical regimen is most important in patients who are prone to developing postinflammatory hyperpigmentation.

bacteria-induced inflammation with antibiotics has limited benefits, and these agents should not be used long term because of their potential to induce bacterial resistance and other side effects.

Administering Procedures: Timing and Selection

Procedure selection and timing should be based on the individual's signs and symptoms of rosacea (Table 6.5), as well as the patient's priorities. Patient priorities play a part in treatment plan selection and timing only when isotretinoin is a part of rosacea treatment. When a patient desires overall improvement in the shortest time possible, the fast protocol is preferred. But if the patient is interested only in improvement of the rosacea, and not in cosmetic improvement at the same time, the slow protocol is preferred.

Rosacea Treatment Protocols

The Fast Protocol   The fast protocol (Table 6.6) allows patients to improve their appearance and correct skin texture with a procedure, such as CO_2 fractional laser or a 26% to 28% TCA peel (ZO Controlled Depth Peel to the immediate reticular dermis [IRD]), as soon as their skin is ready for it (invasive

TABLE 6.6 Fast Treatment Protocol for Rosacea*

Step 1: Prepare Skin	Step 2: Correction	Step 3: Rosacea Treatment
Skin conditioning 6 weeks or longer with:	Treat textural damage and irregularities with:	After healing, treat for three keratinocyte maturation cycles (5 months) with:
Topical agents	CO_2 fractional laser treatment or a ZO Designed Controlled Depth Peel	Topical agents
Disease-specific agents (if necessary)		Low-dose isotretinoin (20 mg/day), if indicated

*Rosacea with excessive sebum.

TABLE 6.7 Slow Treatment Protocol for Rosacea*

Step 1: Treat the Disease (Three KMCs = 5 months)	Step 2: Discontinue Isotretinoin and Begin Maintenance (Three or more KMCs)	Step 3: Skin Conditioning (One or more KMCs to prepare skin)	Step 4: Begin Skin Health Restoration (After 8 to 10 days or When Healing Is Complete)
Skin Health Restoration with:	Continue topical agents as maintenance.	Perform CO_2 fractional laser to improve texture and/or ZO Controlled Depth Peel.	Restart topical agents and disease-specific agents, if needed.
Topical agents	To eliminate isotretinoin effects on skin, wait $\geq$5 months after discontinuing isotretinoin before performing a procedure to improve texture.		Restart another course of low-dose (20 mg/day) isotretinoin for 3-5 months for long-term rosacea control.
Disease-specific agents			
Consider course of low-dose (20 mg/day) isotretinoin or photodynamic therapy.			

*Rosacea with excessive sebum.

procedures are contraindicated in the context of active rosacea). Begin with skin conditioning for one to two KMCs (6 to 12 weeks). When the skin is ready and the rosacea has been adequately controlled, perform the procedure. Allow the patient's skin to heal for 8 to 10 days after the procedure. Then, restart the rosacea topical treatment agents and initiate a 5-month course of daily oral isotretinoin (usually 20 mg/day). The fast method is preferred because it saves time, quickly provides both disease treatment and cosmetic improvement, and restricts the use of isotretinoin to the time after the procedure.

The Slow Protocol First arrest the disease, starting with topical agents and isotretinoin for three KMCs (5 months) (Table 6.7). Then, discontinue the isotretinoin and continue maintaining improvements with topical agents. Continue this regimen for three KMCs (5 months) to eliminate the residual effects of isotretinoin, which could lead to unreliable, suboptimal post-procedure results. A procedure can now be safely performed (CO_2 fractional laser or a ZO Controlled Depth Peel). If rosacea has been activated by the procedure, an additional course of isotretinoin may be needed.

FOLLICULITIS AND PSEUDOFOLLICULITIS BARBAE

Folliculitis refers to a family of skin conditions involving infected and inflamed hair follicles. This inflammation can lead to skin reactions including papulopustular eruptions, eczematous rashes, pruritus, PIH, and scarring.

Of the many forms of folliculitis (eosinophilic pustular folliculitis, folliculitis decalvans, herpetic folliculitis, and more), pseudofolliculitis barbae (PFB) is the one that dermatologists most commonly encounter and treat. As its name implies, PFB is not a true folliculitis because it is not caused by a pathogenic microorganism. Rather, this potentially disfiguring condition results from ingrown hairs, which occur quite commonly, although not exclusively, in African Americans. It also affects other races genetically predisposed to tightly curled hair, such as Hispanics. Caucasians can be affected. In affected individuals, hairs can curl before they exit the follicle and grow under the epidermis, which subsequently induces focal areas of inflammation.

PFB classically presents in groups of small, red, raised folliculocentric papules that may flare after shaving. In men, PFB occurs most often in areas of increased sebum production, such as the cheeks, jawline, chin, and neck. Postmenopausal women can also experience PFB because hormonal changes may enhance facial hair growth. Additionally, PFB can affect other hair-bearing areas (such as the neck, chest, back, arms, and legs) in both genders. Conversely, one rarely sees folliculitis (or acne, for that matter) in hairless, oil-free areas of the skin because these areas lack sebaceous glands and terminal hairs. Figures 6.13 and 6.14 show patients with PFB.

CAUSES OF PSEUDOFOLLICULITIS BARBAE

Causes of folliculitis range from infection, occlusion, and irritation to specific skin diseases, such as discoid lupus erythematosus and lichen planus. In

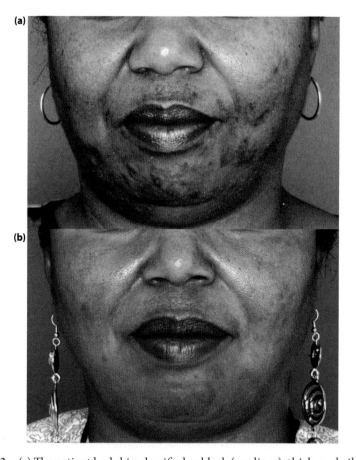

Figure 6.13 (a) The patient had skin classified as black (medium), thick, and oily. She was diagnosed as having pseudofolliculitis barbae, early scarring from skin excoriation and hair plucking with tweezers, and severe postinflammatory hyperpigmentation. (b) Five months later. The patient had HQ-based Skin Health Restoration with emphasis on correction, exfoliation, blending (tretinoin and HQ), epidermal melanocyte stabilization, and acne treatment. She took isotretinoin, 20 mg/day, simultaneously with topical treatment.

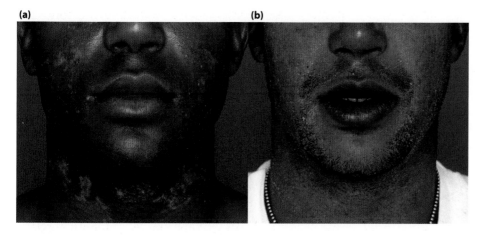

FIGURE 6.14 (a) Before. The patient had skin classified as deviate black (medium black), medium thick, and oily. He was diagnosed as having pseudofolliculitis barbae (PFB), cystic acne, postinflammatory hyperpigmentation, and depigmentation after laser hair removal. (b) On completion of treatment. The patient was treated with aggressive, HQ-based ZO Medical and had extractions of trapped hairs. He was also treated with isotretinoin, 20 mg/day, for 5 months. Notice the restoration of normal color tone and the disappearance of both the acne and the PFB.

PFB, close shaving, as well as tweezing and plucking hairs, can give already curved hair shafts sharp tips that, as they grow, penetrate and reenter the dermis (sometimes extending to the surrounding epidermis). In particular, when someone uses a double-bladed razor, the first blade pulls the hair slightly out of the follicle. The second blade cuts it, but then the now-sharpened hair retracts back into the follicle to continue growing in a curvilinear direction. The same dynamic can occur when someone stretches the skin while shaving for a closer shave. When the hair grows into the skin, a foreign-body reaction, including follicular inflammation and an acne-like eruption, occurs. Over time, infection develops, most often bacterial in cases involving shaving or heavy sweating. The inflammation of folliculitis and PFB destroys hair follicles, leading to the development of focal scars (including hypertrophic scars and keloids), alopecia, and PIH.

DIAGNOSING PSEUDOFOLLICULITIS BARBAE

The diagnosis of PFB rests on the clinical appearance, location, and type of lesions observed. In this regard, characteristic PFB lesions can appear as flesh-colored, erythematous, or hyperpigmented papules occurring in a follicular distribution. Often, one can see the ingrown hair within the papule. To get to the root of the problem, patient histories should investigate any hair-removal methods a patient is using.

PFB and other forms of folliculitis can be somewhat difficult to diagnose because folliculitis commonly occurs concurrently with other skin conditions and systemic disorders. For example, the infectious type of folliculitis can be seen more commonly in patients with impaired immune systems, such as those with underlying diabetes or atopic dermatitis. Similarly, sebum-induced inflammation and acne can aggravate folliculitis, which explains why patients commonly present with both acne and folliculitis. Likewise, on the scalp and chest, folliculitis almost always presents in the context of seborrheic

TABLE 6.8 Preventing Folliculitis and Shaving-Induced Pseudofolliculitis Barbae

Facial pseudofolliculitis barbae—objectives	Actions
1. Reduce bacteria	Cleanse skin thoroughly before shaving.
2. Reduce trauma to the hair	Use shaving creams that soften the hair shaft before shaving with a razor.
3. Eliminate hair entrapment	Scrub with nonirritating formula before shaving to free entrapped hair.
4. Control sebum and bacteria after shaving	Shave with a clean, sharp single-blade razor (or consider an electric clipper or laser hair removal).
5. Avoid occlusion and excess moisture	Avoid very close shaving (including moving the razor in multiple directions).
	Avoid use of blunt or used razor blades.
	Apply antibacterial and sebum-reducing agents after shaving.
	Avoid after-shave moisturizers; use mild exfoliant or barrier repair agent instead.

dermatitis. Additionally, folliculitis (and acne) can occur in the context of hormonal syndromes and after use of systemic steroids.

PREVENTING AND TREATING FOLLICULITIS

In general, prevention of PFB is the best approach (Table 6.8).

To prevent PFB when shaving nonfacial skin (such as the chest, axillae, arms, and legs), patients should take the following steps daily for 3 days before and 3 days after shaving:

- Scrub the area (to free trapped hair)
- Apply astringent (to control sebum and bacteria) AM and PM
- Use a mild exfoliating and barrier repair formulation

To treat an existing outbreak of PFB, instruct patients as in Box 6.14.

Successfully treating PFB also requires treating any coexisting problems, such as acne. Additionally, for seborrheic dermatitis associated with folliculitis in the scalp area, the physician can prescribe appropriate topical agents (including medicated shampoos and mousse preparations) and, in severe cases, isotretinoin.

Box 6.14

Calming Pseudofolliculitis Barbae Outbreaks

- Stop shaving for at least 30 days to free any trapped hair and eliminate ingrown hairs.
- Cleanse and exfoliate the beard area by using a scrub or exfoliating formula daily for 30 days.
- Apply topical retinoid nightly to soften the hair and regulate surface skin keratinization.
- Treat any infected areas with appropriate topical (or in severe cases, systemic) antibiotics, based on the results of sensitivity cultures.

KERATOSIS PILARIS

Keratosis pilaris (KP) is commonly called "chicken skin" because affected areas appear to have persistent "goosebumps" (Figure 6.15). Specifically, KP presents as large patches of small (1 to 3 mm), lightly pigmented papules, each covering a hair follicle. KP usually appears on the upper arms and thighs, often presenting between the ages of 14 and 25 years. It can also extend to the upper back, buttocks, and shoulders and, in rare cases, can affect the cheeks in the form of fine, erythematous patches, usually in young children and teenagers. About 50% of children and 40% of adults experience KP (males and females equally). It is thought to be passed through generations in an autosomal dominant fashion.

KP is a chronic condition that cannot be cured, but it can be kept under control with the regular application of topical treatments. Although KP is usually asymptomatic, patients tend to excoriate the involved areas in their attempts to get rid of them. This tends to worsen the condition and may cause localized discoloration and scarring. If left untreated, the condition usually persists for many years and fades later in life, although it can recur as well.

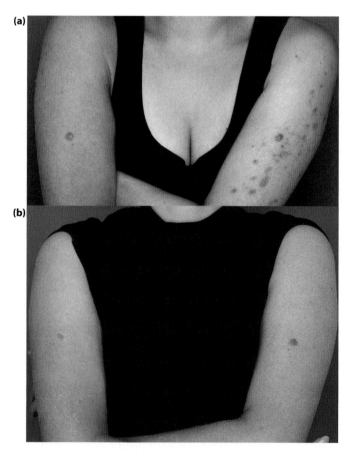

FIGURE 6.15 (a) The patient was diagnosed as having keratosis pilaris. Her right arm was treated aggressively for 6 weeks with a ZO body renewal protocol that consisted of 1) Invisapeel formula applied for 3 hours then washed off in the evening; 2) Oraser Body Emulsion Plus lotion to renew the epidermis applied morning and evening; and 3) Retamax (1% retinol) applied in the evening. Her left arm was untreated. (b) Twelve weeks after treatment with the same program (both arms). Notice the improvement in redness, exfoliation, and texture of the treated arm. On completion, the patient will use only the Oraser Body Emulsion Plus, applied morning and evening.

TABLE 6.9   Keratosis Pilaris: Treatment Steps

Step A. Avoid triggers:	Tight clothing
	Overly hot baths and showers
	Harsh loofah scrubs and washcloths
	Drying soaps
	Scratching and picking
Step B. To stabilize and repair skin, use this topical regimen:	AM: alpha-hydroxy acids, stabilization and barrier repair products
	PM: Tretinoin or retinol stimulation (tretinoin 0.1% or retinol 1% work best), more stabilization and barrier repair
	For patients with postinflammatory hyperpigmentation, add HQ 4% (AM and PM) or non-HQ melanocyte stabilization to restore even skin color tone.

Causes of Keratosis Pilaris

No one knows the exact cause of KP. However, most experts believe it results from a combination of genetic susceptibility, dry skin, hypersensitivity reactions, and friction. The most common factors that cause KP in susceptible individuals include the following:

- Continuous skin friction caused by rough and tight clothing (shirts, jeans)
- Excessive exposure to hot baths and showers
- Obsessive and overly vigorous skin scrubbing (often with loofah scrubs)

Clinically, these factors can stimulate keratin overproduction and accumulation of excess keratin around the opening of hair follicles, creating the individual bumps of KP. Along with hyperkeratosis, microscopic evaluation of lesions reveals mild thickening of the skin and plugging of the hair follicle. Dilation of small, superficial blood vessels also may occur, giving affected skin a red or flushed appearance. Additionally, the red or brown spots that form beneath the excess keratin stem from follicular inflammation.

Treating Keratosis Pilaris

Much like with PFB, treating KP demands that patients eliminate causative factors (Table 6.9, Step A) whenever possible and apply a carefully designed topical regimen regularly (Table 6.9, Step B). KP treatment objectives include softening of the surface keratin, exfoliating the superficial accumulation of hypertrophic corneocytes, and restoring normal skin-surface keratinization, thereby restoring barrier function. In these areas, the stronger the morning and evening stimulation, the stronger the skin's anticipated reactions (such as erythema and exfoliation) will be, and the faster the patient will experience improvement. By following the steps described here, patients should achieve normal-looking skin within two to three KMCs (12 to 18 weeks). For severe cases, adding two to three exfoliative chemical peels during that period can further hasten resolution.

MEDICAL APPLICATIONS
Treating Pigmentation Problems and Photodamage

PIGMENTATION PROBLEMS

Problems with skin pigmentation rank among the most common problems seen by dermatologists. Examples range from melasma and vitiligo to photodamage, postinflammatory hyperpigmentation (PIH), genetic conditions, and various types of nevi. Melanocytes, which actively produce melanin, are the cells responsible for all skin pigmentation problems. The high frequency of pigmentation problems stems largely from the fact that melanocytes are sensitive to a variety of influences from within and outside of the body (Box 7.1).

One could easily write a book on any single pigmentary disorder. The medical literature is rich with information regarding the full spectrum of pigmentary disorders—their causes, comorbidities, differential diagnoses, and treatments. Because this material is extensively reviewed elsewhere, this chapter focuses on a system for classifying and treating pigmentary disorders.

Physicians tend to treat pigmentary disorders on a case-by-case basis, selecting an individualized regimen geared to what they believe are each patient's needs. However, results of this approach have been mixed. Regarding melasma, for example, physicians typically treat with hydroquinone (HQ) concentrations ranging from 2% to 12%, various concentrations of retinoic acid, topical steroids, and exfoliative procedures involving chemical peels, intense pulsed light (IPL), and lasers. Yet some patients improve; others do not. In still others, melasma worsens. To avoid such pitfalls, the proposed classification system (Table 7.1) seeks to standardize the way physicians think about and treat pigmentary disorders so that they may achieve more consistent results.

Box 7.1

Factors that Influence Melanocytes

- Temperatures: excessive heat and cold can stimulate or kill melanocytes.
- Chemicals: exposure to phenols (hydroquinone, resorcinol) and other chemicals can be toxic and fatal to melanocytes. Phenols can also stimulate melanocyte activity, depending on the concentration.
- Mechanical and endogenous stimuli: factors that can easily stimulate melanocytes include skin irritation, inflammation, injury, diseases, sun exposure, hormones, genetic influences, hot baths, and showers.
- Certain medications

TABLE 7.1   Zein Obagi Classification of Pigmentary Problems

Column 1: Etiology	Column 2: Depth	Column 3: Origin
Hormonal	Epidermal	Endogenous
Inflammatory	Dermal	Exogenous
Genetic	Epidermal and dermal	Endogenous and exogenous
Acquired	Epidermal, dermal, and subdermal	

The columns in Table 7.1 are equally important, and it doesn't matter which column or category is considered first. The key is that by using all three columns, we can comprehensively describe any pigmentary disorder. Additionally, columns 1 and 3 provide valuable prognostic information. For example, melasma is a hormonal problem with possible genetic influences (column 1) that usually involves the epidermis, dermis, or both (column 2) and originates endogenously, although it can be exacerbated by exogenous factors (column 3). As a hormonally caused pigment disorder, melasma has an unpredictable long-term course (as do most genetically based disorders).

Conversely, pigment disorders with acquired and inflammatory sources are largely curable—provided one removes these sources. PIH, for instance, is an inflammatory disorder (column 1) that mainly affects the epidermis (column 2) and that stems from endogenous and exogenous factors (column 3). In contrast to the uncertain course of hormonal and genetic pigment disorders, PIH, once treated, can be considered cured—as long as the epidermal inflammation does not return.

THE MYSTERIES OF MELASMA

Clinically, it is difficult to mistake melasma for anything else. It presents as areas of ill-defined brownish or dark macules or patches, usually in a symmetrical pattern, on a sun-exposed area, especially the face. In particular, melasma seems to favor the forehead, nose, cheeks, and upper lip. The skin color change depends on the location of the melanin deposition. Epidermal involvement appears as brown discoloration, whereas dermal deposition appears as blue-gray. Mixed epidermal and dermal depositions appear as brown-gray discolorations. Whether the melanin is deposited in the epidermis or dermis is important therapeutically because dermal hyperpigmentation is much more challenging to treat.

Although melasma strikes all races, it occurs most commonly in darker Fitzpatrick skin types III through V. It is also more common in women. Like most pigment problems, it is clinically benign but psychologically distressing to patients because of the effect it can have on their social and professional lives. Although much is known about melasma, research has not yet identified why the following statements are true of melasma:

- Some melanocytes become hyperactive, whereas other melanocytes nearby do not.
- Some women develop melasma, whereas others who are exposed to the same factors do not.
- Although not exposed to the same hormones as women are, some men develop melasma.
- Melasma appears mainly on the face and very rarely on other body areas, sun-exposed or otherwise.

Likewise, the precise cause of melasma remains a subject of debate. In addition to genetic and hormonal (including pregnancy) influences, researchers have identified several potential factors (Box 7.2).

We do not know exactly how these factors ultimately contribute to increase the synthesis of melanin (within melanocytes) and the deficiency in the even transfer of melanin to surrounding keratinocytes. Increased melanin production by some melanocytes can be explained by two possibilities, which in some cases may work together (Box 7.3).

Genetic predisposition could explain why melasma tends to run in families. In many cases, a mother and daughter (or two sisters) share not only melasma but also a similar distribution and severity level. People with a genetic predisposition to melasma may also require a triggering factor to develop the disease. However, triggers may also operate independently of genetics. In short, internal or external factors may overstimulate melanocyte receptors. When

---

Box 7.2

Potential Causes of Melasma

- Ultraviolet light exposure
- Vascular factors
- Chronic inflammation and inflammatory disorders
- Use of cosmetics and other products
- Phototoxic or photosensitizing agents
- Medications: antiseizure, blood pressure, and antimalarial agents, and tetracycline

Box 7.3

Potential Causes of Melanin Overproduction

■ Genetic factors
■ Internal or external factors that act as triggers
■ Among internal triggers, inflammation is most likely the main cause of dermal melasma.

the receptors reach this hyperexcited state, they respond on subsequent exposure to the trigger by producing more melanin. Or perhaps the trigger might affect the melanocyte receptors, disrupting the melanocytes' ability to regulate melanin production altogether.

Internal Melasma Triggers

Internal triggers of melanin production may include hormones. This might explain why melasma appears after women begin taking birth control pills or hormones or become pregnant. In fact, chloasma, a condition seen commonly during or shortly after pregnancy, is merely epidermal melasma. It usually responds quickly to treatment, although it tends to reoccur.

Among internal triggers, inflammation is most likely the main factor that causes the dermal form of melasma. The potential for inflammation to initiate or worsen melasma is perhaps most evident in that patients with melasma who also suffer from adult acne or rosacea (both of which arise from sebum-induced inflammation) usually have more severe resistant melasma than people with normal or dry skin. When sebum is reduced through topical or oral treatments, these more serious cases of melasma begin responding better and faster to treatment.

Additional internal triggers for melasma may include melanocyte-stimulating hormone (MSH). When a receptor is triggered, the associated melanocyte may become more sensitive to MSH, leading to excessive melanin production.

External Melasma Triggers

External factors, on the other hand, may include everything from ultraviolet (UV) rays and hot water to continuous skin irritation and inflammation caused by improper use of topical drugs. In the latter area, melasma sometimes paradoxically worsens in patients who self-treat with HQ, alpha-hydroxy acids (AHAs), or kojic acid for more than 1 year. Over time, melanocytes can acquire resistance to these treatments and respond by the overproduction of tyrosinase, which leads to rebound hyperpigmentation. Additionally, the reduced melanin levels created by these treatments may result in photosensitivity or phototoxicity, which represent additional sources of UV sensitivity and induced inflammation.

Nevertheless, melanin overproduction represents only half of the melasma story. The other half involves uneven uptake of melanin by certain surrounding keratinocytes. In this regard, we know that each melanocyte provides

Box 7.4

Retinoids and Melanocyte Activity

■ Retinoids regulate keratinocyte activity that leads to more even melanin uptake.

Box 7.5

Suggested Pathophysiology of Melasma

■ Overproduction of melanin by certain melanocytes
■ Uneven uptake of melanin by surrounding keratinocytes with normal or increased production of melanin

melanin to approximately 36 surrounding keratinocytes. But in melasma, perhaps only a few of these keratinocytes take up all the melanin, leaving little or none for the rest. The success of certain retinoids (tretinoin [retinoic acid] and retinol) in treating melasma appears to support this theory. Applying these topical agents can increase keratinocyte activity and turnover and equalize melanin uptake, thereby restoring even color tone and improving the appearance of melasma, not through bleaching, but through more even melanin uptake (Box 7.4). Box 7.5 shows the suggested pathophysiology of melasma.

POSTINFLAMMATORY HYPERPIGMENTATION

Postinflammatory hyperpigmentation presents as generalized or focal dyschromia that can occur after any type of skin injury, disease, or inflammation. It can appear on sun-exposed or sun-protected skin. However, UV exposure usually worsens PIH. We can even consider a suntan a form of generalized, uniform PIH because people who tan evenly and easily have skin that is more prone to develop PIH when exposed to anything that might cause localized skin inflammation.

Postinflammatory hyperpigmentation occurs commonly in all skin types, including deviated (racially mixed) skin, which is more sensitive to the effects of inflammation and dermatologic procedures. As such, this group of patients tends to develop more profound and prolonged PIH than do patients of purely black, Asian, Hispanic, or of any other ethnic or racial descent. Similarly, patients with oily skin often develop more severe, resistant PIH because sebum is a pro-inflammatory substance. Accordingly, reducing sebum, treating inflammatory skin diseases, and conditioning the skin before and after procedures will reduce or prevent post-procedural PIH and make treatment easier and more successful.

TREATING MELASMA AND POSTINFLAMMATORY HYPERPIGMENTATION

The guidelines for treating melasma and PIH are fairly similar, though not identical (Box 7.6). Successful treatment of skin symptoms and the underlying causes essentially cures PIH; however, treated melasma can recur, because of hormonal or other unpredictable influences, months or even years after successful treatment.

Melasma-Specific Steps

When treating melasma, one must first distinguish the epidermal type from the dermal type. In this regard, use a Wood's lamp or a simple skin-stretching test (just stretch the affected skin with your hands—if the pigment appears lighter, it is epidermal melasma; if not, it is dermal) (Box 7.7). Remember that the more stubborn dermal component will require a procedure (e.g., a ZO Controlled Depth Peel) to the papillary dermis (PD) performed after 4 to 6 weeks of skin conditioning.

The best approach to treating melasma or PIH is the aggressive treatment approach that incorporates the following four essential steps:

Step 1. Bleaching. This step arrests melanin production, thereby reducing hyperpigmentation. The regimen involves applying HQ 4% (daily, AM and PM) and AHAs for exfoliation (daily, AM). It is important

---

Box 7.6

Guidelines for Treating Melasma and Postinflammatory Hyperpigmentation

TREAT THE DISEASE AND ITS CAUSES

- Reduce sebum.
  - Sebum induces inflammation and represents a major cause of treatment failure.
- Use topical astringent, and even isotretinoin (in stubborn cases), in patients being treated for melasma or postinflammatory hyperpigmentation.
- Treat any active disease (such as acne) simultaneously.
- Use strong sun protection throughout treatment.

TREATMENT MODALITY

- Treat aggressively.
- Bleaching and blending work best.
- When procedures are needed as part of the treatment, peels are better than heat-generating devices (intense pulsed light lasers).
- Use skin conditioning for one to three keratinocyte maturation cycles (6 to 18 weeks) before and after procedures.

Box 7.7

Dr. Zein Obagi Skin Stretch Test for Melasma

Stretch the affected skin with your hands—if the pigment appears lighter, it is epidermal melasma; if not, it is dermal.

Box 7.8

Pulsed Hydroquinone Therapy

To avoid HQ side effects, use pulsed therapy:

■ Five months of bleaching and blending
■ Two to 3 months of rest
■ Resumption of hydroquinone, if needed

not to use HQ for too long and to discontinue use at an appropriate time to avoid serious side effects. HQ adverse effects can be avoided with pulsed therapy. This entails 5 months of bleaching and blending, 2 to 3 months of rest, then resumption of HQ, if needed. Pulse therapy is explained in Box 7.8.

Figures 7.1, 7.2, and 7.3 show patients with epidermal and dermal melasma, and Figure 7.4 shows a patient with dermal melasma; all

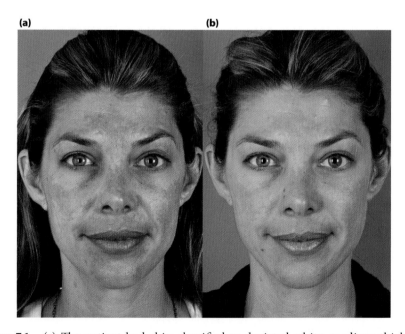

FIGURE 7.1   (a) The patient had skin classified as deviated white, medium thick, and oily. She was diagnosed as having epidermal and dermal melasma. (b) One year later. The patient was treated with aggressive HQ-based Skin Health Restoration for 6 months, during which she had three monthly treatments with a ZO Retinol Stimulation Peel. The dermal melasma on her forehead remained after treatment and required a ZO Controlled Depth Peel to the papillary dermis.

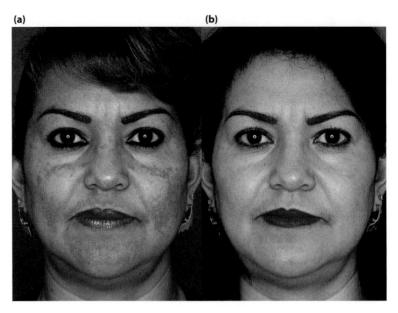

Figure 7.2 (a) Before. The patient had skin classified as deviated (dark), thick, and oily. She was diagnosed as having epidermal and dermal melasma by means of Dr. Zein Obagi Skin Stretch Test. (b) One year later. The patient was treated with an aggressive HQ-based ZO Medical Skin Health Restoration program for 6 weeks followed by a ZO Controlled Depth Peel to the papillary dermis. This peel was repeated 6 weeks before the end of treatment. Maintenance consisted of non-HQ-based Skin Health Restoration.

were treated with ZO programs. Figure 7.5 shows a patient with PIH and melasma, Figure 7.6 shows a patient with rosacea and PIH, and Figure 7.7 shows a patient with rosacea, discoloration, large pores, and laxity who was treated with ZO programs and a combination of a ZO Designed Controlled Depth Peel and a CO_2 fractional laser procedure. Figure 7.8 shows a patient with PIH who was successfully

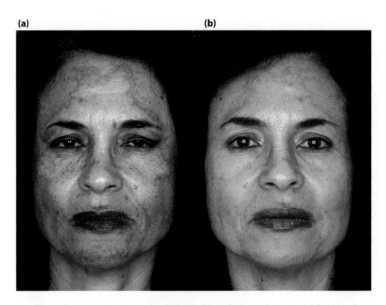

Figure 7.3 (a) Before. The patient had skin classified as deviated (dark) white, medium thick, and oily. She was diagnosed as having epidermal and dermal melasma. (b) One year later. The patient was treated with four courses of HQ-based ZO Medical. Each course consisted of Skin Health Restoration for 6 weeks followed by a ZO Controlled Depth Peel to the papillary dermis. To prevent HQ resistance, non-HQ-based ZO Medical was used between each course for 3 months. Notice the residual of dermal melasma in the forehead area that may require deeper peels or pigment laser treatment.

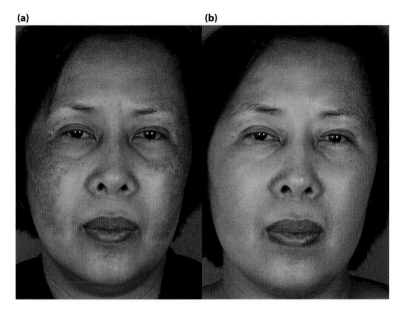

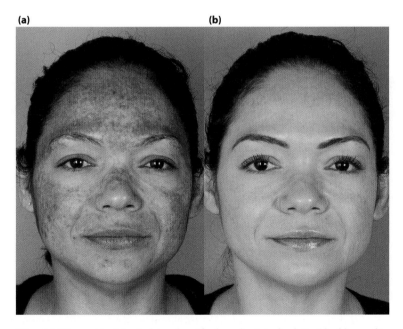

FIGURE 7.4 (a) Before. The patient had skin classified as deviated (medium) Asian, thick, and nonoily. She was diagnosed as having dermal melasma. (b) One year later. The patient was treated for 5 months with HQ-based ZO Medical followed by a ZO Controlled Depth Peel to the papillary dermis. Maintenance consisted of non-HQ-based Skin Health Restoration.

treated with Skin Health Restoration and a ZO Controlled Depth Peel to the PD for PIH, after previous unsuccessful treatment with other peels.

Step 2. Stabilization. After stopping the bleaching step, patients should start the stabilization step (as described in Chapter 2), using anti-inflammatory topical agents (antioxidants) and retinol (in a high concentration) to stabilize melanocytes and make them less responsive to

FIGURE 7.5 (a) The patient had skin classified as deviated white (dark), medium thick, and oily. She was diagnosed as having severe postinflammatory hyperpigmentation and melasma. (b) One year later. The patient was treated with aggressive HQ-based Skin Health Restoration for 5 months. Six weeks after starting Skin Health Restoration, she underwent a ZO Controlled Depth Peel to the papillary dermis. After healing, isotretinoin was added to the Skin Health Restoration regimen.

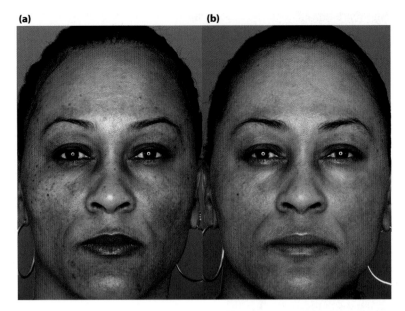

FIGURE 7.6 (a) Before. The patient had skin classified as black (medium), medium thick, and oily. She was diagnosed as having rosacea and postinflammatory hyperpigmentation. (b) One year later. The patient was treated with aggressive HQ-based ZO Medical Skin Health Restoration for 5 months along with isotretinoin, 20 mg/day. She also had two treatments with a ZO 3-Step Peel. Maintenance consisted of non-HQ-based Skin Health Restoration.

external and internal stimulation and inflammation, while starting the blending regimen (step 3).

Step 3. Blending. To force even melanin distribution and increase uptake by surrounding keratinocytes, patients should use a fresh mixture of HQ 4% and tretinoin (retinoic acid), in proper proportions, as discussed in Chapter 2, for three keratinocyte maturation cycles (KMCs) (18 weeks). Start with a moderate or mild approach and build to the aggressive approach as soon as the patient's skin can

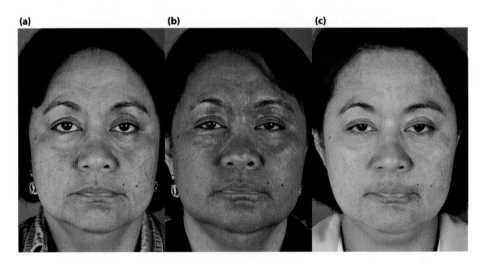

FIGURE 7.7 (a) Before. The patient had skin classified as deviated Asian (medium), thick, and oily. She was diagnosed as having rosacea, discoloration, large pores, and laxity. (b) Eight days after a combined procedure of a ZO Designed Controlled Depth Peel and a CO_2 fractional laser procedure. The patient had been treated with 6 weeks of aggressive, HQ-based skin conditioning before the procedures. After the procedures, she followed the same topical regimen along with 20 mg/day isotretinoin for 3 months. (c) One year later.

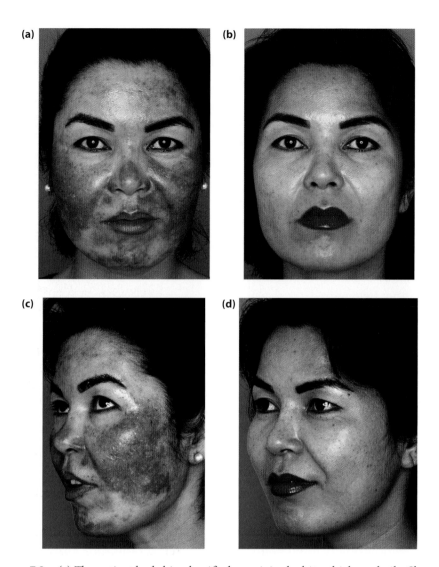

Figure 7.8 (a) The patient had skin classified as original white, thick, and oily. She was diagnosed as having PIH. Six months earlier, she had undergone a TCA peel at another clinic. The PIH did not respond to topical HQ and two Cosmelan peels, and her condition worsened. (b) The patient at one year. She was treated with non-HQ-based Skin Health Restoration for three months for epidermal and melanocyte stabilization, followed by five months of aggressive HQ-based Skin Health Restoration. Six weeks after starting the second course of Skin Health Restoration, a ZO Controlled Depth Peel to the PD was performed. After healing, isotretinoin 20 mg/day was added to her Skin Health Restoration regimen. (c) Before. Side view. (d) After. Side view.

tolerate it. Melanocytes do not build resistance to blending as quickly as they do to HQ alone, and patients can use the blending regimen longer than the bleaching regimen. As with bleaching, however, patients should discontinue HQ blending as soon as their color tone has been corrected. This helps prevent photosensitivity, resistance, rebound hyperpigmentation, and ochronosis (discussed later).

Step 4. Continue stabilization/begin maintenance. After stopping the bleaching and blending steps, an HQ-free approach is ideal for maintaining skin improvements and preventing future recurrences of PIH or melasma. This means using retinol, antioxidants, anti-inflammatory agents, and non-HQ skin lighteners to provide continuous correction, stabilization, and stimulation. If melasma starts to recur, patients can return to the bleaching and blending steps.

TREATING MELASMA AND POSTINFLAMMATORY HYPERPIGMENTATION WITH HYDROQUINONE

HQ is a popular and effective topical agent used extensively to treat a wide variety of skin pigmentation problems. It is approved by the U.S. Food and Drug Administration (FDA) for the treatment of melasma, and when used in reasonable concentrations (4% is best) and under physician supervision, it is the gold standard for treating pigmentation disorders. Unfortunately, HQ is often used in an arbitrary and dangerous manner. It can be easily obtained from doctors' offices, pharmacies, the Internet, and the black market, and individuals often self-treat with high concentrations for long periods of time. Continuous use in this manner can lead to medical and aesthetic disasters that cannot be repaired.

HQ acts in two ways: 1) by reversibly inhibiting tyrosinase, the main enzyme involved in the conversion of tyrosine to melanin; and 2) by selectively damaging melanosomes and melanocytes. Therefore, the mechanism of action of topical HQ is through prevention of new melanin production. Pigmented areas do not disappear immediately with HQ treatment: as skin cells mature, the melanin-containing keratinocytes within the epidermis are shed, and new keratinocytes are formed with less pigmented melanosomes.

Hydroquinone Side Effects

In recent years, we have encountered an increasing frequency of unexplained side effects induced by HQ and noticed several commonalities in these patients (Box 7.9). The side effects in these patients included rebound hyperpigmentation, photosensitivity or phototoxicity, tolerance or resistance, and exogenous ochronosis.

Rebound Hyperpigmentation

The best concentration of HQ for treating pigmentation problems is 4%, and more benefits or faster results do not follow use of higher concentrations. On the contrary, patients who use 6%, 8%, or 12% concentrations tended to develop more stubborn, difficult-to-treat hyperpigmentation, which often appeared more prominent than their original problem. The exact mechanism

---

Box 7.9

Commonalities Seen in Patients Who Experienced Hydroquinone Side Effects

- HQ was used without medical supervision and without stopping for 1 year or longer.
- A high concentration (6% to 12%) of HQ was used.
- A combination of HQ with tretinoin (retinoic acid) and corticosteroid (Tri-Luma Cream, Galderma: fluocinolone acetonide 0.01%, HQ 4%, tretinoin 0.05%) was used.

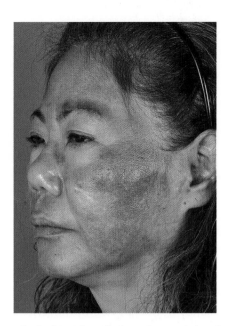

FIGURE 7.9 The patient had skin classified as deviated (medium) Asian, thick, and oily. She was diagnosed as having melasma, postinflammatory hyperpigmentation, and rebound hyperpigmentation. She had been treated with 4%, 8%, and 10% hydroquinone (HQ) in various clinics for 1 year, but the melasma progressively worsened. This indicated resistance to both HQ and HQ-induced sensitivity and inflammation.

responsible for rebound hyperpigmentation associated with the use of topical hydroquinone has yet to be fully elucidated. However, the most likely explanation is that higher concentrations 1) induce toxic or shocking effects on melanocytes, forcing cells to rebound and increase melanin production (rebound hyperpigmentation); or 2) provoke skin inflammation (because HQ is a known inflammatory agent), which leads to melanocyte hyperactivity that overpowers the tyrosinase-suppressing effect of hydroquinone. Figure 7.9 shows a patient with rebound hyperpigmentation.

Photosensitivity and Phototoxicity

The skin-damaging effects of UV light exposure are well known and include DNA damage, an increased incidence of skin cancer, and accelerated signs of aging. Medications, both topical and systemic, can increase skin sensitivity to UV exposure, with subsequent damage being seen with shorter yet repeated exposure. Thus, it is surprising that photosensitivity to HQ is rarely mentioned. By reducing the amount of melanin (which has a natural sun protection factor of 4 to 8), HQ weakens or eliminates the skin's natural ability to protect itself. Without proper protection from the sun, skin may be damaged by inflammation, which can then ultimately *stimulate* overproduction of melanin.

Exogenous Ochronosis

Exogenous ochronosis is a paradoxical hyperpigmentation caused by the overuse of HQ and is the worst side effect of its use because many cases of ochronosis cannot be successfully treated (Figure 7.10). Although triggering factors for exogenous ochronosis are known, there is no scientific explanation for why this condition develops in certain individuals and not in others who share the same HQ history and triggering factors.

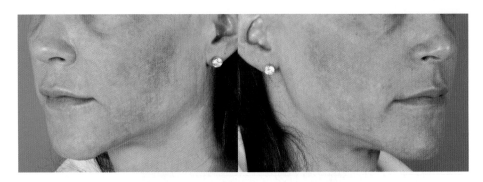

FIGURE 7.10 The patient had skin classified as white, medium thick, and oily. She was diagnosed as having early exogenous ochronosis that was more severe on her left cheek. The condition developed 2 years after she had used 4% HQ in an unsupervised manner in an attempt to induce skin lightening.

Endogenous ochronosis, in contrast to exogenous ochronosis, is due to a patient's inherent deficiency in the enzyme homogentisic acid oxidase (HAO), which ultimately leads to the accumulation of homogentisic acid in multiple organs, including the skin, in affected patients. Photosensitivity induced by HQ may cause deficiency of HAO, leading to an accumulation of homogentisic acid, which forms complexes with melanin in the skin that manifest macroscopically as bluish patches. These patches are indicative of exogenous ochronosis. Exogenous ochronosis may also be triggered by the phototoxic effect of HQ, ultimately leading to the production of chemically altered, bluish melanin compounds, which are again characteristic of exogenous ochronosis.

Exogenous ochronosis was once thought to be a problem limited to people within certain tribes in Africa, and its etiology was thought to be partially due to the prolonged use of HQ in patients with this genetic predisposition. At that time, neither photosensitivity nor phototoxicity was considered to be a major factor in causing this problem. However, within the past few years, we have observed a higher incidence of exogenous ochronosis not only in African Americans but also in Caucasian brunettes, Asians, and Hispanics. The common variable among these patients was that each had been using HQ in various concentrations (sometimes compounded to strengths as high as 20% to 30%) for years. Another commonality was that they had each been using HQ without adequate medical supervision and had obtained it from repeated unsupervised physician prescription refills, the Internet, or the black market. Often these patients were also not properly protected from daily sun exposure because the areas of the face with the most sun exposure were also those most likely to show exogenous ochronosis.

Tolerance or Resistance

When treating melasma, we have observed no further improvement from HQ application in some patients after 4 to 5 months of good response. Furthermore, the bleaching effects from HQ application were more pronounced in the areas not affected by melasma, whereas the affected dark areas showed no further improvement. We could only conclude that active melanocytes in the affected areas were becoming resistant to HQ and that the patient's hyperpigmentation became worse from the prolonged use of HQ.

When such resistance is observed, HQ use should be immediately discontinued to prevent rebound pigmentation. To reverse HQ resistance, patients

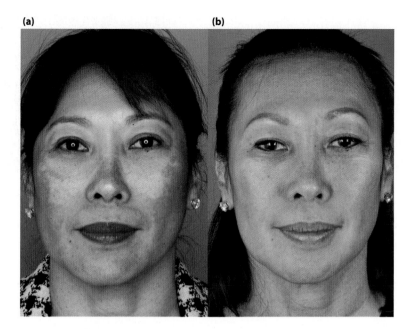

(a) **(b)**

FIGURE 7.11 (a) Before. The patient had skin classified as deviated Asian (light), medium thick, and oily. Her history showed 6 years of unsupervised HQ use. She was diagnosed as having melasma and rebound hyperpigmentation due to HQ resistance. (b) One year later. The patient underwent 3 months of nonmedical Skin Health Restoration with an emphasis on epidermal, melanocyte, and dermal stabilization. She underwent two treatments with a ZO 3-Step Peel and had a ZO Controlled Depth Peel to the papillary dermis. Maintenance consisted of non-HQ-based Skin Health Restoration.

should stop HQ use for 2 to 3 months to allow melanocytes to stabilize. This process makes melanocytes more resistant to negative stimuli that could trigger their activity. After such rest, patients can resume HQ use if needed—under proper supervision. Figure 7.11 shows a patient who developed melasma and rebound hyperpigmentation due to HQ resistance.

Of note, HQ has also been used in combination with a topical corticosteroid and retinoic acid (Kligman formula, Tri-Luma) with the rationale that the steroid suppresses inflammation that excites melanocytes and subsequently results in an increased production of melanin with associated patches of skin showing hyperpigmentation. This is only true for pigmentation induced by injury or disease, such as PIH. In some patients, long-term use of this combination formulation has been shown to result in skin atrophy, the appearance of telangiectatic matting, more stubborn pigmentation, and photosensitivity. A general rule of thumb is that, regardless of the condition being treated, topical steroids should only be used for short durations (or "pulses") of 5 to 7 days in a row. The long-term use of topical steroids to treat melasma should be avoided because melasma is induced by factors other than inflammation alone.

Treating Melasma and Postinflammatory Hyperpigmentation with and without Hydroquinone

After many years of experience, we developed two approaches for treating melasma and PIH: 1) the HQ-based approach (Table 7.2) and 2) the non-HQ-based approach (Table 7.3). Most important, we recognized the limitations of HQ treatment and developed pulsed HQ therapy (as was shown in Box 7.8) that avoids the development of ochronosis and other undesirable effects. We also developed guidelines for discontinuing the use of HQ (Box 7.10).

TABLE 7.2   The Hydroquinone Approach for Treating Melasma and Postinflammatory Hyperpigmentation[*†]

Step	Function
1. Bleaching	To minimize or stop melanin production, 4% HQ (AM and PM) works best.
	Alternative agents, including arbutin, kojic acid, vitamin C, retinol, and tretinoin, are weak bleaching agents without therapeutic value.
2. Epidermal exfoliation	To reduce epidermal melanin and provide mild blending benefits, use a formulation of alpha-hydroxy acid and anti-inflammatory agents (once daily).
3. Stabilization	This step does the following: • Increases skin tolerance (strengthens barrier function) • Repairs damaged DNA • Provides anti-inflammatory benefits • Reduces melanocytes' response to negative factors (such as ultraviolet light or hormones) A formulation available from ZO Skin Health can provide all these benefits.
4. Blending	To stimulate keratinocyte activity and turnover so that all active keratinocytes phagocytize melanin evenly (to be done once or twice daily, AM and PM). This ensures more even color tone without bleaching effects.

[*]These steps should be performed in the order above: 1, 2, 3, 4.
[†]Many of the formulations recommended are not readily available except from ZO Skin Health.

TABLE 7.3   The Nonhydroquinone Approach to Melanocyte Stabilization[*]

Step	Function
1. Accelerate epidermal turnover (to unload epidermal melanin): the Invisapeel	To decrease epidermal pigmentation by accelerating natural epidermal exfoliation, which reduces epidermal melanin and provides beneficial blending effects The Invisapeel (an enzymatic invisible peel) is used for this purpose. (See formulation and use in Chapter 9) To be applied once daily
2. Stabilizing melanocytes: Brightenex-F	To suppress abnormal melanin production by melanocytes that have been exposed to internal or external stimuli. The stabilizing process makes melanocytes more resistant to such stimuli so that they produce only normal melanin (maintaining normal color tone without bleaching effects). Use Brightenex-F in AM. This product is a non-HQ-blending agent that does not bleach the skin. It helps only in restoring an even color tone.
3. Epidermal stabilization: Retamax-F	This step is similar to step 3 in the section "Melasma-Specific Steps"
4. Stimulation	To activate keratinocyte phagocytosis of melanin in order to blend for an even color tone This step requires a special formulation of encapsulated retinol (apply in PM)

[*]The non-HQ approach will prove more effective if one performs a special peel 1 month after using the program above for one keratin maturation cycle (6 weeks). Recommended peels include the ZO Retinol Stimulation Peel and the ZO 3-Step Peel (see Chapter 9).

PHOTODAMAGE

Photodamage is a universal problem that can affect any skin type. It starts at an early age (2 to 3 years old) and is undetectable initially. However, as a person experiences more sun exposure over the years, damage becomes clinically significant, as localized and generalized pigmentation increases and texture (wrinkling, loss of elasticity) become apparent.

Box 7.10

Guidelines for Discontinuing Hydroquinone

To avoid HQ overuse, discontinue HQ:

■ After achieving an even skin tone (one to three KMCs, 6 to 18 weeks) in most skin types

■ After three KMCs (18 weeks) to avoid resistance that can lead to rebound hyperpigmentation

■ After one to two KMCs (6 to 12 weeks) in black skin to avoid hypopigmentation and photosensitivity

■ Whenever HQ stops delivering further improvement

Unfortunately, many physicians and the majority of the public do not recognize sun damage until it becomes severe and extensive (e.g., actinic keratoses [AKs] and skin cancers appear). Thus, they ignore the early signs of photodamage, such as tanning, freckles, and lentigines. One of the key messages of this chapter is that recognizing and treating photodamage in its earliest stages will help patients avoid the more severe and clinically troublesome types of photodamage and perhaps, more important, to prevent all photodamage, which is our ultimate goal. Figure 7.12 shows a patient with severe photodamage treated with ZO Programs. Figure 7.13 shows a patient with early signs of photodamage.

Prevention of Photodamage

The best way to address photodamage is not to have it occur in the first place. This requires going beyond basic sun protection and incorporating principles of Skin Health Restoration (Box 7.11).

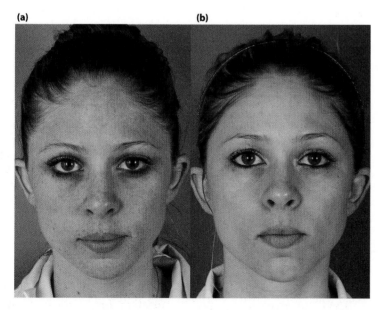

FIGURE 7.12 (a) Before. The patient had skin classified as original white, medium thick, and oily. She was diagnosed as having severe photodamage with lentigo, freckles, and actinic keratoses. She was treated with HQ-based ZO Medical for 5 months. (b) Six months later.

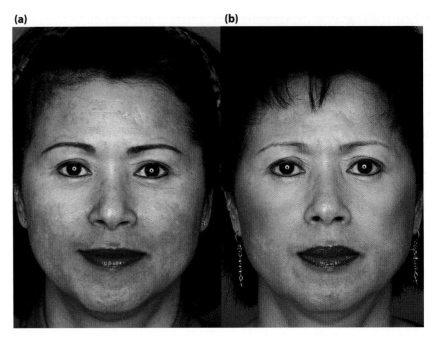

(a) **(b)**

FIGURE 7.13 (a) Before. The patient had skin classified as deviated Asian (medium), medium thick, and oily. She was diagnosed as having skin dullness, sensitivity, and nonspecific discoloration (early signs of sun damage). (b) One year later. The patient was treated for 2 to 3 months with non-HQ-based Skin Health Restoration to treat the skin sensitivity, followed by 3 months of HQ-based ZO Medical treatment and two ZO Retinol Stimulation Peels.

Box 7.11

Preventing Photodamage

- Avoid tanning: physicians must educate the public so that they know that tanning reflects DNA damage and a host of unhealthy skin changes that can have major consequences over time.
- Do not rely on sunscreens alone: regardless of how high the sun protection factor is, chemical and physical sunscreens wear off after 1 to 2 hours. Research shows consistently that people underapply sunscreen and fail to reapply it often enough.
- Practice sun avoidance: wear protective clothing (hats, long pants, and sleeves); pursue outdoor activities before 10 AM or after 4 PM, and use adequate sunscreen and protective clothing.
- Adopt a healthy skin protection program as part of a daily routine:
    - Load the skin with antioxidants (four to six types) in a proper formulation that also provides DNA protection and repair agents.
    - Enhance skin barrier function by using appropriate concentrations of retinol and alpha-hydroxy agents daily, and before applying sunscreens.
- Increase the skin's ability to repair and renew itself by following a skin care program that provides effective stabilization of the epidermis (keratinocytes and melanocytes) and the dermis (fibroblasts).

Along with the prevention and treatment of all early signs of photodamage, this chapter addresses the treatment of textural photodamage and solar elastosis because these conditions are part of skin aging and respond to rejuvenation therapies. This chapter also covers longer term forms of photodamage, such as photosensitivity and dyschromias. Additionally, the chapter addresses the advanced forms of photodamage (AKs and skin cancers), but only briefly. Much of this material can be found in more specialized skin cancer texts.

Aging Effects of Photodamage

Photodamage is a form of extrinsic aging (Box 7.12) and represents direct damage to the skin, whether the damage occurred superficially or at deeper levels.

Photosensitivity

Photosensitivity deserves special mention because it accelerates the onset and severity of many types of photodamage. The process begins with alterations in the skin's barrier function caused by problems ranging from dermatitis and other skin diseases to injury, allergy, infection, and excessive use of moisturizers or exfoliants. This altered barrier function causes skin sensitivity, which manifests as irritation, itching, burning, erythema, dryness, exfoliation, and/or intolerance to many topical cosmetic products.

People rarely consider the sun as a cause of skin sensitivity. However, dermatologic literature recognizes photosensitivity as an allergic or immune response to UV light. Photosensitivity is more widespread than previously recognized and plays a major role in aggravating all other causes of skin sensitivity. Additionally, because UV light can trigger skin inflammation, UV light alone can cause barrier function abnormalities.

Similarly, medications, including hydrochlorothiazide, antimalarials, tetracycline, and minocycline, and agents such as resorcinol, kojic acid, and salicylic acid (as well as HQ, discussed previously) can themselves cause skin sensitivity and are known to increase skin photosensitivity. Accordingly,

---

Box 7.12

Intrinsic versus Extrinsic Aging

INTRINSIC AGING

- A normal, progressive phenomenon characterized by skin atrophy.
- Proper treatment can correct, reverse, or at least slow down this process.

EXTRINSIC AGING

- Abnormal, progressive changes in skin appearance and texture that occur in response to factors such as cigarette smoking and sun exposure.
- With sun exposure, fair skin experiences more profound, aggressive changes, whereas darker skin undergoes milder changes.
- Avoiding harmful exposures is the key to preventing extrinsic aging.

Box 7.13

Treating Photosensitivity

■ Treat irritated areas with topical corticosteroids and/or oral antihistamines.
■ Avoid sun exposure, use sunscreens, and wear sun-protective clothing.
■ For best results, patients should also avoid photosensitizing chemicals and treat any skin sensitivity these chemicals may have caused.

photosensitivity can be considered the sole cause or an aggravating factor for all patients with sensitive skin. Treatment recommendations follow (Box 7.13).

Progressive Forms of Photodamage

No one wakes up one day with full-blown skin cancer. Rather, research has established conclusively that skin cancer tends to develop gradually, sometimes decades after a person's most harmful sun exposures. And the process begins with benign-looking initial changes (Box 7.14).

In Zein Obagi Skin Classification System, tanning, freckles, and most lentigines are acquired, epidermal, and endogenous (although one cannot rule out genetic causes in lentigines). Lentigo maligna, melanoma, and skin cancers may combine acquired and genetic causes and reside in the epidermis and dermis.

Tanning

Sometimes you hear people say that a golden tan is a healthy sign of beauty and vitality. In the Western world, some associate tanned skin with an active lifestyle and the pursuit of relaxation and recreation. Tanning accelerators and tanning salons are big business; in fact, the U.S. indoor tanning industry makes an estimated $5 billion annually.

Moderate sun exposure (no more than 15 minutes daily on exposed face and arms) does provide real benefits—it helps the body to synthesize vitamin D, which is necessary for bone health and perhaps prevents various diseases,

Box 7.14

Stages of Visible Skin Damage

■ Tanning
■ Freckles (ephelides)
■ Lentigines
  ■ Solar
  ■ Senilis
■ Lentigo maligna, lentigo maligna melanoma
■ Actinic keratoses
■ Skin cancers

Box 7.15

Tanning

Tanning is the body's attempt to protect itself by increasing pigment production; it is actually a sign of DNA damage.

such as multiple sclerosis and certain cancers. These preventive effects have yet to be proved beyond doubt, though. And even if they are substantiated, for people concerned about their vitamin D levels, it is much safer to take oral vitamin D supplements than to deliberately tan the skin.

In reality, tanning is a sign of DNA damage (Box 7.15). It is the skin's way of screaming for help and an attempt to protect itself by increasing pigment production. Both the World Health Organization and the U.S. Department of Health and Human Services have declared natural and artificially generated UV rays as known carcinogens. Exposure to these rays—especially early in life—has been shown to increase rates of melanoma and nonmelanoma skin cancer. Therefore, for health reasons, Westerners should emulate the approach to sun safety taken by women in Asia, Africa, and the Middle East. In these regions, people consider darker skin less desirable, a sign of lower social standing. These women faithfully apply sunscreens, wear hats, use parasols, and avoid peak midday sun exposure.

Freckles

Freckles (ephelides) are small, flat macules with a smooth surface and uniform color (light tan to brown). They occur predominantly on the face and nose, mainly in fair-skinned individuals, but can also involve other sun-exposed areas. Freckles result from increased activity of melanocytes in response to repeated sun exposure. As such, the sun darkens them, whereas HQ application can lighten them.

Freckles are more dangerous than a tan because their presence indicates that the person's skin cannot tolerate sun exposure (Box 7.16). More specifically, the focal areas where freckles actually appear will suffer somewhat less damage because the melanin content of the freckles provides some protection. However, the surrounding areas, which are unable to tan, will suffer the greatest damage, including textural changes, photoaging, actinic keratoses, and possibly skin cancer. Although freckles themselves rarely develop into skin cancer, it is important not to misdiagnose skin cancer as a freckle or vice versa, which could lead to unnecessary treatment and

Box 7.16

Freckles

Freckles are more dangerous than a tan because their presence indicates that the person's skin cannot tolerate sun exposure.

(a)   (b)

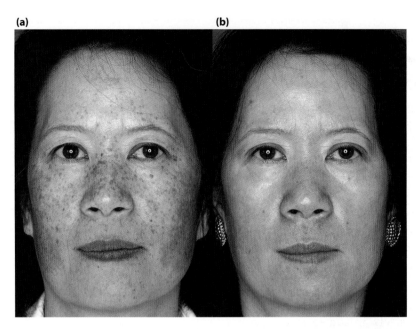

Figure 7.14   (a) Before. The patient had skin classified as deviated Asian (light), medium thick, and nonoily. She was diagnosed as having disseminated ephelides and melasma. (b) One year later. The patient was treated for 5 months with aggressive HQ-based ZO Medical, followed by a ZO Controlled Depth Peel 6 weeks later.

anxiety for the patient. Figure 7.14 shows a patient with disseminated ephelides and melasma.

Lentigines

Larger than freckles, lentigines are small (5 to 10 mm), round or oval macules of a light tan to brown color. Their surfaces can be smooth and flat or hyperkeratotic. Though usually the result of sun exposure, lentigines can appear on sun-exposed and on sun-protected skin (Box 7.17). Except for solar lentigines, lentigines do not darken in response to further sunlight exposure, and once formed, they generally persist in the absence of sunlight. Figure 7.15 shows a patient with multiple lentigos solares treated with a ZO Skin Health program and two treatments with the ZO Retinol Stimulation Peel.

Actinic Keratoses and Skin Cancer

Appearing on sun-exposed areas, AKs present as rough, scaly, often asymptomatic reddish macules measuring 2 to 15 mm. They can be atrophic or hypertrophic, appearing in relative isolation or in clusters. AKs may enlarge slowly and carry a greater than 20% risk for transforming into skin cancer (basal cell carcinoma, squamous cell carcinoma, de novo melanoma, and melanoma arising from lentigo maligna or from mutated nevi). The color and surface characteristics of AKs can help one distinguish them from solar lentigines. Figure 7.16 shows a patient with disseminated AKs and rosacea.

Diagnosing Early Photodamage

Distinguishing all types of lentigines and lentigo-like lesions can be done with a simple, gentle scratch test with a #15 blade. The scratch test produces the results shown in Box 7.18.

Box 7.17

Types of Lentigines

1. **Solar lentigines (lentigo solaris).** These lesions tend to have rougher, hyperkeratotic surfaces and appear on sun-exposed areas, indicating severe focal sun damage. Compared with freckles, solar lentigines historically show more dyskeratosis and DNA damage. This means that, over time, they can transform into lentigo maligna (see #3 below). Accordingly, dermatologists must closely follow patients with lentigo solaris and treat these lesions aggressively if they appear to have the potential to transform into lentigo maligna.

2. **Lentigo senilis.** Often called liver spots, these lesions actually reflect local areas of melanocyte proliferation and hyperactivity. They can have irregular borders, and they occur mainly, though not exclusively, in sun-exposed areas. As with solar lentigines, patients with lentigo senilis require monitoring to make sure these lesions do not develop into lentigo maligna.

3. **Lentigo maligna.** These premalignant areas of dark pigmentation, often found on the neck and face of older patients, show characteristic cancerous features, including enlargement, ill-defined borders, and color variations within individual lesions. They require biopsy and vigorous treatment because they are highly likely to develop into lentigo maligna melanoma (invasive melanoma).

(a)   **(b)**

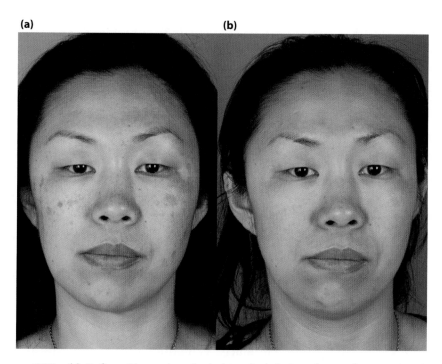

FIGURE 7.15 (a) Before. The patient had skin classified as deviated Asian (medium), medium thick, and nonoily. She was diagnosed as having skin dullness and multiple lentigo solares. (b) One year later. The patient was treated for 5 months with the ZO Skin Health program and had two treatments with a ZO Retinol Stimulation Peel.

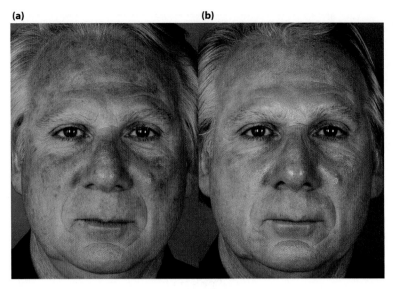

(a) **(b)**

Figure 7.16 (a) Before. The patient had skin classified as white (light), thick, and oily. He was diagnosed as having disseminated actinic keratoses and rosacea. (b) Three months later. The patient was treated for 5 months with aggressive HQ-based ZO Medical treatment.

Box 7.18

Scratch Test Results

- Freckles: no bleeding or scarring
- Lentigo solaris, lentigo senilis: fine scaling, lightening of lesions, no bleeding
- Lentigo maligna: lesion may or may not scale, does not lighten, and may bleed easily
- Actinic keratoses: scaling, bleeding

It is crucial to identify any lentigo maligna, dysplastic lentigines, and AKs because they require aggressive treatment.

Treating Visible Photodamage

As sun damage progresses, it requires increasingly aggressive treatments (Table 7.4).

Other Changes Indicating Textural Damage

Physicians and patients also must watch for longer term changes indicating that sun exposure is damaging the skin's texture (Box 7.19).

Solar Elastosis

Over time, damage to dermal collagen and elastin leads to the appearance of wrinkles that gradually become deeper, indurated, and unstretchable (see Box 7.7). Severe photodamage produces a condition known clinically as solar elastosis, in which damaged collagen and elastin accumulate in bulk in the dermis. This causes the skin to appear yellowish and to have a leathery texture and deep furrows and wrinkles. Figures 7.17 and 7.18 show patients with solar elastosis treated with a ZO Designed Controlled Depth Peel.

TABLE 7.4   Treatments for Visible Photodamage

Condition	Treatment
Freckles	Bleaching and blending
	Exfoliative peels and HQ treatment
	Sun protection to prevent recurrences
Lentigines:	
Lentigo solaris and lentigo senilis	Scraping with blade or curette, followed by TIA 30%
	Electrodessication
	Laser resurfacing (CO_2, erbium)
	ZO Retinol Stimulation Peel or ZO 3-Step Peel
	Correction, stimulation, and sun protection to prevent recurrences
Lentigo maligna	Proper surgical excision
Actinic keratoses	Treat topically (options include 5-fluorouracil, imiquimod, diclofenac, and ingenol mebutate)
	Cryosurgery (for isolated or small numbers of lesions)
	Photodynamic therapy, dermal peels
Skin cancer	Perform an accurate biopsy
	Diagnose properly
	Treat promptly with appropriate surgical and/or nonsurgical modalities

---

Box 7.19

Signs of Skin Textural Damage

- Solar elastosis
- Dyschromia
- Poikiloderma of Civatte

(a)   (b)

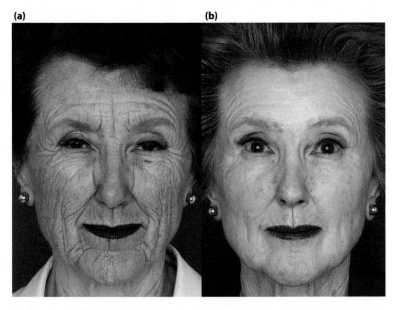

FIGURE 7.17   (a) Before. The patient had skin classified as original white (light), medium thin, and nonoily. She was diagnosed as having solar elastosis. (b) One year later. The patient had aggressive non-HQ-based Skin Health Restoration with emphasis on epidermal stabilization and stimulation, as well as a medium-depth ZO Designed Controlled Depth Peel.

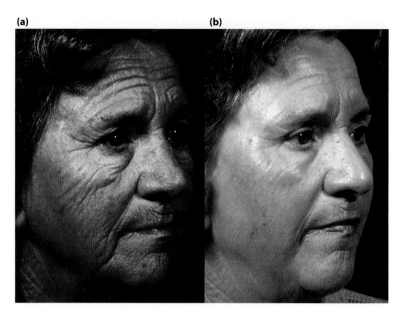

(a) **(b)**

FIGURE 7.18 (a) Before. The patient had skin classified as white (medium) thick, and nonoily. She was diagnosed as having severe solar elastosis. (b) One year later. The patient was treated for 2 to 6 months with aggressive, HQ-based Skin Health Restoration, followed by a medium-depth ZO Designed Controlled Depth Peel performed after 6 weeks of skin conditioning.

Dyschromia

Dyschromia refers to nonspecific pigmentation problems that can appear in sun-exposed areas, either alone or along with other forms of photodamage (e.g., lentigines, freckles, or uneven tanning). The identifying features of dyschromia include round focal areas of depigmentation surrounded by ill-defined patches of hyperpigmentation. The sharply demarcated depigmented lesions stem from the focal death of melanocytes and the presence of epidermal atrophy. The surface of these lesions may also display roughness and hyperkeratosis. Above all, dyschromia indicates that early textural (epidermal and dermal) damage has occurred.

Additionally, physicians sometimes misdiagnose dyschromia because it can look similar to other pigmentary changes, at least superficially. To avoid such misdiagnoses, consider the dyschromia look-alikes (Table 7.5). Figure 7.19 shows a patient with dyschromia.

Poikiloderma of Civatte

Poikiloderma of Civatte is a form of erythema associated with mottled pigmentation that appears on both sides of the neck, usually below the hairline. It

TABLE 7.5 Conditions that May Resemble Dyschromia

Condition	Differentiating Factors
Vitiligo	Dyschromia has surrounding circles of hyperpigmentation; vitiligo does not.
Postinflammatory hyperpigmentation (PIH)	Dyschromia affects only sun-exposed skin; unexposed adjacent areas appear normal, whereas PIH can affect sun-protected skin.
	If the patient has no associated condition that might cause PIH (e.g., acne, rosacea, injury, or dermatitis), it is dyschromia.

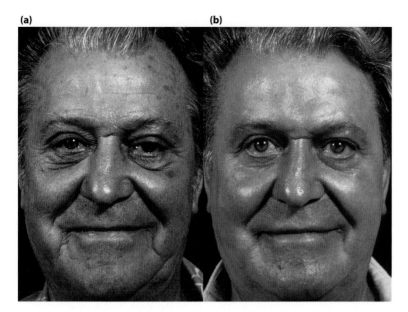

(a) **(b)**

FIGURE 7.19 (a) Before. The patient had skin classified as white, thick, and oily. He was diagnosed as having lentigos, actinic keratoses, and nonspecific discoloration (dyschromia). (b) One year later. The patient was treated with aggressive HQ-based Skin Health Restoration, followed by a medium-depth ZO Designed Controlled Depth Peel performed after 8 weeks of Skin Health Restoration.

typically strikes women, involving the upper lateral part of the neck, while the surrounding skin, which is equally sun-exposed, shows minor changes due to direct photodamage, but no apparent changes due to photosensitivity. It can prove somewhat difficult to diagnose and treat because it combines several elements:

- Dyschromia (hyperpigmentation and hypopigmentation)
- Photo-induced textural atrophy (dermal and epidermal)
- Telangiectasias
- Guttate dermal lumpiness (solar elastosis)

First characterized in 1923, poikiloderma of Civatte proves refractory to treatment unless the photosensitizing offender is eliminated. This offender is often perfume, which women tend to apply on both sides of the upper neck. With repeated application, the perfume photosensitizes the area, leading to much more severe photodamage than that found in perfume-free areas. After a patient stops using the perfume, the condition is more likely to respond to treatment.

Treating Deeper Photodamage
As with earlier forms of photodamage, treating textural changes induced by the sun requires matching therapeutic modalities with causative factors (Table 7.6).

NEVI

Nevus of Ota
Essentially a hamartoma of dermal melanocytes, this congenital nevus presents as a blue, blue-black, or gray patch on the temples, forehead, or periocular

TABLE 7.6   Treating Textural Changes

Solar elastosis (and textural damage)	Activate skin (correction, stimulation, bleaching and blending for three keratin maturation cycles [KMCs] [18 weeks]).
	For conditions that show improvement on skin stretch test, perform a trichloroacetic acid or ZO Controlled Depth Peel to the immediate reticular dermis.
	For conditions that do not show improvement with the stretch test, perform tightening procedures (e.g., CO_2 fractional laser or a custom-designed ZO Controlled Depth Peel).
Dyschromia (dermal and epidermal)	Use essential topical agents (tretinoin, hydroquinone, alpha-hydroxy acids), ideally using the aggressive approach for three KMCs (18 weeks).
	In the meantime, add a ZO Controlled Depth Peel to the papillary dermis.
	Consider laser resurfacing for dermal dyschromia.
	For pigmentation too deep to reach with laser resurfacing, a pigment laser treatment may be indicated.
	For focal depigmentation, a simple 2- to 3-mm epidermal punch graft can be used. (Topical agents and peels cannot correct focal depigmentation.)
Poikiloderma of Civatte	Discontinue application of perfume (or other irritants) on the neck, and instead apply perfume to hair-bearing areas on either side of the lower scalp.
	Add topical agents (aggressive approach) for three KMCs, plus peels and vascular laser treatment, if needed.

area. These nevi also can involve conjunctival and ocular tissue, as well as mucous membranes of the mouth and nose. Usually appearing unilaterally (and occasionally bilaterally), these lesions are present at birth and can darken and enlarge with age. They mainly affect Asian persons (usually women), though they can occur in black skin.

A biopsy of nevi of Ota reveals heavy deposits of melanin in the dermis and subepidermis caused by aberrant melanocytes located throughout the dermis. When considered as a whole, the foregoing factors dictate that Zein Obagi Skin Classification System groups them among genetic, endogenously caused disorders that can affect any layer of the skin. Figure 7.20 shows a photo of a patient with nevus of Ota and Figure 7.21 a patient with nevus of Hori.

Nevus of Hori

These brown-gray to brown-blue nevi look much like congenital bilateral nevi of Ota, except nevus of Hori typically involves the malar area. And although these nevi are present from birth, they usually become apparent in a patient's 40s or 50s (most often in women). Histologically, the abnormal melanocytes that cause these nevi reside in the papillary and middle portions of the dermis (not the subcutaneous tissue, or the conjunctiva and mucous membranes), causing dot-like or speckled patches of hyperpigmentation. As such, Zein Obagi Skin Classification System considers them to be genetic, endogenous, and dermal.

Diagnosis and Treatment of Congenital Nevi

The striking appearance of both nevi of Ota and Hori means that often they can be diagnosed based on clinical findings alone. However, these lesions may require careful follow-up; nevi of Ota in particular have been associated with comorbidities ranging from malignant melanoma to increased intraocular pressure. Additionally, neither type of nevus responds well to topical treatment with HQ. However, they typically respond well to four to six treatments

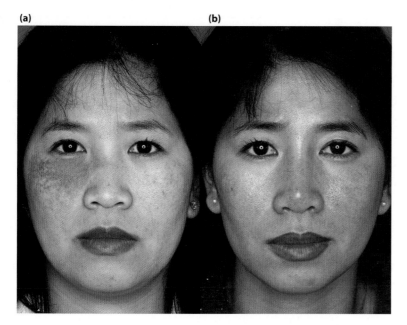

Figure 7.20 (a) Before. The patient had skin classified as deviated Asian (light) and medium thick. She was diagnosed as having nevus of Ota. (b) One year later. The patient was treated with moderate HQ-based Skin Health Restoration to prevent postinflammatory hyperpigmentation and stabilize her skin. She also underwent five Q-switched Nd:YAG 1,064-nm laser treatments.

with pigment-targeting lasers such as the Q-switched ruby, alexandrite, or Nd:YAG laser.

Nonspecific Dermal Melanosis

This condition presents as hyperpigmented patches occurring usually on areas that come in contact with scalp hair: the forehead, ears, and upper neck.

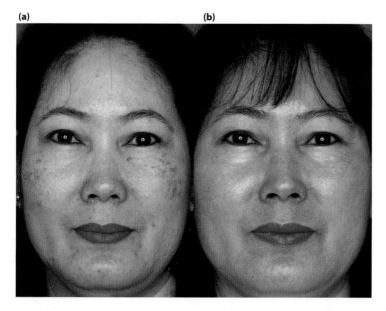

Figure 7.21 (a) Before. The patient had skin classified as deviated (medium) Asian, thick, and oily. She was diagnosed as having dermal pigmentation on the zygoma for many years that did not lighten with Dr. Zein Obagi Skin Stretch Test. She had failed to respond to previous treatments with HQ, exfoliative peels, and intense pulse laser treatments in different clinics. (b) One year later. The patient was treated for 2 to 5 months with aggressive HQ-based Skin Health Restoration. Four Q-switched Nd:YAG 1,064-nm laser treatments were performed at monthly intervals during Skin Health Restoration treatment.

Box 7.20

Treating Nonspecific Dermal Melanosis

■ Stop using the offending products (which may include heavy facial creams).
■ Undergo a series of peels to the papillary dermis.
■ Consider topical stabilization and stimulation through Skin Health Restoration. In some patients, however, this approach may worsen the condition.

It most commonly afflicts individuals who frequently treat their hair with chemical straighteners or apply oily products to help style or hold it in place. Zein Obagi Skin Classification System characterizes nonspecific dermal melanosis as a dermal condition with acquired, endogenous inflammatory causes (hair-treating agents induce chronic skin inflammation).

Unfortunately, this condition does not respond to any known treatments, including HQ or pigment-targeting lasers. However, patients may experience some improvement if they take the measures shown in Box 7.20.

OCHRONOSIS

Exogenous or acquired ochronosis develops gradually and progresses slowly, in response to external factors, such as HQ application. It typically presents as asymptomatic blue-black or blue-gray macules of varying intensity on sun-exposed areas such as the cheeks, temples, and neck (Box 7.21). Figures 7.22 and 7.23 show patients with ochronosis. Ochronosis occurs more frequently in black skin, particularly in regions such as Africa, where people try to lighten their skin color with HQ to achieve a higher social status. Recently, however, this condition has become a problem in other skin types, including skin of Asians, Hispanics, and Caucasians.

Performing Dr. Zein Obagi Stretch Test reveals the root of ochronosis to be guttate or pinpoint pigmentation in the dermis. Based on all these factors, Zein Obagi Skin Classification System characterizes this condition as exogenous, acquired, inflammatory, and dermal.

Alkaptonuria is an example of an endogenous cause of ochronosis. This autosomal recessive disease results from a deficiency of the enzyme HAO, which helps to metabolize the amino acids phenylalanine and tyrosine. The

Box 7.21

Ochronosis

Ochronosis typically presents as asymptomatic blue-black or blue-gray macules of varying intensity on sun-exposed areas.

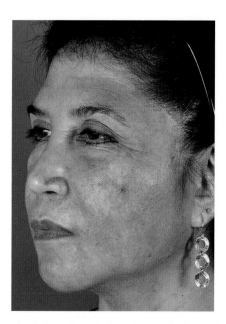

FIGURE 7.22 The patient had skin classified as deviated white (dark), thick, and oily. She had used 4% HQ for melasma, unsupervised, for 10 years. She was diagnosed as having ochronosis.

result is an accumulation of homogentisic acid (a byproduct of phenylalanine and tyrosine metabolism) in the dermis and other organs.

In both exogenous and endogenous ochronosis, the pigmentation level and severity are identical. But although exogenous ochronosis occurs mainly on sun-exposed skin, the pigmentation in endogenous ochronosis can also involve skin that is not exposed to the sun. The proposed pathophysiology of ochronosis is shown in Box 7.22.

Diagnosing, Managing, and Preventing Ochronosis

Because ochronosis affects only HQ-treated areas, diagnosing it and distinguishing it from other types of hyperpigmentation (e.g., induced by drugs or systemic diseases such as Addison's disease) are relatively simple. Similarly, biopsy findings and patient histories of prolonged HQ use can confirm the presence of ochronosis. However, no successful treatments for ochronosis exist. Exfoliative peels and non-HQ skin lighteners prove useless against it.

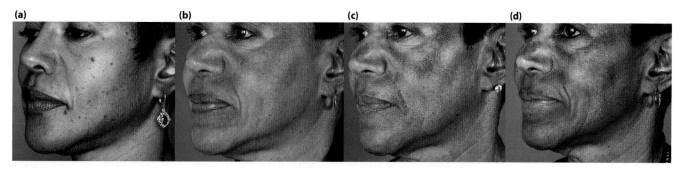

FIGURE 7.23 (a) Before. The patient had skin classified as deviated black (medium), medium thick, and normally oily. She was diagnosed as having postinflammatory hyperpigmentation and dermatosis papulosa nigra. She was seen in 1995 and treated with hyfrecation and bleaching and blending for 3 months with good results. (b) The patient in 2010 (15 years later). She was self-treating with 4% HQ (purchased online) without supervision. Notice the ochronosis on her left cheek. (c) The patient in 2012 (2 years after development of ochronosis). Two months after discontinuing HQ-based treatment, she started treatment with non-HQ-based blending with Brightenex-F and stimulation with Retamax-F. (d) The patient in 2013 (after 1 year of treatment). She is being treated with non-HQ-based blending and stimulation (as in 2012). Notice that the restoration of normal skin color tone is masking the ochronosis.

Box 7.22

Proposed Pathophysiology of Ochronosis

- A paradoxical increase in tyrosinase production causing rebound hyperpigmentation and pigment migration to the dermis
- Skin photosensitivity or phototoxicity, causing severe inflammation that leads to structural alteration in dermal melanin synthesis
- Resistance to HQ, possibly causing melanocytes to produce an altered form of melanin. Combined with photosensitivity, this creates a photoreaction and the appearance of classic ochronotic pigment in the dermis
- Suppression of homogentisic acid oxidase, leading to the accumulation of homogentisic acid in the dermis, as in alkaptonuria

Box 7.23

Addressing Ochronosis

- A topical regimen involving rigorous sun protection, melanocyte stabilization, and anti-inflammatory agents
- Repeated ZO Controlled Depth Peel to the papillary dermis
- Pigment laser therapy
- CO_2 fractional laser resurfacing (may be useful for mild ochronosis)

One may achieve partial success by stopping the patient's HQ use immediately, then choosing one or more of the measures shown in Box 7.23.

Recommendations

All cosmetic companies should refrain from using the word "whitening" on any of their products. As we all know, "whitening" the skin requires killing all the melanocytes. Medically, this is an extreme, high-risk measure for a purely aesthetic goal. Physicians sometimes try to do this in severe cases of vitiligo, using specific drugs (not HQ), all the while knowing that such patients will suffer the rest of their lives from severe photosensitivity.

Simultaneously, every effort should be made to regulate and restrict HQ use by persons without a proper medical indication and medical supervision. This approach includes efforts to end Internet and black-market sales of HQ. Additionally, manufacturers should make HQ available only in small packages that suffice to treat small, well-defined areas of skin, and these packages should carry a hefty price tag to discourage overuse.

Furthermore, HQ should carry an FDA-mandated "black box" warning against its dangers like many dermatologic drugs such as isotretinoin do. In short, physicians should make every effort to prevent HQ abuse and to prescribe it only in a safe manner, for specific medical indications, under medical supervision, and for a specified period of time.

OVERVIEW OF CHEMICAL PEELING AGENTS

HISTORY OF CHEMICAL PEELS

Although the ancient Egyptians used various herbs and chemical extracts as treatments to rejuvenate and beautify the skin,[1] peeling agents such as salicylic acid, resorcinol, phenol, and trichloroacetic acid (TCA) were not scientifically described until 1882 by the work of German dermatologist P. G. Unna.[2] Furthermore, the use of phenol to treat soldiers with gunpowder burns during World War I strengthened the knowledge base of this chemical peeling agent, which was used predominantly for the next 30 years.

MacKee used full-strength (88%) phenol for the treatment of acne scars as early as 1903; his biopsy findings 1 year after surgery showed compact collagen bundles and fibers arranged parallel to the surface.[3] In 1960, Ayres[4] essentially confirmed MacKee's findings when he reported a subepidermal band of new collagen with parallel fibers arranged horizontally following application of phenol to actinically damaged skin of the neck. Litton, in 1962, described an increase in the number and thickness of collagen fibers following a phenol peel.[5]

From the 1920s to the 1940s, TCA peels and sulfur and resorcinol pastes, salicylic acid, carbon dioxide snow, and 13-naphthol peels were described in the literature.[6-9] In the 1960s, the introduction of the Baker-Gordon formula for the phenol peel eclipsed other phenol peel protocols.[10-12] This formula penetrated deeper (to the mid-reticular dermis) than full-strength (88%) phenol, while also eliminating severe photodamage as well as deep rhytides. Baker, Stuzin, and Baker[13] believe that phenol peeling produces the most predictable degree of dermal penetration followed by a predictable degree of neocollagen formation and dramatic, long-term clinical improvement (Box 8.1, Table 8.1).

However, the striking clinical results of phenol peels came at the price of potential for serious systemic toxicity (cardiac, renal, and hepatic), toxicity to melanocytes that caused permanent hypopigmentation and a "china-doll" skin color,[14-21] conspicuous lines of demarcation between treated and untreated areas, and a prolonged post-procedure recovery period. Furthermore, phenol peels were not suitable because of the greater potential for scarring. Despite its toxicity, phenol was considered the gold standard for facial chemical peels[22] and was widely used. In a 1981 survey, 74% of plastic surgeons reported using

Box 8.1

Baker-Gordon Formula

- 3 mL 88% USP phenol
- 8 drops liquid soap (Septisol)
- 3 drops croton oil
- 2 mL distilled water

phenol for facial peeling.[23] In the 1990s, however, the phenol peel fell out of favor because of its reported complications.

To prevent potential complications such as systemic toxicity and hypopigmentation, only fair-skinned patients should undergo phenol peels, and the treatment needs to be applied slowly and cautiously.[24] Brody recommended dividing the face into five to eight segments, with application of phenol to each of the segments at 10- to 20-minute intervals.[25] Heart rhythm had to be monitored during the procedure and intravenous fluids administered.[26]

A number of safer and equally effective alternatives to phenol peels are now available. Dermabrasion is very effective for treating coarse rhytides and scars in the perioral, cheek, and forehead regions and does not have the same bleaching effect. However, it is not recommended for all skin types, cannot be used to treat rhytides around the eyes, and is a difficult procedure to master. CO_2 fractional laser resurfacing and deeper TCA peels such as the ZO Controlled Depth Peel, with a TCA concentration of 28%, can produce very effective results with full-face treatment and are replacing phenol peels for the treatment of deeper wrinkles and scars in most patients. These modalities produce more predictable results in terms of fewer changes in facial pigmentation because the depth of penetration of the peeling agent is controlled and can thus treat a wider spectrum of skin-color types.

The sharing of knowledge from multiple disciplines such as dermatology, plastic surgery, and cosmetic surgery has resulted in the availability of many techniques and makes it possible for us to improve the appearance of all skin types and colors, in facial and nonfacial areas, with a quality of results and safety not imagined 20 years ago. The methods that have been used for medium to deep chemical peels are shown in Box 8.2, and the mechanism of action of chemical peeling agents is shown in Table 8.2.

TABLE 8.1	Suggested Timing and Sequence for Full-Face Baker-Gordon Peel
Time	*Activity*
8:30 AM	Perioperative preparation: skin cleaning, analgesia, intravenous access, cardiac monitoring
9:00 AM	Solution applied to forehead
9:15 AM	Solution applied to first cheek
9:30 Am	Solution applied to contralateral cheek
9:45 AM	Solution applied to nose and glabella
10:00 AM	Solution applied to perioral and vermillion areas
10:15 AM	Solution applied to lower eyelids
10:30 AM	Solution applied to upper eyelids
11:00 AM	Patient monitored for 30 minutes before dressing of wound

Box 8.2

Methods Used for Medium to Deep Chemical Peels

- Phenol
- Conventional TCA, 35% to 50%
- 35% TCA augmented with solid CO_2
- 35% TCA augmented with Jessner's solution (resorcinol, salicylic acid, lactic acid, and ethanol)
- 35% TCA augmented with 5% to 10% methylsalicylate, 1% polysorbate 20

TABLE 8.2   Mechanism of Action of Chemical Peeling Agents

Agent	Mechanism of Action
Trichloroacetic acid (TCA)	Coagulation of dermal and epidermal proteins resulting in desquamation (keratolytic)
Phenol	Coagulation of dermal and epidermal proteins
Jessner's solution	Breaking of intercellular bridges to enhance effects of keratolytic agents
Alpha-hydroxy acids (AHAs)	Low concentrations (5%-10%) decrease corneocyte adhesion; high concentrations (50%-70%) produce epidermolysis

TRICHLOROACETIC ACID PEELS

The feasibility of performing a chemical peel that was less deep than a phenol peel became apparent in the 1980s as TCA peel techniques were refined to increase their efficacy and safety. Stagnone showed the absence of toxicity of 50% TCA.[11] Other investigators demonstrated the histologic changes that correlated with peel penetration depth in humans and in animal models[27-29] and provided clinical descriptions of patient peels.[30-32] Following these and other reports, the clinical spectrum of TCA skin peeling came to be recognized, ranging from exfoliation to eradication of lines, wrinkles, elastotic deposits, and mottled pigmentation (now called skin rejuvenation) by penetration to the papillary dermis or below.

Today, chemical peels using TCA are widely practiced techniques for superficial penetration depths (exfoliation) to deep penetration depths (mid-dermal penetration). These chemical peels are currently performed in a variety of ways, including the following:

1. Used alone in concentrations ranging from 30% to 50%
2. Combined with augmenting agents, such as glycolic acid or solid CO_2, for increased penetration
3. Use of the Designed and Medium-Depth ZO Designed Controlled Depth Peel with TCA, which can be performed to reach the papillary dermis (PD), the immediate reticular dermis (IRD), and the upper reticular dermis (URD). These peels have specific, clinically apparent

depth signs indicating that the desired proper depth has been reached. Specifically, a blue coloring agent is used as a guide for even application, and the TCA concentration is fixed at 20% or 26% to 28%, as needed.

This book emphasizes the ZO Controlled Depth Peel with TCA mentioned previously, as well as new exfoliative (epidermal) peels that provide dermal benefits (stimulation).

TRICHLOROACETIC ACID 30% TO 50%, USED ALONE

Although conventional TCA peels have produced good results in the hands of certain physicians, many others have experienced poor depth control and variable results. The properties of TCA vary with its concentration. However, at any concentration, TCA penetrates the skin quickly. Therapeutic effects dominate at low (≤30%) concentrations, producing protein coagulation and rapid self-neutralization, made apparent by the slow formation of a skin frost (see Figure 10.1). At high concentrations (>45%), the caustic effects of TCA dominate, producing protein denaturation and slow neutralization that allow deep and dangerous penetration to the dermis. Permanent textural damage, hypopigmentation, or even depigmentation and scarring are continuing concerns with higher concentrations. Other problem areas are a generally poor understanding of the mechanism of a TCA peel and poor control of the many variables involved, such as thin, fragile skin, where excessive dermal depth can be reached rapidly in concentrations of 35% or higher (strong caustic effects). Conventional, deeper TCA peels are difficult to perform and are not recommended for anyone but the most experienced physician.

The most important variable in the quality of outcome and safety of a TCA peel procedure is the depth of acid penetration (Box 8.3). Light penetration (to the basal layer) generally improves the epidermis and evens out superficial hyperpigmentation. If the upper papillary dermis is reached, improvement in texture, increased tightness, removal of fine lines, and correction of deeper pigmentation problems and some scars can be expected. Medium-depth wounding (reaching the URD to the mid-dermis) generally improves deeper wrinkles and scars, softens the texture, corrects deep discoloration, and increases skin firmness. Deep wounding (below the URD to the lower reticular dermis) should be avoided.

TCA peels in concentrations of 10%, 30%, and 50% have been erroneously classified as superficial, medium, and deep, respectively, with the assumption that a certain concentration penetrates to a certain depth.[33] As will be explained later, TCA concentration determines only the speed at which the acid penetrates the skin and the amount of skin protein needed to neutralize such a concentration. Specifically, higher concentrations penetrate faster and denature larger amounts of protein, leading to deeper peels, as well as a higher risk for scarring from the caustic effect. However, any concentration can be made to penetrate to any depth.

As with other rejuvenation procedures, TCA complications are correlated with depth; deeper TCA peels have a higher incidence of complications

Box 8.3

Peel Depth

- Skin thickness and fragility must be determined before the peel is performed, and only a proper safe depth should be considered.
- Peel depth is the most important variable in peel safety and quality of outcome.
  - Light penetration (to the basal layer) generally improves the epidermis and corrects superficial hyperpigmentation.
  - Penetration to the PD or the IRD leads to improvement in skin tightness and stretchable scars (removes fine lines), and corrects deeper pigmentation problems.
  - Penetration to the URD provides both tightening and leveling (corrects deeper wrinkles and scars, softens texture, corrects deep discoloration, and increases skin firmness).
- Deep wounding (below the URD) should be avoided.

than lighter TCA peels. Two common misconceptions about TCA peels are that high concentrations cause scarring, implying that lower concentrations are thus safer and that lower concentrations cannot penetrate deeply. Table 8.3 shows the general characteristics of the TCA peels known today, and Table 8.4 shows the problem areas of conventional, nonstandardized TCA peels. Box 8.4 shows the prevailing misconceptions about TCA peels. The Designed and Standard ZO Controlled Depth Peel was developed to address and prevent these problems. The ZO Peels are discussed in depth in subsequent chapters.

TABLE 8.3	Characteristics of Trichloroacetic Acid Peels
Characteristic	**Comment**
Histology	Upregulate production of collagen and elastin in the dermis, while maintaining the natural three-dimensional alignment of collagen
Neutralization	Self-neutralizing
Penetration	Higher concentrations penetrate skin faster
	Penetration can be increased with additional applications
	With continuous application, deep penetration can be achieved with any concentration
Quality of results	Depth reached generally determines the postpeel quality of skin texture and color
Skin conditioning	Conditioning before and after a TCA peel—through the patient's home use of topical agents—improves the quality of skin after the peel and expedites healing
Complications	Related to depth; deeper procedures have a higher risk for complications, such as keloids and hypopigmentation

TABLE 8.4   Variables Associated with Conventional, Nonstandardized Trichloroacetic Acid Peels

Variable	Characteristic
Concept of depth	Not consistent—a "superficial peel" can range from penetration to the stratum corneum to the papillary dermis
Skin type	Not properly classified for proper patient selection
Before and after skin conditioning programs (patients applying topical agents to treatment areas at home)	Erratic and arbitrary
Trichloroacetic acid concentration can vary from 20% to 50%	Optimal concentration is not identified
Depth-monitoring signs	Nonexistent

Box 8.4

Misconceptions about Trichloroacetic Acid Peels

Misconceptions	Reality
High concentrations cause scarring.	Scarring is related to depth.
Lower concentrations are safer because they cannot penetrate deeply.	With continuous application, low concentrations can penetrate to any depth.

ELIMINATING TRICHLOROACETIC ACID PEEL VARIABLES

The practitioner must keep in mind that a 100% safe chemical peel or procedure does not exist; however, risk can be significantly lowered with procedures that give the physician more control of the variables associated with the peel. Eliminating the variables provides more predictable penetration and depth, thus reducing complications, increasing peel safety, and ensuring the best results.

Many peeling methods have been devised to increase the penetration of TCA into the skin by using various agents mixed with TCA or applied to the skin before the application of TCA. These augmented peels are not necessary, however, because TCA does not need any enhancement to penetrate deeper (Box 8.5). These peels are mentioned here for historical value.

SOLID CARBON DIOXIDE PLUS TRICHLOROACETIC ACID

Adjunctive agents have been combined with 35% TCA to increase the depth of penetration, thus augmenting its action.[22,34] In 1986, Brody and Hailey reported satisfying clinical results with the application of solid carbon dioxide, followed by application of 35% TCA, to enhance the penetration of the

Box 8.5

Trichloroacetic Acid

■ Trichloroacetic acid (TCA) is a versatile peeling agent that can be used for a peel depth ranging from superficial (the stratum corneum) to deep (the lower reticular dermis).
■ The ability of TCA to correct skin conditions is controlled by two factors: 1) the depth of the problem, which is especially important in the case of scars; and 2) the depth of the peel that is performed.

TCA solution.[35] Specifically, actinic damage, appearance of atrophic scars, fine rhytides, and irregular hyperpigmentation were improved with this "medium-depth" peel. Histological specimens showed an expanded papillary Grenz zone (neocollagen formation in the subepidermal region of the dermis) and a mid-reticular dermal band consisting of elastic fibers and collagen. This technique was reported to penetrate to the upper reticular dermis, a depth that was similar to that previously reached with full-strength phenol, and to be more effective than Jessner's solution plus TCA in the treatment of scars.[36]

Solid carbon dioxide should not be used with TCA for several reasons:

1. It will produce edema with poorly defined boundaries at the site of application that can result in uncontrolled deeper penetration in certain areas.
2. It can destroy melanocytes not only in the epidermis but also in the adnexal structures, leading to hypopigmentation, especially in darker skin.
3. There are no clear endpoints for using the agent along with TCA.

This form of TCA peel is poorly controlled and yields unpredictable and variable results. It should be considered a questionable variation of a TCA peel until clinical studies demonstrating its value are available.

PEELS USING JESSNER'S SOLUTION, METHYLSALICYLATE, OR GLYCOLIC ACID PLUS TRICHLOROACETIC ACID

Jessner's Solution plus Trichloroacetic Acid

Monheit developed a medium-depth peel that incorporated Jessner's solution (resorcinol 14 g, salicylic acid 14 g, lactic acid 14 mL, and ethanol 100 mL), an agent that destroys the epidermal barrier function by breaking the intercellular bridges between keratinocytes.[37,38] His procedure involved vigorous degreasing with Septisol and acetone, then application of Jessner's solution to remove the stratum corneum and "open" the epidermis to TCA penetration, followed by application of 35% TCA. Formation of a white frost indicated protein coagulation. According to Monheit, the application of Jessner's solution allows TCA to penetrate to the papillary dermis and leads to the formation of new collagen that clinically decreases wrinkles and improves skin texture. Treatment with Jessner's solution plus TCA has been shown to reach the same depth and achieve similar results as solid carbon dioxide (CO_2) plus TCA, with the exception of the treatment of scars, for which solid carbon dioxide plus TCA has shown superior results.

Methylsalicylate plus Trichloroacetic Acid

Fulton[39] developed a hot-rod TCA peel that contained 35% TCA with 5% to 10% methylsalicylate to augment penetration and 1% polysorbate 20 as a surfactant. Dermabrasion was suggested 4 to 6 weeks after the peel to remove scars or remaining perioral and periorbital wrinkles.

Glycolic Acid plus Trichloroacetic Acid Peels

Glycolic acid 70% has also been applied before the application of 35% TCA. This is believed to allow TCA to frost more evenly and to penetrate deeper.[49] After 2 minutes of contact with the skin, the glycolic acid is removed with water, and the 35% TCA solution is applied. The skin sloughs between the fourth and sixth postoperative day, and after 7 days, the patient can usually wear makeup. Postoperative histology specimens showed effects similar to those of other medium-depth peels. According to the investigators, this peeling method has the advantage of not requiring storage of solid CO_2, the precise mixing of components needed for Jessner's solution, or vigorous pre-peel scrubbing with acetone.

Jessner's Solution, Methylsalicylate, or Glycolic Acid plus Trichloroacetic Acid

Removing the stratum corneum before the application of 35% TCA to enhance TCA penetration appears to have no clear advantage, and histological studies have not shown results to be any different from those obtained after a peel in which TCA alone was used. Subjecting the skin to two injurious agents is not necessary when TCA as a single agent can penetrate very well, and the second agent simply complicates the penetration issues. Acid penetration depth with peels that use augmenting agents is arbitrary, and the peels do not have clear endpoints indicating when application of the peeling agent should stop. Furthermore, papillary dermis peels performed with augmenting agents have erroneously been labeled "medium-depth" peels. Peels to this depth are in reality "superficial" peels (see recommended terminology in Chapter 10). Augmentation of TCA by removing the stratum corneum with methylsalicylate (the Fulton hot-rod peel) is similar to using Jessner's solution, and both techniques of augmentation are unnecessary.

GLYCERIN AND POLYSORBATE PLUS TRICHLOROACETIC ACID

In 1994, Dinner reported good cosmetic results with less irritation and easier and more even application when using a mixture of 40% TCA and glycerin that was emulsified with the surfactant polysorbate 20.[42] He believed that the concentration of TCA used for a peel was actually of limited importance and that factors such as volume of the acid, the force of application, and the susceptibility of the skin determined the depth of penetration and subsequent tissue destruction. He attributed the beneficial clinical effects and ease of application to the emollient action of glycerin.

Collins[44] reviewed the variables that affect penetration of TCA, including concentration of the acid, technique of application, prior use of retinoic acid, pre-peel skin degreasing, sebaceous gland density and activity, and application of pre-peel keratolytic agents and solutions. He believed a 15% to 25% TCA concentration would produce mild epithelial sloughing, whereas a 45% TCA concentration would produce necrosis of the epidermal proteins and a dermal, inflammatory infiltrate. With vigorous rubbing, however, a 35% solution could penetrate to the same depth as a 45% solution. Similarly, he stated that repetitive application of TCA would increase penetration, so that several TCA peels with a lower concentration, separated by intervals of weeks to months, could be as effective as a single, more concentrated peel.

Glycerin plus Polysorbate plus Trichloroacetic Acid

Dr. Dinner's peel follows Dr. Obagi's original principles and techniques to a certain extent, but his use of polysorbate 80, a well-known penetrating agent, makes it necessary to categorize this peel in the augmented TCA peel group. TCA penetrates skin very well, and agents that increase its penetration, such as polysorbate 20, lead to a faster appearance of frost and give the physician less time to observe depth signs.

ALPHA-HYDROXY ACID PEELS

Alpha-hydroxy acids (AHAs) have been extolled by manufacturers and the media as products that dramatically improve skin appearance and texture, despite a lack of well-controlled studies. Numerous daily-use skin care products contain AHAs in concentrations of 2% to 10%, and "refresher" or "lunchtime" low-concentration (e.g., 30%) glycolic acid peels are being performed by medical personnel as well as aestheticians for "rejuvenation." These procedures cannot live up to their rejuvenation claims because they remove only the stratum corneum for a simple exfoliation effect. They can produce smoother skin and improve comedogenic acne, but they have minimal effects on wrinkles or scars and cannot tighten lax skin. Unsubstantiated and inaccurate claims, however, are prevalent.

Although the mechanism of action is not fully known, glycolic acid is believed to thin the stratum corneum and thicken the stratum granulosum.[49-55] The effects are pH dependent; solutions with a pH between 2.8 and 3.5 are the most effective for inducing desquamation. Whether the therapeutic effects are merely a result of pH-induced irritation has not been demonstrated.

AHAs have also been used in concentrations of 50% to 70% for true chemical peeling to the level of the papillary dermis, usually using glycolic acid. A higher concentration, as well as an increased length of time the acid is left in contact with the skin, results in deeper penetration because these agents are not self-neutralizing like TCA. However, these peels rarely penetrate to the epidermal-dermal junction, and, if they do, penetration can be uneven. A 70% glycolic acid concentration in contact with the skin for up to 7 minutes

Box 8.6

Results with Glycolic Acid Peels

Clinical results with glycolic acid peels are subtle and hard to validate scientifically.

may not penetrate into the PD. Deeper penetration into the dermis, however, can occur if the peel is not monitored or neutralized properly, especially in thin skin. Cases of significant irritation and hypertrophic scarring have been reported. Fifty percent glycolic acid solutions, considered "safer" than the 70%, can also penetrate the dermis if left long enough on the skin.

Glycolic acid agents need to be neutralized by washing off with large amounts of water to terminate their action when they have penetrated to the desired depth. However, there are no clear endpoints for when to stop the peel. After application, the skin appears pink and then progressively redder, indicating penetration of the epidermis. If the solution has penetrated to the epidermal-dermal junction, small gray-white patches will appear, and with significant dermal involvement, some white frosting may be seen.

Uneven penetration and highly variable results from patient to patient have been reported with glycolic acid peels. Although a high concentration (>50%) of glycolic acid used repeatedly (over multiple sessions) can stimulate the dermis to form new collagen and increase glycosaminoglycans in the upper dermis, the process has to be repeated a number of times for beneficial effects to be realized. Patients often drop out before completion of the sequence, feeling dissatisfied with the limited improvement and inconvenience. Clinical results have been described as "subtle" and hard to validate scientifically (Box 8.6). As expected, more superficial beneficial skin changes, including surface texture, superficial hyperpigmentation, acne, and xerosis, can improve following a glycolic acid peel. Fine wrinkles may be improved, but deeper wrinkles are not.

A clinical study conducted to evaluate short-contact (3- to 6-minute) 70% glycolic acid peels used on a monthly basis showed no benefit in the treatment of photodamaged skin.[56] The investigators concluded that the value of glycolic acid "refresher peels" should be questioned as a "value-added" treatment for aging skin and that topical retinoids and low-concentration TCA peels are a better value for the consumer. Another study, however, of 50% glycolic acid applied for 5 minutes once weekly for 4 weeks showed mild improvement of some skin photoaging signs.[57] AHA research is currently in its infancy, and there is not yet enough scientific evidence to support AHAs as true therapeutic agents.[58]

REFERENCES

1. Bryan CP, trans. *Ancient Egyptian Medicine: The Papyrus Ebers.* Chicago: Ares Publishers; 1974:158-161.
2. Marmelzat WL. A historical review of chemical rejuvenation of the face. In: Kotler R, ed. *Chemical Rejuvenation of the Face.* St. Louis: Mosby; 1992:934-938.

3. MacKee GM, Karp FL. The treatment of post-acne scars with phenol. *Br J Dermatol.* 1952;64:456.

4. Ayres S. Dermal changes following application of chemical cauterants to aging skin. *Arch Dermatol.* 1960;82:578.

5. Litton C. Chemical face lifting. *Plast Reconstr Surg.* 1962;29:371.

6. Roberts HL. The chloroacetic acids: a biochemical study. *Brit J Dermatol.* 1926;38:323-391.

7. Monash S. The use of trichloroacetic acid in dermatology. *Ural Cut Rev.* 1945;49:119.

8. Ayres S. Superficial chemosurgery in treating aging skin. *Arch Dermatol.* 1962;82:125.

9. Eller JJ, Wolff S. Skin peeling and scarification. *JAMA.* 1941;116:934-938.

10. Baker TJ, Gordon HL. The ablation of rhytides by chemical means: a preliminary report. *J Fla Med Assoc.* 1961;48:541.

11. Baker TJ. Chemical face peeling and rhytidectomy. *Plast Reconstr Surg.* 1962;29:199.

12. Baker TJ, Gordon HL, Seckinger DL. A second look at chemical face peeling. *Plast Reconstr Surg.* 1966;37:487-493.

13. Baker TJ, Stuzin JM, Baker TM. Histologic effects of photoaging and facial resurfacing. In: *Facial Skin Resurfacing.* St. Louis: Quality Medical Publishing; 1998:12-28.

14. Wexler MR, Halon DA, Teitelbaum, et al. The prevention of cardiac arrhythmias produced in an animal model by the topical application of a phenol preparation in common use for face peeling. *Plast Reconstr Surg.* 1984;73:595-598.

15. Kligman AM, Baker TJ, Gordon H. Long-term histologic follow-up of phenol face peels. *Plast Reconstr Surg.* 1985;75:652-659.

16. Warner MA, Harper JV. Cardiac dysrhythmias associated with chemical peeling with phenol. *Anesthesiology.* 1985;62:366-367.

17. Stagnone JJ, Orgel MB, Stagnone GJ. Cardiovascular effects of topical 50% trichloroacetic acid and Baker's phenol solution. *J Dermatol Surg Oncol.* 1987;13:999-1002.

18. Lober CW. Chemexfoliation-indications and cautions. *J Am Acad Dermatol.* 1987;17:109-112.

19. Asken S. Unoccluded Baker-Gordon phenol peels: review and update. *J Dermatol Surg Oncol.* 1989;15:998-1008.

20. Alt TH. Occluded Baker-Gordon chemical peel: review and update. *J Dermatol Surg Oncol.* 1989;15:980-993.

21. Klein DR, Little JH. Laryngeal edema as a complication of chemical peel. *Plast Reconstr Surg.* 1983;71:419-420.

22. Beeson WH. Chemical peeling: a facial plastic surgeon's perspective. *Dermatol Surg.* 1995;21:389-391.

23. Litton C, Trinidad G. Complications of chemical face peeling as evaluated by a questionnaire. *Plast Reconstr Surg.* 1981;67:738-744.

24. Baker TJ, Stuzin JM, Baker TM. Histologic effects of photoaging and facial resurfacing. In: *Phenol Peels.* St. Louis: Quality Medical Publishing; 1998:118-143.

25. Brody HJ. Complications of chemical peeling: a variation of superficial chemosurgery. *J Dermatol Surg Oncol.* 1989;15:1010-1019.

26. Hopping SB. Chemical peeling in 1996: what have we learned? *Int J Aesthetic Restor Surg.* 1996;4:73-80.

27. Stegman SJ. A study of dermabrasion and chemical peels in an animal model. *J Dermatol Surg Oncol.* 1980;6:490-497.

28. Stegman SJ. A comparative histologic study of the effects of three peeling agents and dermabrasion on normal and sundamaged skin. *Aesthetic Plast Surg.* 1982;6:123-135.

29. Brodland DG, Cillimore KC, Roenigk RK. Depths of chemexfoliation induced by various concentrations and application techniques of trichloroacetic acid in a porcine model. *J Dermatol Surg Oncol.* 1989;15:967-971.

30. Resnick SS, Lewis LA, Cohen BH. Trichloroacetic acid peeling. *Cutis.* 1976;17:127-129.

31. Resnik SS, Lewis LA. The cosmetic uses of trichloroacetic acid peeling in dermatology. *South Med J.* 1973;66:225.

32. Brodland DG, Roenigk RK. Trichloroacetic acid chemexfoliation (chemical peel) for extensive premalignant actinic damage of the face and scalp. *Mayo Clin Proc.* 1988;63:887.

33. Brody HJ. *Chemical Peeling and Resurfacing.* 2nd ed. St. Louis: CV Mosby; 1997:109-136.

34. Collins P. Trichloroacetic acid peel revisited. *J Derm Surg Oncol.* 1989; 15:933-940.

35. Brody HJ, Hailey CW. Medium depth chemical peeling of the skin: a variation of superficial chemosurgery. *J Dermatol Surg Oncol.* 1986;12: 1268-1272.

36. Brody HJ. Variations and comparisons in medium-depth chemical peeling. *J Derm Surg Oncol.* 1989;15:953-963.

37. Monheit G. The Jessner's + TCA peel: a medium depth chemical peel. *J Dermatol Surg Oncol.* 1989;15:945-952.

38. Monheit GD. The Jessner's-trichloroacetic acid peel: an enhanced medium-depth chemical peel. *Cosmet Dermatol.* 1995;13:277-283.

39. Fulton JE. Step-by-step skin rejuvenation. *Am J Cosmet Surg.* 1990;7:199-205.

40. Coleman WP, Futrell JM. The glycolic acid-trichloroacetic acid peel. *J Dermatol Surg Oncol.* 1994;20:76-80.

41. Fulton, JE. Paper presented at American Academy of Aesthetic and Restorative Surgery, World Congress, Los Angeles, 1997.

42. Dinner MI, Artz JF. Chemical peel: what's in the formula? *Plast Reconstr Surg.* 1994;94:406-407.

43. Laub DR. Polysorbate as an adjunctive chemical in the trichloroacetic acid peel [letter]. *Plast Reconstr Surg.* 1995;95:425.

44. Collins PS. Trichloroacetic acid revisited. *J Dermatol Surg Oncol.* 1989;15:933-940.

45. Johnson JB, Ichinose H, Obagi ZE, Laub, DR. Obagi's modified trichloroacetic acid (TCA)-controlled variable depth peel: a study of clinical signs correlating with histological findings. *Ann Plast Surg.* 1996;36:225-237.

46. Obagi ZE, Sawaf MM, Johnson JB, et al. The controlled depth trichloroacetic acid peel: methodology, outcome, and complication rate. *Int J Aesthetic Restor Surg.* 1996;4:81-94.

47. Duffy D. Alpha hydroxy acids/trichloroacetic acids risk/benefit strategies: a photographic review. *Dermatol Surg.* 1998;24:181-189.

48. Baker TJ, Stuzin JM, Baker TM. *Facial Skin Resurfacing.* St. Louis: Quality Medical Publishing; 1998:88.

49. Van Scott EJ, Yu RJ. Alpha hydroxy acids: therapeutic potentials. *Can J Dermatol.* 1989;1:108-112.

50. Matarasso ST, Salman SM, Glogau RG, et al. The role of chemical peeling in the treatment of photodamaged skin. *J Dermatol Surg Oncol.* 1990;16:945-954.

51. Moy LS, Murad H, Moy RL. Glycolic acid peels for the treatment of wrinkles and photoaging. *J Dermatol Surg Oncol.* 1993;19:243-246.

52. Moy LS, Murad H, Moy RL. Glycolic acid therapy: evaluation of efficacy and techniques in treatment of photo damage lesions. *Am J Cosmet Surg.* 1993;10:1.

53. Murad H, Shamban AT, Premo PS. The use of glycolic acid as a peeling agent. *Dermatol Clin.* 1995;13:285-307.

54. Daniello NJ. Glycolic acid controversies. *Int J Aesthetic Restor Surg.* 1996;4:113-116.

55. Draelos ZD. Dermatologic considerations of AHAs. *Cosmet Dermatol.* 1997;10:14-18.

56. Piacquadio D, Dobry M, Hunt S, et al. Short contact glycolic acid peels as a treatment for photodamaged skin: a pilot study. *Dermatol Surg.* 1996;22:449-452.

57. Newman NN, Newman A, Moy LS, et al. Clinical improvement of photoaged skin with 50% glycolic acid. *Dermatol Surg.* 1996;22:455-460.

58. Brody H, Coleman WP, Piacquadio D, et al. Round table discussion of alpha hydroxy acids. *Dermatol Surg.* 1996;22:475-477.

EXFOLIATING CHEMICAL PEELS

ELIMINATING THE GUESSWORK

Chemical peels have been used for decades to improve the skin's appearance by addressing problems ranging from sun damage and minor wrinkling to specific dermatologic conditions, such as melasma and postinflammatory hyperpigmentation (PIH). Until recently, all chemical peels on the market were based on one simple concept: application of one or more acid solutions directly onto the skin surface. These agents would remove variable levels of the epidermis and dermis, after which the patient's skin would heal by replacing the treated or damaged skin with fresh-looking, new skin. In general, the deeper the peel was allowed to penetrate, the longer the treated area took to heal.

Exfoliative peels improve only the epidermis, a fact not often explained to the patient. These superficial, exfoliative peels, currently the most popular type of chemical peel being performed, do not have a uniform lexicon in terms of their active ingredients, percentage strength of each component, and overall efficacy. Many contain active ingredients of questionable efficacy. Results of many currently available exfoliative peels are unpredictable—some exfoliative peels are effective in inducing epidermal exfoliation, whereas others are not. Similarly, deeper penetrating, dermal peels, as discussed in Chapter 10, also tend to be poorly defined, have multiple difficult-to-control variables, and produce unpredictable results. Furthermore, the terms "light," "medium," and "deep," when used to describe chemical peels, are virtually meaningless because peel ingredients, percentage concentrations, and ultimate efficacy of these peels vary greatly, depending on the active ingredients, the physician's skill level, and other patient-related factors (Boxes 9.1 and 9.2).

AGENTS USED FOR EXFOLIATING CHEMICAL PEELS: MECHANISMS OF ACTION AND OTHER PROPERTIES

TRICHLOROACETIC ACID

Trichloroacetic acid (TCA) works by coagulating epidermal and dermal proteins and can be used for both epidermal and dermal peels. A few days after application of TCA, the affected cells in each skin layer that is reached by the acid will

---

Box 9.1

Variables Related to Peeling Agents that Affect Outcome

Currently, there is no generalized consensus regarding the following:

- Suitable active ingredients in terms of peeling agents for penetrating to specific depths (exfoliative agents are not suitable for dermal peels)
- Ideal concentrations of acids used for peels penetrating to specific depths
- Ideal volume of acid solution for specific size of skin surface areas
- Methods for ensuring even application, absorption, and interaction of the peeling agents with the skin.

---

peel off as sheets. Repeated application causes the peel to penetrate more deeply as the TCA coagulates more protein. In other words, the concentration and volume of TCA determine the TCA peel depth (Box 9.3). After application, a frost usually forms and gradually progresses. TCA is not absorbed systemically, and it self-neutralizes following interaction with skin proteins. Thus, unlike several other chemical peeling agents (e.g., glycolic acid), the treatment site does not have to be treated with sodium bicarbonate or another neutralizing agent

---

Box 9.2

Patient-Related Variables that Affect Peel* Outcome

- Poor or uneven skin hydration†
  - Properly hydrated skin (through proper and adequate skin conditioning) allows consistent, even acid penetration and distribution because well-hydrated skin shows a quick, visible, quantifiable response (frosting) after acid application and heals evenly and relatively quickly.
- Poorly hydrated skin (due to improper or inadequate skin conditioning) shows little to no visible or quantifiable response initially. This delayed response can lead the physician to administer additional layers of acid, which yield a deeper than intended peel penetration and can ultimately lead to adverse events.
- Skin sensitivity (innate or acquired)
  - Sensitive skin is indicative of skin having an impaired barrier function.
  - Sensitive skin is unsuitable for any resurfacing procedure because of its propensity toward developing strong post-procedural irritation, inflammation, and suboptimal healing.

*This box uses trichloroacetic acid as the example of the peeling agent, but most of the principles can be applied to other chemical peeling agents as well.

†Adequate and even skin hydration are achieved by at least 6 weeks of consistent daily topical use of products to precondition skin (see Chapter 2).

---

continued

211

AGENTS USED FOR
EXFOLIATING CHEMICAL
PEELS: MECHANISMS
OF ACTION AND OTHER
PROPERTIES

Box 9.2

Patient-Related Variables that Affect Peel Outcome
(Continued)

■ Presence of certain active diseases (including autoimmune disorders)
  ■ Those with active lesions or simply a history of autoimmune condi-
    tions such as systemic lupus erythematosus, discoid lupus erythe-
    matosus, or bullous disorders, and those with vascular dysfunction,
    such as stasis dermatitis or vasculitis, should not undergo chemi-
    cal peels or other resurfacing procedures because these disorders
    are associated with compromised healing and occasional flares of
    otherwise latent disease.
  ■ In contrast, those with disorders related to pilosebaceous units (acne,
    rosacea, and seborrheic dermatitis) can benefit from exfoliative peels
    as part of a treatment protocol, even when their disease is active.
    Of note, these conditions should be controlled before these patients
    undergo more deeply penetrating procedures, such as dermal peels or
    other resurfacing procedures.

Box 9.3

The concentration and volume of trichloroacetic acid determine the
peel depth.

following application of the TCA. Of note, TCA penetrates through the skin
rapidly (within 1 to 2 minutes), and *its effects cannot be reversed* by washing skin
with water or sodium bicarbonate after the cutaneous proteins have coagulated.

ALPHA-HYDROXY ACIDS

Used for epidermal exfoliation, alpha-hydroxy acids (AHAs) break apart bonds
between skin cells (desmosomes), which allows epidermal exfoliation to occur
through the shedding of single cells. AHAs are water soluble. The main AHAs
used in dermatology are glycolic, lactic, and mandelic acid. There is no generally accepted consensus regarding the ideal concentration of AHAs needed
to achieve an optimal epidermal exfoliating effect. Typically, concentrations of
glycolic acid used for this purpose vary broadly, usually ranging from 30% to
70%. AHAs are not absorbed systemically and *do not* self-neutralize. Thus, areas
treated with AHAs must be neutralized after several minutes by the application of a basic solution like sodium bicarbonate or diluted by the application of
water; the approximate time that the AHA should be in contact with the skin
(before dilution or neutralization) usually ranges from 3 to 5 minutes. Without
subsequent neutralization or dilution, the AHAs and their associated effects will
penetrate deeper than intended (occasionally into the dermis). AHAs penetrate
slowly through the epidermis. However, the amount of time that the AHAs are

allowed to sit on the skin needs to be carefully monitored because they are very caustic to collagen and elastin and will cause scarring if permitted to penetrate to the depth of dermis. The practitioner should expect some redness and little to no frost to appear on treatment sites after application of AHAs.

BETA-HYDROXY ACIDS

Also effective in inducing epidermal exfoliation, beta-hydroxy acids (BHAs) essentially "melt" cells with which they come in contact (acantholysis), leading to epidermal shedding and exfoliation. The most commonly used BHA in dermatology is salicylic acid. Of note, *unlike TCA and AHAs, BHAs are lipophilic and are thus systemically absorbed.* Thus, BHAs have the potential to yield both allergic and toxic reactions. Salicylate toxicity, though rare, can affect the central nervous system (e.g., confusion, dizziness, psychosis) as well as the gastrointestinal system (nausea and vomiting). Consequently, in general, physicians should avoid using BHAs in concentrations greater than 30% because higher concentrations not only are more likely to induce negative side effects but also have not been shown to offer additional benefit compared with solutions of less than 30%. Similar to AHAs, BHAs are not self-neutralizing and also penetrate the epidermis quickly. The practitioner must use caution when determining how much time to allow the BHA solution to be in contact with the skin before dilution and neutralization (optimal times typically range from 3 to 5 minutes). Also similar to what is observed with AHA application, little to no frost will appear after the application of a BHA to the skin.

RESORCINOL

Resorcinol is used for epidermal action. Its mechanism of action is much like that associated with phenol, which is a deeper dermal peel solution that has lost its popularity because of its potential for serious systemic side effects. Specifically, both resorcinol and phenol induce epidermal acantholysis as well as coagulation and precipitation of cellular proteins. With resorcinol, protein coagulation is limited to keratinocytes within the epidermis, whereas with phenol, penetration is deeper, and proteins within the dermis are coagulated. Although serious systemic side effects are more likely to occur with phenol, resorcinol is much less likely to induce systemic effects. Of note, resorcinol is absorbed systemically and can lead to methemoglobinemia, especially when used on children or on large areas of the body.

A NOVEL APPROACH TO CHEMICAL PEELS

The lack of predictability and efficacy of previously available chemical peels inspired the development of new principles and applications. The result is a comprehensive spectrum of chemical peels that address and minimize the previously mentioned uncertainties (e.g., optimal concentration of the active ingredients in the peeling solution, optimal total volume of the acid solution administered, and ideal duration of time between when the acid and the diluting and neutralizing agent are subsequently applied, when the solution is not self-neutralizing). Specifically, this new approach has fine-tuned the art of administering chemical peels to make them safer to perform and easier to learn through the following measures:

- Adopting a skin classification system (see Chapter 4) that takes into account the effect of skin thickness, color, and suitability for peels to various depths
- Conditioning the skin before the peel to eliminate skin sensitivity, restore proper hydration, and activate the skin's ability to renew itself
- Establishing that TCA is the gold-standard peeling agent to be used when one wants to perform a chemical peel that penetrates down to the level of the dermis. TCA offers superior, predictable results; short-lived activity (seconds); and a self-neutralizing capability. Because of the latter, it does not need to be washed off or buffered with a basic solution.
- Incorporating a color guide (blue dye) into the peeling solution, which penetrates into the dermis, to ensure that an even application and intended depth are reached
- Standardizing optimal concentrations and formulations of TCA used in chemical peels, as well as the appropriate volumes for specific surface areas and intended depths of penetration
- Obtaining not only superficial, exfoliating benefits of more superficial peels but also the deeper, dermal benefits following such peels
- Allowing physicians to accurately determine the depth of dermal penetration by providing clearly identifiable, clinical depth signs
- Establishing safe, yet effective, peel depths for all skin types (determined by observing clinical depth signs). This way, peels will not alter one's original skin color or texture, and the chances of serious complications are minimized.

These innovations include three highly safe and reliable exfoliative peels, as well as a universal dermal peel (Table 9.1) that offers clearly identifiable depth signs. More specific details regarding this dermal peel are given in Chapter 10. Through this comprehensive spectrum of chemical peels, characterized by the

TABLE 9.1 ZO Peels: Penetration Depths and Their Associated Objectives

Peel	*Penetration Depth*	*Objective*
ZO Retinol Stimulation Peel (home application)	Epidermis	Light exfoliation and stimulation (epidermis and upper dermis)
ZO Invisapeel	Epidermis	Near-invisible (microscopic) exfoliation
ZO 3-Step Peel	Epidermis	Deep exfoliation and stimulation (epidermis and upper dermis)
ZO Controlled Depth Peel	Papillary dermis	Mild skin tightening
	Immediate reticular dermis	Strong skin tightening
	Upper reticular dermis	Maximal skin tightening and some skin leveling

intended and maximal depth of penetration, physicians are now able to offer a peel that precisely reaches whichever of the following four main levels that one desires: the epidermis, the papillary dermis (PD), the immediate reticular dermis (IRD), and the upper reticular dermis (URD).

NEW ZO EXFOLIATING PEELS

To simplify the exfoliating peel process and increase its benefits, the new exfoliating peels—ZO Retinol Stimulation Peel, Invisapeel, and ZO 3-Step Peel—combine agents that induce epidermal exfoliation and strongly stimulate the epidermis and dermis simultaneously. This is not generally characteristic of other exfoliating peels on the market. The ZO exfoliating peels are delivered in easy-to-administer packages with clear instructions. They are remarkably safe, resulting in little to no side effects *when performed properly on compliant patients*.

ZO RETINOL STIMULATION PEEL

Retinol is a powerful acid that can be very irritating and chemically unstable. Vehicles and formulations that include water or oil significantly diminish retinol's activity. The concentration of retinol must be 1% or greater in chemical peels and greater than 0.3% in topical cosmetic products. However, most retinol-containing products currently on the market contain only trace amounts of retinol (below a 0.3% concentration), and the retinol may be delivered in a neutralized form by manufacturers trying to reduce irritation. The efficacy of these products is therefore highly questionable (Box 9.4).

The ZO Retinol Stimulation Peel, a home peel that entails several consecutive days of twice-daily application of a specified amount of Ossential Advanced Radical Night Repair, avoids the previously mentioned problems through its unique anhydrous formulation as well as its 1% concentration of retinol. The retinol is encapsulated in microspheres and liposheres to reduce potential irritation. The microspheres and liposheres allow absorption of retinol into skin cells and prevent contact of free retinol with the skin extracellularly. This ultimately reduces the potential for irritation. When applied nightly, the retinol in Ossential Advanced Radical Night Repair functions as an anti-aging agent, delivered in a stabilized formulation. The cream is applied to the face each night (4 pumps, the equivalent of 1 gram). For a milder approach,

---

Box 9.4

Most retinol-containing products currently on the market contain only trace amounts of retinol (below a 0.3% concentration), and the retinol may be delivered in a neutralized form by manufacturers trying to reduce irritation. The efficacy of these products is highly questionable.

patients may begin with two pumps, which is the equivalent of ½ gram, once to twice weekly and gradually increasing, as tolerated, to a goal of nightly application of 4 pumps (1 gram).

When used twice daily as a peeling agent, it can induce exfoliation through dehydration and forced exfoliation of the surface epidermis for 2 to 3 days, leading to much deeper and more powerful stimulation and anti-aging effects. This stimulation also improves skin strength and texture by increasing the production of collagen, elastin, and glycosaminoglycans.

Use of Retinol versus Tretinoin

For direct application to the skin, retinol is preferred over tretinoin (Table 9.2). Tretinoin is extremely irritating and, as a free agent, penetrates through the epidermis intercellularly before exerting its benefit intracellularly. Any excess tretinoin that remains extracellularly within the epidermis will continue to cause severe irritation. It is virtually impossible to predict the optimal amount of tretinoin for any given treatment area of skin. In contrast, the retinol in Ossential Advanced Radical Night Repair penetrates down to the dermis, while causing exfoliation of only the upper portion of the epidermis.

Home Application

The specially formulated retinol (with an anhydrous base) allows Ossential Advanced Radical Night Repair to be used nightly as part of a basic skin care regimen and twice daily as a peeling agent that provides strong stimulation and benefits. This was demonstrated in 100 patients of all skin types and with various skin disorders. After completion of the ZO Retinol Stimulation Peel, all experienced healing times of 3 to 4 days, without occurrence of significant irritation, redness, or sensitivity. Subsequently, patients experienced continuous improvement for 2 to 3 weeks after the peel, which other current commercially available exfoliating peels cannot provide.

TABLE 9.2 Properties of Retinol versus Tretinoin as Peeling Agents

Properties	Retinol	Tretinoin
Formulation	1% Anhydrous	0.4% in oil
Volume/size of treatment area	Controlled	Uncontrolled
Penetration	Even and effective	Variable and poor
Stabilization benefits	Strong	None
Anti-aging effects	Strong	Weak (poor penetration)
Irritation	Minimal and short lived	Strong and dominant
Use of applied amount	Complete	Partial (unused portion causes continuous irritation)
Healing	Three to 4 days, with no residual redness	Five to 6 days, with redness for 1 week or more
Indications	Prevention, anti-aging, and textural benefits	Not popular; no clear indications
Person performing the peel	Patient, at home	Physician, in clinic

Mechanism of Action

In the upper epidermis, the stratum corneum and the stratum granulosum (down to the upper mid-epidermis) are composed of keratinocytes that are rich in keratin granules and are significantly less hydrated than the keratinocytes in the lower epidermis. The less-hydrated upper epidermis, on contact with the retinol in the anhydrous base, dries up completely and exfoliates, whereas the hydrated lower portion of the epidermis is unaffected because of its higher level of hydration.

In the lower epidermis, well-hydrated keratinocytes offer no barrier resistance to the penetration of retinol within the Ossential Advanced Radical Night Repair formula. This explains why the encapsulated retinol is able to penetrate through the lower portion of the epidermis into the PD. After daily application of Ossential Advanced Radical Night Repair, exfoliation starts on about day 3 and is completed by days 6 to 7. Figure 9.1 illustrates the penetration of the ZO Retinol Stimulation Peel according to day of application.

Course Duration

The reactions experienced by patients undergoing a standard duration (5 consecutive days of application) or a short duration (3 consecutive days of application) of the ZO Retinol Stimulation Peel are shown in Table 9.3. For both the standard and the short duration course, the patient is to apply Ossential Advanced Radical Night Repair twice daily; the strength of treatment can be further adjusted to light, medium, or strong based on the total amount of

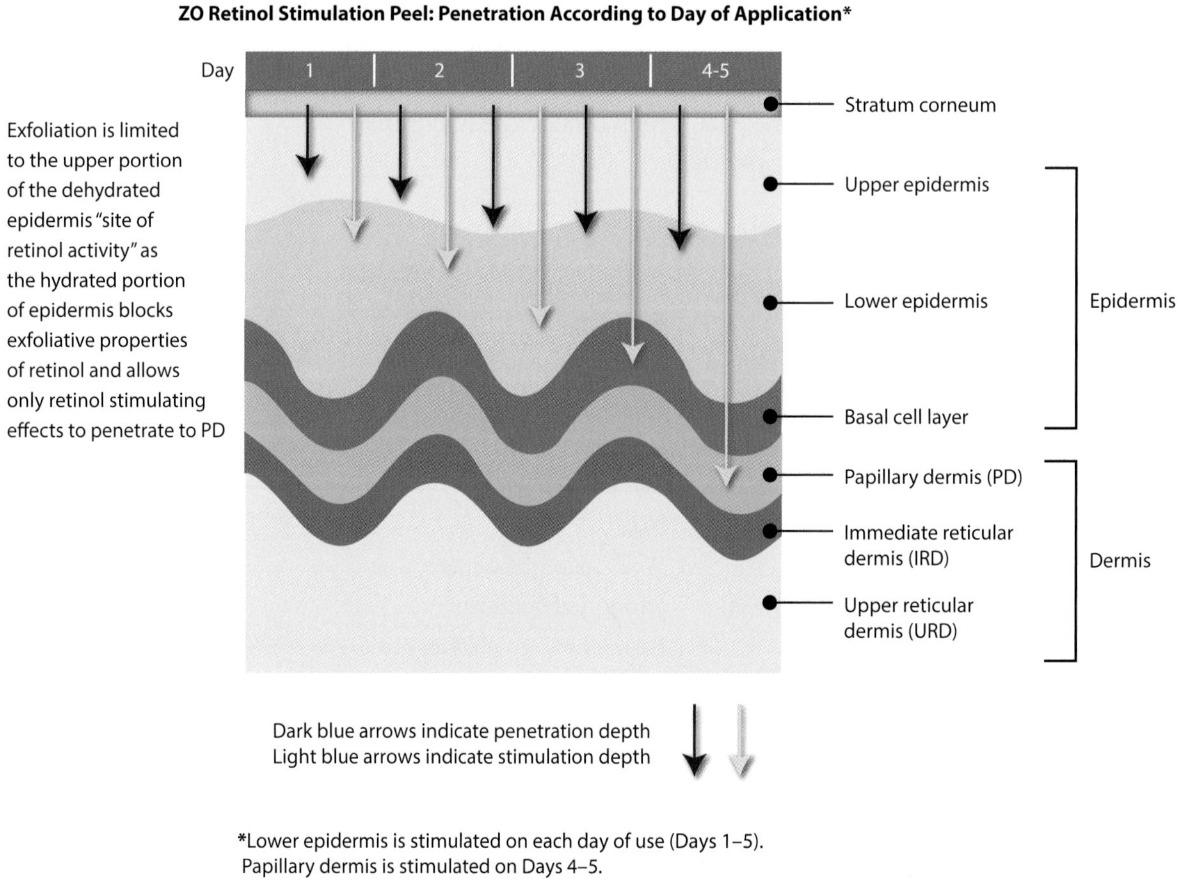

ZO Retinol Stimulation Peel: Penetration According to Day of Application*

Exfoliation is limited to the upper portion of the dehydrated epidermis "site of retinol activity" as the hydrated portion of epidermis blocks exfoliative properties of retinol and allows only retinol stimulating effects to penetrate to PD

Day 1 2 3 4-5

Stratum corneum
Upper epidermis
Lower epidermis — Epidermis
Basal cell layer
Papillary dermis (PD)
Immediate reticular dermis (IRD) — Dermis
Upper reticular dermis (URD)

Dark blue arrows indicate penetration depth
Light blue arrows indicate stimulation depth

*Lower epidermis is stimulated on each day of use (Days 1–5).
Papillary dermis is stimulated on Days 4–5.

FIGURE 9.1 Penetration according to day of application during the ZO Retinol Stimulation Peel.

TABLE 9.3 Anticipated Sensations and Reactions during the ZO Retinol Stimulation Peel (Standard and Short Duration)

	Standard Duration ZO Retinol Stimulation Peel (5 Days)
Day	**Reactions**
1	Begin application—no reaction or a mild, stinging sensation
2	Tightness and/or a mild, stinging sensation
3	Tightness and stinging sensation; exfoliation begins
4	More intense exfoliation
5	Same or slightly less exfoliation (last day of treatment/application)
6	No longer applying Ossential Advanced Radical Night Repair Begin anti-inflammation treatment and hydration, four to five times daily
7	Continue anti-inflammation treatment and hydration, four to five times daily Expect complete healing
8	Patient should be instructed to return to his/her pretreatment topical regimen
	Short Duration ZO Retinol Stimulation Peel (3 Days)
Day	**Reactions**
1	Begin application—no reaction or a mild, stinging sensation
2	Tightness and/or a mild, stinging sensation
3	Tightness and/or stinging sensation; exfoliation begins Final day of application of Ossential Advanced Radical Night Repair
4	Begin anti-inflammation treatment and hydration, four to five times daily Expect complete healing
5	Patient should be instructed to return to his/her pretreatment topical regimen

TABLE 9.4 Variable Strengths of the ZO Retinol Stimulation Peel and Associated Ultimate Responses

Strength	Amount Applied* (No. of Pumps)	Anticipated Response[†]
Light	5	Mild exfoliation, mild stimulation
Medium	8	Moderate exfoliation, moderate stimulation
Strong	10-12	Intense exfoliation, strong stimulation

*Regardless of which treatment strength category is chosen, the Ossential Advanced Radical Night Repair should be applied twice daily.

[†]The physician may have the patient change to ZO Retinol Stimulation Peel strength Ossential Advanced Radical Night Repair. To shorten the exfoliation and healing phase, the physician may recommend that the patient perform the ZO Retinol Stimulation Peel for 3 days and then perform the 5-day peel at a later time.

Ossential Advanced Radical Night Repair applied at each application (between 5 and 12 pumps) (Table 9.4). Patients ultimately decide on their desired ZO Retinol Stimulation Peel strength and peel duration (3 or 5 days), depending on their motivation and lifestyle.

Application Steps

Patients should undergo the ZO Retinol Stimulation Peel only after using a basic (preventive) or therapeutic ZO Skin Health or ZO Medical program for at least 4 to 6 weeks. During this pre-peel conditioning stage, patients should use Ossential Radical Night Repair Plus every night to activate skin renewal and strengthen the skin's barrier function. Patients must not perform the

ZO Retinol Stimulation Peel (increasing the amount of Ossential Advanced Radical Night Repair applied or change the frequency from once to twice per day) until their skin can tolerate the nightly application of 3 pumps of Ossential Advanced Radical Night Repair (this usually takes 2 to 4 weeks). The ZO Retinol Stimulation Peel can be performed only after skin is properly activated and repaired.

With AHA, BHA, Jessner's solution, and other currently available exfoliators, the peeling agent is applied during one visit, and the skin exfoliates for 2 to 3 days thereafter. Such peels result in limited, short-lived improvement of the skin's surface, with no stimulating effects. In contrast, the ZO Retinol Stimulation Peel is an ongoing process of total epidermal repair that provides dermal benefits that no other epidermal peels can offer. This peel consists of multiple steps (Table 9.5) that users must follow sequentially for 3 to 5 days to maximize the procedure's benefits and therapeutic efficacy. Patients should perform this peel every 2 to 3 months as an anti-aging strategy, which will keep skin looking its best indefinitely.

Additionally, patients can perform the ZO Retinol Stimulation Peel at variable strengths, providing variable levels of stimulation and epidermal renewal and exfoliation. The amount of Ossential Advanced Radical Night Repair peeling formula applied determines the procedure's strength. The peeling formula comes in a 1-fluid-ounce (30-mL) tube that includes a pump from which the formula is dispensed.

Patients who are just beginning the peeling process should start with the light level and progress to the moderate and strong levels for their second and third peels, respectively. The optimal time between peels is 3 to 4 weeks. After patients have experienced all levels of the ZO Retinol Stimulation Peel, they can choose whichever level they prefer for future peels. Figures 9.2, 9.3, and 9.4 show patients who underwent a ZO Retinol Stimulation Peel for various conditions.

Alternately, patients can also use the ZO Retinol Stimulation Peel to accelerate and accentuate overall response to separate treatment programs for conditions such as melasma, textural damage, actinic keratoses, acne, and rosacea. When the ZO Retinol Stimulation Peel is used in this fashion—as merely a portion of a broader treatment protocol—the moderate or strong levels should be used when feasible. Benefits of the ZO Retinol Stimulation Peel are shown in Box 9.5.

TABLE 9.5 ZO Retinol Stimulation Peel: Daily Steps

Step	*Function*	*Instructions*
1. Cleanse*	Remove surface impurities, dead skin cells, and excess sebum	AM and PM[†]
2. Apply Ossential Daily Power Defense	Reduce inflammation, support DNA repair, and restore barrier function	AM and PM
3. Apply Ossential Advanced Radical Night Repair Plus	Stimulate and exfoliate	AM and PM

*Disease-specific topical agents can be added after skin cleansing.
†Recommended: for oily skin—Oilacleanse; for normal skin—Normacleanse, Foamacleanse, or the Offects Exfoliating Cleanser; and for dry skin—the Offects Hydrating Cleanser.

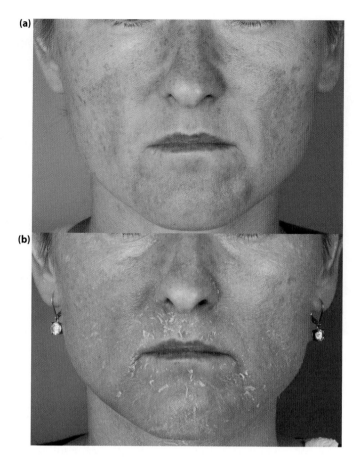

FIGURE 9.2 (a) The patient had skin classified as deviated white (light) skin, medium thick, and oily. She was diagnosed as having photodamage and rosacea. (b) Five days after the peel. The patient underwent 6 weeks of treatment with the ZO Skin Health program and also had a ZO Retinol Stimulation Peel. Notice the exfoliation and overall textural improvement on day 5 of the peel.

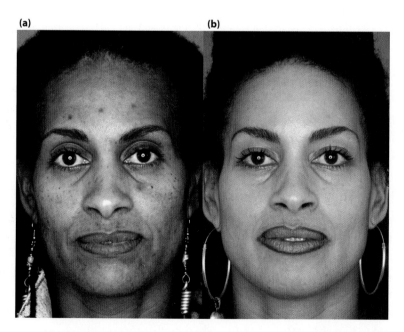

FIGURE 9.3 (a) The patient had skin classified as deviated black (light) skin, medium thick, and oily. She was diagnosed as having acne, rosacea, and postinflammatory hyperpigmentation. (b) Six months later. The patient followed an aggressive hydroquinone-based Skin Health Restoration program during which she underwent three monthly ZO Retinol Stimulation Peel applications. Dermal melasma on the forehead remained after the peels that necessitated a ZO Controlled Depth Peel to the papillary dermis.

(a) (b)

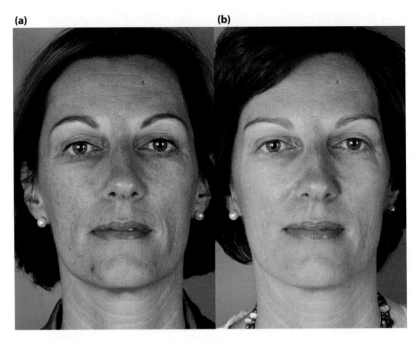

Figure 9.4 (a) The patient had skin classified as original white, medium thin, and oily. She was diagnosed as having photodamage, fine wrinkles, and mild laxity. (b) Eight months later. The patient followed a non-hydroquinone-based Skin Health Restoration program for 6 months with emphasis on epidermal and melanocyte stabilization. She also underwent two ZO Retinol Stimulation Peel applications.

Box 9.5

Benefits of the ZO Retinol Stimulation Peel

- Epidermal renewal and dermal stimulation
- Thicker epidermis
- Powerful anti-aging benefits (collagen and elastin stimulation)
- Faster and more effective results in treating various skin conditions
- Stabilization of melanocytes (evens color tone)
- Stabilization of keratinocytes (yields softer keratin and a stronger barrier function)
- Repair and reversal of photodamage (actinic keratoses, dullness, and dyschromia) through enhanced DNA repair
- Epidermal and dermal hydration (glycosaminoglycans regulate trans-epidermal water loss)
- Improved overall results of skin resurfacing procedures (e.g., ZO Controlled Depth Peel, CO_2 fractional laser resurfacing) as well as surgical procedures, such as facelifts. In such cases, the ZO Retinol Stimulation Peel is performed after patients' skin has re-epithelialized (when skin is tolerant and when healing is complete), as a part of the Skin Health Restoration program
- Maximal safety (no allergies, dermal damage, postinflammatory hyperpigmentation, scars, or infections) when properly performed

Healing occurs quickly—in 2 to 3 days—after stopping the ZO Retinol Stimulation Peel formula and starting the calming and hydrating creams (ZO Medical Calming Creme). During and after stopping the peel, patients must be instructed to refrain from picking, peeling, or overly manipulating actively exfoliating skin because these could lead to PIH and secondary skin infections.

Rarely, reactions including redness, stinging, and excessive exfoliation may occur during the peeling process following inadequate pre-peel conditioning (not reaching tolerance with the once-daily use of Ossential Advanced Radical Night Repair before the peel). In such cases, patients can be instructed to 1) stop the peel at any time or 2) apply calming and hydrating creams *before* applying the ZO Retinol Stimulation formula (never after or on top of it) to increase skin tolerance. Of note, application of calming and hydrating creams on top of (after) the application of the ZO Retinol Stimulation Peel formula is discouraged because this would reduce the activity and the penetration of the Ossential Advanced Radical Night Repair.

INVISAPEEL

Invisapeel, the only peel that does not require prior skin conditioning, is a universal peel that can be applied to any skin surface, on any skin type, and as part of treatment for any condition. It is applied by the patient at home, usually to the target areas daily or two to three times per week. Invisapeel is intended to maximize the benefits and accelerate the results of any treatment program, medical or nonmedical, because it enhances penetration of topical agents, stimulates epidermal renewal, and maintains the skin's smoothness and natural healthy glow. It is called Invisapeel because patients who undergo this peel experience no visible exfoliation or reactions. Without visible peeling or symptoms, patients need not worry about the appearance of exfoliating skin.

This peel delivers proteases and fruit enzymes from papain and bromelain together with glycolic acid. It is enriched with bio-preventative and immune-regulatory factors that eliminate burning or stinging sensations, inflammation, redness, and the skin dryness and irritation that are encountered with currently available exfoliating peels. In contrast to other peels, Invisapeel preserves the barrier function while maintaining natural hydration and is not associated with any symptoms. Patients can use Invisapeel on the face or the body.

Indications
Because of its keratolytic activity, Invisapeel is ideal for treating hyperkeratotic disorders that commonly affect the skin of the arms, knees, and elbows. Daily application of Invisapeel can also be beneficial for the following:

- To even skin tone after healing from ablative and nonablative laser or chemical resurfacing procedures
- To maximize the benefits of Skin Health Restoration programs (especially the mild types in which patients want little to no visible reactions)
- To improve skin texture and treatment results (enhanced penetration of other topically applied agents) for all forms of acne and rosacea therapies

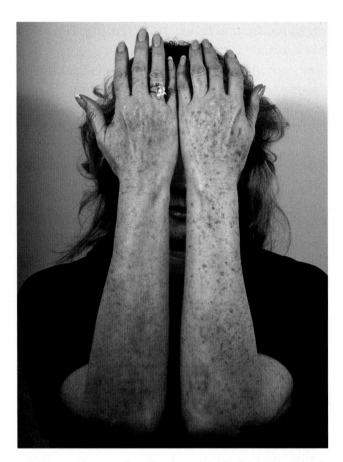

FIGURE 9.5   A patient with skin classified as original white showing photodamage on arms. Her right arm was treated with Invisapeel Intensive Resurfacing Peel in the PM, Oraser Body Emulsion in the AM and PM, Retamax Active Vitamin A Micro Emulsion in the PM, and three treatments with the ZO Retinol Stimulation Peel.

Figures 9.5, 9.6, and 9.7 show successful treatment of arms with Invisapeel. Table 9.6 gives instructions on applying Invisapeel to the face and body.

Invisapeel is well tolerated by nearly all patients. For that reason, it can be left on (without washing off) before each patient's application of the individual components of his or her specific ZO Program without any interruption. However, certain patients who have sensitive skin may complain of a burning sensation from Invisapeel. In these cases, patients need to wash off the Invisapeel before subsequent application of their ZO Program.

ZO 3-STEP STIMULATION PEEL

Compared with the ZO Retinol Stimulation Peel, the ZO 3-Step Peel is a deeper exfoliating peel that provides much stronger stimulation. The ZO 3-Step Peel must be performed in the office because there is a small chance the peel solution could penetrate down to the PD, especially in patients with thin skin. If this occurs, the situation requires more intense, dermal peel management.

The ZO 3-Step Peel can be performed as part of a treatment program to expedite and improve results in the conditions shown in Box 9.6. The ZO 3-Step Peel can be safely repeated at monthly intervals. Of note, certain cases or conditions may require two to three peels to achieve optimal

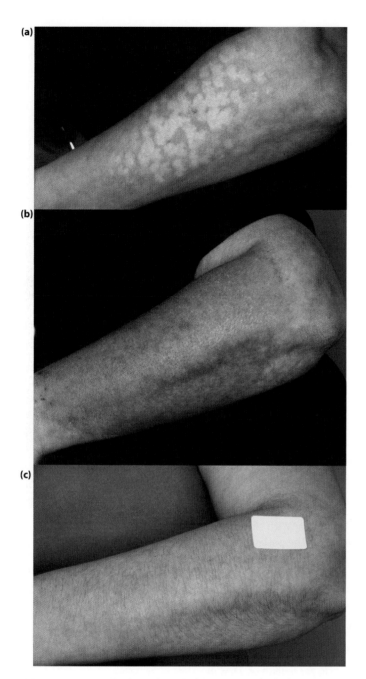

FIGURE 9.6 (a) A patient with skin classified as deviated (dark) white. He was diagnosed as having hypopigmentation on his arm 6 months after laser hair removal. (b) Four weeks after Invisapeel applied in the PM, Oraser Body Emulsion Plus in the AM and PM, and Retamax Active Vitamin A Micro Emulsion in the AM and PM. Notice redness and mild exfoliation. (c) Skin on arm showing complete recovery 3 months later.

benefit. Characteristics of the ZO 3-Step Peel are shown in Box 9.7. Figures 9.8 and 9.9 show patients who underwent a ZO 3-Step Peel for various conditions.

Components

The ZO 3-Step Peel includes the following components (Figure 9.10):

- Eight milliliters of an acid cocktail (TCA, salicylic acid, and lactic acid mixed with a saponin-like cofactor for rapid neutralization) in a sealed bottle for individual use

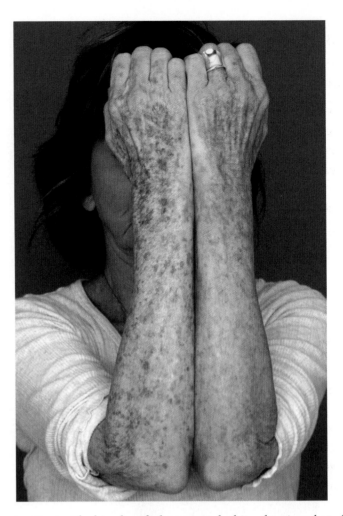

Figure 9.7 A patient with skin classified as original white, showing photodamage and lentigines on arms. The patient's left arm was treated with Invisapeel in the PM, Oraser Body Emulsion Plus in the AM and PM, Retamax Active Vitamin A Micro Emulsion in the PM, and two treatments with the ZO 3-Step Stimulation Peel.

Table 9.6 Applying Invisapeel	
For the Face	*For the Body*
(Mild Approach, for Sensitive, Dry, or Thin Skin)	*(Strong Approach Preferred)*
Cleanse the skin. Apply the peel solution, two or three times per week; leave on for 2 to 3 hours, then wash. Proceed with the specific ZO Program that was recommended to you.	Prepare the skin. Apply peel lotion (do not wash it off). Follow with the specific ZO Program that was recommended for you.
Three to 4 pumps of the peel lotion are sufficient for 5% of body surface skin.	

- Five grams of 6% retinol in a microsphere formulation with a highly penetrating base
- Two-ounce tube of calming and hydrating lotion with powerful anti-irritative and anti-inflammatory properties

The volume of the "acid cocktail" was specifically calculated to provide limited action and penetration to keep it as an "exfoliating" peel. Each acid component will therefore be neutralized by epidermal proteins before reaching

Box 9.6

Indications for the ZO 3-Step Peel

- Melasma
- Postinflammatory hyperpigmentation
- To improve and even out the results of past resurfacing procedures
- Textural damage and irregularity (enlarged pores or fresh, early acne scars—before fibrosis)
- Diffuse photodamage (including solar lentigines and poikiloderma)
- Aging signs (mild wrinkles, laxity)

Box 9.7

ZO 3-Step Peel Features

- Fast healing time (3 to 4 days of exfoliation)
- Easily performed by the clinician with minimal patient discomfort
- Lack of swelling, crusting, or oozing, as is commonly seen in dermal peels
- Strong epidermal stimulation (renewal) and repair
- Dermal (anti-aging) benefits and dermal textural repair

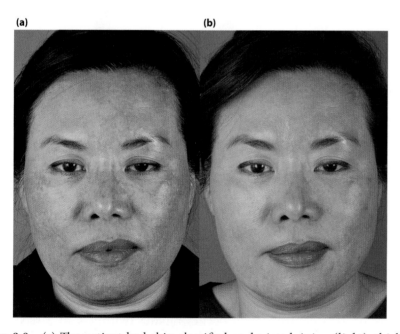

(a)   **(b)**

FIGURE 9.8   (a) The patient had skin classified as deviated Asian (light), thick, and oily. She was diagnosed as having melasma and postinflammatory hyperpigmentation. (b) Eight months later. The patient followed a hydroquinone-based Skin Health Restoration program and underwent two treatments with the ZO 3-Step Peel. Currently, she is on a maintenance program with the non-hydroquinone-based ZO Skin Health program.

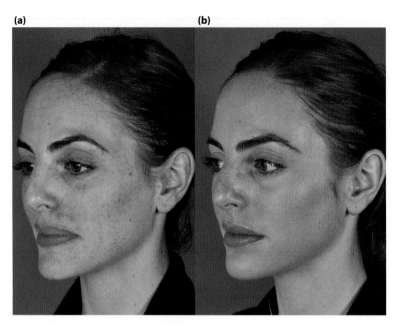

(a)   **(b)**

FIGURE 9.9   (a) The patient had skin classified as original white, medium thick, and oily. She was diagnosed as having photodamage, freckles, and early wrinkles. (b) Six months later. The patient used a non-hydroquinone-based Skin Health Restoration program, followed by two treatments with the ZO 3-Step Stimulation Peel and one ZO Retinol Stimulation Peel.

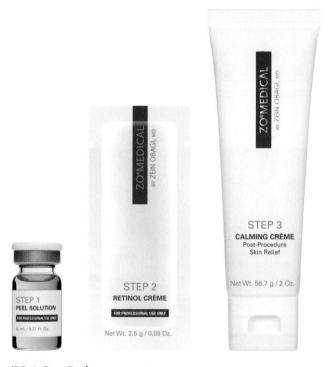

FIGURE 9.10   ZO 3-Step Peel components.

the lower portion of the epidermis. Because of the presence of the saponin-like cofactor, this neutralization occurs rapidly (within 4 to 5 seconds), as evidenced by the appearance of a powdery film on the skin surface that represents the denatured protein.

Each of the three acids in the acid cocktail of this peel works on epidermal protein through a distinct mechanism. Specifically, TCA coagulates and dehydrates epidermal proteins, lactic acid demonstrates an exfoliating phenomenon by breaking the bonds between individual keratinocytes, and salicylic acid demonstrates acantholytic activity by breaking down the cell membranes of keratinocytes. The combined action of these three acids allows for a rapid interaction with the epidermal proteins. Furthermore, the saponin-like agent in the cocktail acts as a cofactor in initiating and accelerating neutralization of the acids. After the acid cocktail has been applied to the skin, the saponin agent, the skin's epidermal proteins, and the acids are chemically altered and converted to a powdery film visible on the surface of the treated skin. The precipitation of this powder indicates the completion of acid activity and full neutralization of the acid solution.

As is the standard in most chemical peels, skin must first be prepared before administration of the ZO 3-Step Peel solution. This preparation involves removing all lotions, sunscreen, and makeup from the area to be treated. The skin in the treatment areas is then stripped of sebum ("degreased") with acetone or alcohol. Degreasing insures that the activity of each acid is intact to exert its action on the epidermis. Because the saponin-like agent in the peel is deactivated on contact with water or oil, the skin must also be completely dry before administering the acid cocktail to the treatment area.

As in the ZO Retinol Stimulation Peel, variations in hydration of the epidermis affect the activity of the acids and the saponin-like agent on the epidermal proteins in the ZO 3-Step Peel. Specifically, the hydration level is high in the lower epidermis and the papillary dermis, which makes these areas resistant to the action of the acids. Accordingly, the activity of the acids is maximal in the upper portion of the epidermis where epidermal hydration is relatively low and keratin protein content is high. In contrast, the activity of the acids is minimal in the lower portion of the epidermis (Box 9.8). This characteristic is beneficial in providing maximal safety because all the acids are neutralized in the upper epidermis, thus preventing unwanted dermal penetration and accidental injury.

Mechanism of Action

The acids in the ZO 3-Step Peel initially denature epidermal proteins, leading to the elimination of the skin's barrier function. This facilitates the activity of the second step, the application of retinol directly over the treatment areas and its penetration through the lower part of the epidermis to the papillary dermis. The basal cells of the epidermis respond with accelerated mitosis and epidermal renewal, melanocyte stabilization, and fibroblast stimulation (which

---

Box 9.8

Acid Cocktail Activity in the Epidermis

- Acid cocktail activity is maximal in the upper portion of the epidermis, where epidermal hydration is low and keratin protein content is high.
- Acid activity is minimal in the lower portion of the epidermis, where epidermal hydration is high and the protein content is low.

yields increased collagen, elastin, and glycosaminoglycans) in the PD (stimulation). The third step involves application of a calming cream that provides triple benefits: anti-inflammatory and anti-irritation effects and increased hydration benefits.

Performing the Peel

All peels require skin conditioning and herpes simplex prophylaxis based on patient history. On the day of the peel, degrease and dry the skin surface with rubbing alcohol. Empty the acid bottle's contents into a cup. Fold the supplied round gauze pad twice to create a quarter of a circle, then dip it in the solution and start painting the face (gently, to prevent any solution from moving freely on the skin surface) (Figure 9.11). Apply the solution evenly, in different directions, and observe the powdery film to ensure that it has been applied over the entire intended treatment area.

Approximately 4 to 5 seconds after the application, a powdery film will begin appearing on the painted areas. Continue painting until all 8 mL of solution have been painted on 5% of the skin surface (usually the face). Finishing the entire bottle requires painting the whole face multiple times. The only exceptions include patients with small faces or thin skin. For these patients, one may use half or more of the total volume of the solution to avoid accidental dermal penetration, which would induce a PD peel in certain areas.

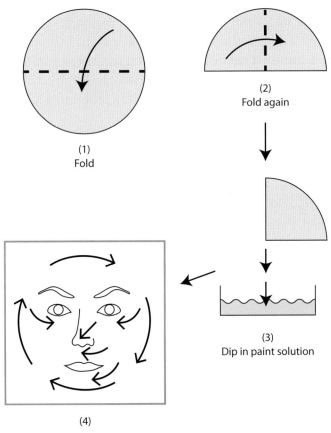

(1)
Fold

(2)
Fold again

(3)
Dip in paint solution

(4)
- Paint, avoid dripping
- Paint on top of powder
- You will circle the face multiple times
- Paint the eyelids (avoid the eyes)

FIGURE 9.11 Folding of gauze and application of the ZO 3-Step Peel to a patient's face.

The powder does not have to be wiped off; one can simply continue the acid application on top of the powdery film.

Using scissors, open the sealed packet of retinol at one corner, then vigorously massage half of the content over the entire face (again, on top of the powdery film) until all the applied retinol (half of the package) is completely absorbed.

To complete the peel, open the sealed tube of calming cream, apply enough to cover the face, and massage it in until it is completely absorbed (Figure 9.12). That completes the peel. The burning sensation that occurs when one applies the acid solution is well tolerated by patients. Using a fan or cold air machine can minimize the discomfort. Avoid topical anesthetics (EMLA or others) because they hydrate the skin surface and can weaken the peel or cause uneven penetration. The steps of the ZO 3-Step Peel are shown in Box 9.9. Figure 9.13

(a) **(b)**

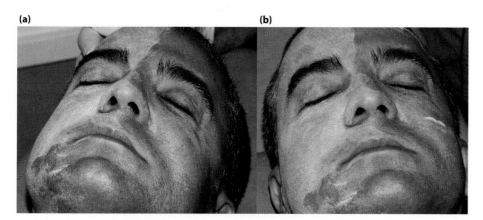

FIGURE 9.12 (a) Patient's right side immediately after application of the acid cocktail of the ZO 3-Step Peel. Notice the powdery film. (b) Patient's left side after the application of the second step (the stimulation step). Notice disappearance of the powdery film.

Box 9.9

Performing the ZO 3-Step Peel

- Degrease and dry the skin surface with rubbing alcohol or acetone.
- Empty the contents of the acid bottle into a cup.
- Dip the supplied sponge into the solution and start painting the face gently.
- Apply the solution evenly, in different directions.
- Using scissors, open the sealed packet of retinol at one corner, and vigorously massage half the content over the entire face (again, on top of the powdery film) until all the applied retinol (half of the package) is completely absorbed.
- Keep the remaining half of the retinol packet for use the next morning.
- Open the sealed tube of calming cream and apply enough to cover the face and massage it in until completely absorbed.

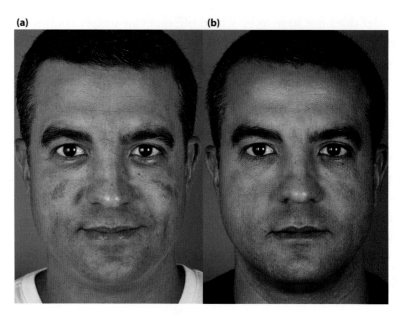

Figure 9.13 (a) Before. The patient had skin classified as deviated white (dark), thick, and oily. He was diagnosed as having dermal pigmentation and postinflammatory hyperpigmentation due to photosensitivity. (b) Twelve weeks later. The patient was treated for 5 months with aggressive hydroquinone-based Skin Health Restoration. Two treatments with the ZO 3-Step Retinol Stimulation Peel were performed at weeks 6 and 10 during the treatment.

Table 9.7 Home Instructions

Day	Activity
Day 1 (day of the peel)	Do not wash the face for 5 hours after the peel. Washing the face sooner will interrupt retinol stimulation. When showering, avoid having the shower water hit the face directly. Apply small amount of calming creams whenever the treated skin feels dry. Excessive application of calming creams could lead to premature exfoliation.
Day 2 in AM	Wash face gently (pat the skin; do not scrub or rub). Apply second half of the retinol packet (used the day before) and massage gently until completely absorbed. Apply calming creams in small amount to maintain comfortable hydration; repeat as needed.
Days 3–5	When skin starts to exfoliate, do not assist the exfoliation by rubbing or peeling the skin. Apply calming cream, as needed. Healing is complete, on average, in 4 to 5 days.

shows a patient who was treated with two ZO 3-Step Retinol Stimulation Peels for dermal pigmentation problems.

Home Instructions

Table 9.7 shows home care instructions for the patient who has a ZO 3-Step Peel.

ZO CONTROLLED DEPTH TRICHLORO-ACETIC ACID PEELS

ZO TRICHLOROACETIC ACID PEELS

This chapter addresses three highly effective variations of the ZO Controlled Depth Peel: the ZO Controlled Depth Peel to the papillary dermis (PD), the ZO Controlled Depth Peel to the immediate reticular dermis (IRD), and the medium-depth ZO Designed Controlled Depth Peel. An illustration in Chapter 5 (Figure 5.1) depicts the skin layers reached by each of these peels.

The ZO Controlled Depth Peel comprises highly controlled skin rejuvenation procedures with precise, standardized variables not commonly seen with other types of trichloroacetic acid (TCA) peels (Box 10.1). The ZO peels were created to eliminate the confusion, limitations, and risks associated with current TCA-based peels and can be performed by virtually any physician who has received adequate training in dermal chemical peels.

SAFETY, EFFICACY, AND EASE OF USE

The ZO Controlled Depth Peel is exceptionally versatile and can be used on all skin types and ethnicities. Moreover, the ZO Controlled Depth Peel has no systemic toxicity and can be performed in a timely manner.

When a fixed concentration of TCA (20% or 26% to 28%) is combined with the blue base dye, the ZO Controlled Depth Peel penetrates the skin and forms frost at a slower rate than other types of TCA peel. Physicians have enough time to observe the development of standardized clinical endpoints that indicate the peel's specific depth of penetration and therefore

Box 10.1

Standardized Variables in a ZO Controlled Depth Peel

1. TCA concentration used: fixed at 20% or 26% to 28%
2. Total volume applied: fixed at 6 mL or 10 mL
3. Surface area treated: 5% of total body surface area
4. Depth control: visible, well-defined clinical endpoints
5. Color of solution: blue tint added to quantify the penetration depth, highlight the location of solution application, and ensure even application
6. Application method by a "coat" system
7. Preprocedure skin conditioning required. Skin quality and thickness are considered when selecting the appropriate peel, which results in faster healing and higher safety margins.

increase the procedure's safety (Box 10.2). The ZO Controlled Depth Peel approach eliminates guesswork for the physician and provides a teaching framework. For several other chemical peels, the techniques are vague and haphazard and are acquired through casually observing others or learning from one's own mistakes. Box 10.3 shows variables associated with other (not ZO) TCA peels.

Transforming TCA chemical peels into a precise science entailed several years of researching, collecting, and analyzing data. Wherever possible, the variables associated with existing TCA peels were minimized or eliminated. This resulted in a unique ZO Controlled Depth Peel, the only TCA-based peel currently available that offers maximal safety and reliability (Box 10.4).

CHOOSING A ZO CONTROLLED DEPTH PEEL

A variety of peeling options are available to satisfy the physician's goals for any given patient. The most commonly performed peel is the ZO Controlled

Box 10.2

ZO Controlled Depth Peel Advantages

ZO Controlled Depth Peel with TCA mixed with blue base:

1. Allows the TCA to act more slowly on the skin (i.e., a smaller amount penetrates the skin at any given time). This increases the practitioner's awareness and control over the peel depth.
2. Penetrates more evenly
3. Causes less irritation through its anti-inflammatory properties

---

Box 10.3

Variables Associated with Other Trichloroacetic Acid Peels

1. Lack of consensus regarding the optimal trichloroacetic acid (TCA) concentration and solution volume needed to peel a fixed skin surface area to the desired depth
2. Lack of definitive penetration depth signs (clearly observable clinical endpoints), which allow physicians to accurately determine peel depth at any given time
3. Lack of a common consensus regarding the safe depths for peels on both facial and nonfacial skin
4. High speed of TCA penetration in current TCA-based peels, which is both risky and troublesome
5. Lack of attention to the significance of skin thickness as a determinant of depth safety
6. Lack of attention to skin quality to determine patient suitability for chemical peels
7. Lack of standardized methods of solution application to ensure even coverage of TCA

Depth Peel to the PD. If a deeper peel is desired, the practitioner can choose the ZO Controlled Depth Peel to the immediate reticular dermis (IRD). The physician skilled in peels may also choose the ZO Designed Controlled Depth Peel, which allows the peeling solution to reach multiple depths within the same treatment. In some areas, the PD will be reached, whereas in other areas, it may be the IRD or upper reticular dermis (URD). This allows the physician to skillfully design and tailor the patient's peel.

Box 10.4

ZO Controlled Depth Peel Advantages

1. Methodological and simple for physicians to learn and perform
2. Clear-cut, easily recognizable endpoints, which allow the practitioner to control penetration depth and reduce the potential for complications
3. Standardized protocol (concentration, volume, surface area, and number of coats), which eliminates peel variables
4. Capability of improving a wide range of cosmetic and medical skin conditions
5. Suitable for all skin types and for facial and nonfacial skin
6. Consistent results with exceptional skin tightening and some skin leveling
7. Design modification that allows physicians to enhance the tightening effect by increasing the peel's depth in precise areas

TABLE 10.1   Tightening and Leveling Characteristics of the ZO Controlled Depth Peel

Aim of Peel	Type of Peel	Penetration Depth	Clinical Indication	Comment
Skin tightening	ZO Controlled Depth Peel	Papillary dermis or immediate reticular dermis	Stretchable scars or wrinkles (those that disappear with light stretching of skin), photodamage, melasma, skin laxity	A gradual, noninvasive effect that reduces skin laxity and other problems without altering skin texture
Skin leveling	ZO Designed Controlled Depth Peel	Upper reticular dermis, focally or largely	Nonstretchable scars or wrinkles	A more invasive effect that can change skin texture to varying degrees

The primary clinical objectives for the ZO Controlled Depth Peel are skin tightening and correcting stretchable rhytides, scars, and other skin problems located within the PD or IRD. The peel is remarkably safe and effective for these purposes. The ZO Designed Controlled Depth Peel provides a further advantage: skin leveling (smoothing of texture). This is accomplished through correction of skin problems located in the URD (deeper than the IRD) (Table 10.1). Because a ZO Controlled Depth Peel to the PD and the IRD does not penetrate to the URD, its leveling effects are limited to only stretchable wrinkles and scars (those that disappear when one gently stretches the skin during Dr. Zein Obagi Skin Stretch Test).

Factors Affecting the Outcome of a ZO Controlled Depth Peel

Performing a successful chemical peel requires identification of key characteristics in each patient's skin before performing the procedure. Box 10.5 shows the three primary skin factors that affect the outcome of a ZO Controlled Depth Peel and resurfacing procedures. Skin quality can be greatly improved through proper skin conditioning and treatment in the weeks or months before the procedure. Although skin thickness and color are fixed variables, they play a fundamental role in determining the safe depth in all skin types for any resurfacing procedure including ZO Controlled Depth Peel.

IMPORTANCE OF TRICHLOROACETIC ACID CONCENTRATION, VOLUME, AND SIZE OF TREATMENT AREA

Importance of Trichloroacetic Acid Concentration

Unlike phenol or alpha-hydroxy acid (AHA) peels, the concentration of TCA alone does not determine the depth to which a TCA peel will penetrate the skin. Concentration determines only the *speed* at which the acid penetrates.[1,2] (Box 10.6). To determine the depth of penetration for any given TCA concentration, the volume (number of coats applied/total amount used) is also important. These conclusions contrast those of Brody, who classifies 10% to 35% TCA as concentrations that reach a superficial depth and 35% TCA combined with other agents, or 50% TCA alone, as concentrations that reach a medium depth.[3]

Depending on its concentration, a TCA peel can produce therapeutic effects, followed by proper healing, or caustic effects, leading to impaired healing. Therapeutic effects result from using a carefully controlled TCA

Box 10.5

**Factors Affecting the Outcome of the
ZO Controlled Depth Peel**

- Skin quality
- Sensitivity (indicates damaged barrier function)
- Hydration status* (dry or poorly hydrated skin will not allow for even acid penetration and will thereby generate an irregular skin response and possibly serious complications)
- Skin thickness
- Skin color

*Hydration status also affects the response to laser resurfacing because water is the chromophore for both modalities.

concentration and volume to produce a consistent and reliable penetration depth. This approach preserves enough dermal adnexal structures and fibroblasts to allow re-epithelialization and dermal regeneration postoperatively (Box 10.7). Conversely, caustic effects damage the dermal adnexal structures to the extent that hypopigmentation, fibrosis, scarring (atrophic as well as hypertrophic), and/or abnormal, prolonged skin healing occur. These effects resemble those seen following second- and third-degree burns.

TCA concentrations above 49% are primarily associated with caustic effects, which can be detrimental in thin, fragile, or dark skin (Figure 10.1). For these particular skin types, even 30% to 40% TCA concentrations can be caustic when a large total volume of TCA is applied (e.g., too many coats).

TCA concentrations greater than 30% can quickly coagulate large amounts of protein. This leads to the inability of proteins in the epidermis and PD to neutralize the TCA. Then, if the concentration of the solution is high enough, even a small volume can penetrate deeper to reach the lower reticular dermis relatively quickly. In contrast, a lower TCA concentration can reach the same desired depth and do so more slowly and only with a higher solution volume. Therefore, repeated applications (yielding higher total volume of TCA applied)

Box 10.6

Trichloroacetic Acid Concentration

- Trichloroacetic acid (TCA) concentration determines the *speed* at which the acid penetrates; it is not the sole determinant of the *depth* reached in the skin. Volume must also be considered when establishing peel *depth*.
- Depending on concentration, a TCA peel can produce therapeutic effects, associated with proper healing, or caustic effects, associated with impaired healing.

Box 10.7

Control of Trichloroacetic Acid Depth of Penetration

■ The importance of using a carefully controlled *trichloroacetic acid (TCA) concentration and volume* to result in a consistent depth of penetration cannot be overstated.

■ Control over TCA concentration and total volume applied preserves enough dermal adnexal structures and fibroblasts to allow re-epithelialization and dermal regeneration.

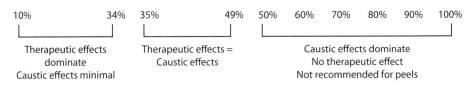

FIGURE 10.1 The therapeutic and caustic effects of trichloroacetic acid (TCA) are related to concentration. At 10% to 34% concentration, the therapeutic effects of TCA dominate, and the caustic effects are minimal. At 35% to 49%, the therapeutic effects equal the caustic effects. Concentrations higher than 49% are caustic and are not recommended for peels.

will allow for any TCA concentration to penetrate to any intended depth. The effects of concentration versus speed are shown in Box 10.8.

TCA concentrations of 20% or 26% to 28% were carefully chosen for the ZO Controlled Depth Peel because, at these concentrations (with a predetermined volume and size of the area to be peeled), TCA is optimally neutralized by proteins within the epidermis and papillary dermis. TCA at these percentages will not penetrate deeply unless one applies a large volume over a long time. This is unlikely to happen, however, because the ZO Controlled Depth Peel parameters, such as the total volume applied and the suggested speed of application, are set to control such variables.

Importance of Trichloroacetic Acid Volume and the Size of Treatment Area

To maximally standardize the TCA chemical peel, the ZO Controlled Depth Peel uses a fixed-volume approach to the TCA solution. This is termed a "coat." The coat system helps to ensure safe and controlled application of the

---

Box 10.8

Concentration versus Speed

Given the same volume, the higher the concentration of trichloroacetic acid used, the faster the peel will penetrate into the dermis.

ZO Controlled Depth Peel solution. This is achieved by carefully applying a fixed TCA concentration and volume to a predetermined size of skin surface using a sponge or gauze and a cotton swab.

A coat application is complete when the entire fixed volume of acid has been evenly applied to the predetermined surface area. This treatment size should constitute 5% of the entire body's skin surface area (Figure 10.2). Typically, this is the face, although the same principle applies to any area of the body that constitutes approximately 5% of the skin's total surface area. One predetermined total volume of TCA (at a 20% or 26% to 28% concentration) should be applied evenly, by multiple applications, until all the volume is consumed. The depth signs should be monitored concurrently. Usually more than one coat is needed to reach the desired depth, and the number of coats or volume needed depends on skin thickness and depth desired.

The 6 mL of 20% TCA prepared ZO Controlled Depth Peel solution, or the 10 mL of the 26% to 28% solution, will reach the desired depth: the PD, the IRD, and/or the URD (Table 10.2). To achieve a greater depth of penetration, the physician will need to apply more than one coat of the fixed-concentration TCA solution. The PD is the ideal level that the ZO Controlled Depth Peel aims to reach because it may correct more than 80% of skin problems that involve the PD. However, more coats (a higher total volume of

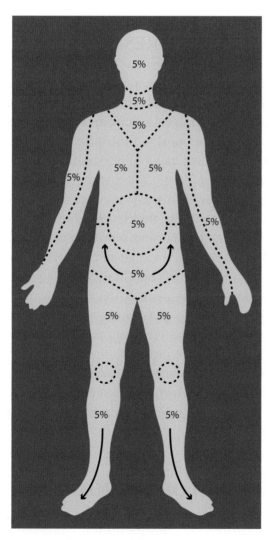

FIGURE 10.2 Diagram of 5% body surface areas.

TABLE 10.2 The Coat System for ZO Controlled Depth Trichloroacetic Acid Peels on Facial Skin

Type/Depth of ZO Controlled Depth Peel	Solution Concentration for Coat	Thin Skin	Thick Skin
Papillary dermis (PD)	20%	Up to 1 coat	Up to 2 coats
	26%-28%	Not used	1 coat
Immediate reticular dermis (IRD)	20%	Up to 2 coats	Up to 2 coats
	26%-28%	1 coat	1 coat ± a partial coat
Designed PD, IRD, upper reticular dermis (URD)			
• Designed peel when URD is minimally and focally involved	26%-28% is best 20% can be used	20% only Up to 2 coats	26% to 28%, up to 2 coats
• Designed medium-depth peel when URD is generally involved; deeper and larger areas	26%-28% is best	Not recommended	Up to 2 coats

Depth signs are more important than coats to determine the depth of any ZO Controlled Depth Peel.

A higher concentration is more suitable for the designed peel because it reaches the depth faster and is better for monitoring the short-lived depth signs. A lighter concentration takes longer to reach the IRD and URD as the depth signs start to disappear.

the TCA solution) can be applied to the treatment site if one intends for the peel to reach deeper into the IRD for maximal tightening or the URD for tightening and some leveling.

PERIOD OF RELATIVE RESISTANCE

The period of relative resistance refers to the length of time that the skin resists penetration of TCA, or the time it takes for TCA to be neutralized. This period can be short or long, depending on specific factors: 1) concentration—a high concentration needs much more skin protein to neutralize the applied TCA (more depth); and 2) volume—rapid application of a larger volume has the same effect.

When one applies an acid to the skin, natural defenses are mobilized to counteract its penetration. In the first line of defense, epidermal protein (keratin) begins to neutralize and arrest the penetration of acid. When this epidermal defense has been exhausted, applying further acid allows for deeper penetration (to the PD and beyond). The second line of defense consists of a cessation of TCA penetration through the following dermal components: collagen, elastin, glycosaminoglycans, blood vessels, blood, and other proteins. After these elements have been used, applying more TCA will result in deeper penetration (to the URD or deeper). A physician should respect the period of relative resistance (1 to 2 minutes) and, when performing the peel, never return to the same area that has been painted with TCA before the required minutes have passed in order to avoid unnecessary additional depth.

NEUTRALIZATION OF TRICHLOROACETIC ACID

TCA is a self-neutralizing acid. This means it is not necessary for the practitioner to apply bicarbonate or another basic solution to the treatment site after the chemical peel solution has been applied. The patient's own skin neutralizes the TCA. The factors that influence the ability of skin's defenses to neutralize TCA include the TCA concentration, the total volume of solution applied (in relation to the size of the skin area being treated), and the thickness of the skin at the application site.

To further clarify, a higher concentration of TCA will rapidly consume a large amount of skin proteins and penetrate faster and deeper than a lower concentration. Similarly, a larger volume of TCA solution (of any concentration) will consume a larger amount of skin proteins, resulting in deeper penetration. In current uncontrolled-depth peels (plain or augmented), TCA penetrates the skin much faster than the TCA within the ZO Controlled Depth Peel. It is therefore relatively impossible to view the crucial depth signs with the uncontrolled peels because the signs develop rather slowly and disappear quickly. Skin thickness also affects the efficacy of TCA neutralization because thicker skin is richer in protein and is capable of neutralizing a larger volume of TCA compared with thin skin.

ADMINISTERING THE ZO CONTROLLED DEPTH PEEL

SELECTION OF PEEL CONCENTRATION

Before administering the ZO Controlled Depth Peel, the physician must make several choices. First, when choosing a TCA concentration, the practitioner must choose a peel appropriate to his or her experience with TCA peels (Table 10.3) and also must consider the importance of depth sign in this choice (Box 10.9). Depth signs are discussed in detail later in this chapter.

TABLE 10.3 Matching Physician Experience with Trichloroacetic Acid Concentration

Physician Skills	20% TCA + Blue Base	26% to 28% TCA + Blue Base	Comment
Novice	X	Not recommended	
Skilled		X	
Facial skin	X	X	
Nonfacial skin	X	Not recommended	
Skin type:			
• Thin	X	Not recommended	
• Thick	X	X Preferred	
Peel depth:			
• Papillary dermis	X "Novice"	X "Skilled"	
• Immediate reticular dermis	X	X Preferred	
• Upper reticular dermis	Not recommended	X Best	
Conscious or general sedation	X	X Preferred	

> **Box 10.9**
>
> **Peel Concentration and Depth Signs**
>
> ■ A low concentration is good for PD- and IRD-level peels because depth signs are easily recognized. However, with a low concentration, depth signs tend to disappear before the URD is reached because of the slow penetration.
> ■ A higher concentration is preferred for IRD and URD depth because depth signs appear faster and indicate to the physician when to end the peel.

Concentration and Skin Thickness

With the appropriate volume (number of coats), the 20% and the 26% to 28% concentration of the peel can achieve any desired depth of penetration (as previously shown in Table 10.1). Skin thickness, however, is an important additional consideration. To further clarify, the standard volume of solution (6 mL) for 20% TCA will penetrate to the PD or IRD in thin skin. In thick skin, however, the same 6-mL volume of the 20% solution may only exfoliate the epidermis to the basal layer. Thick skin may require a greater volume of the 20% solution to penetrate to the same depth as thin skin. The 26% to 28% solution is ideal for the ZO Designed Controlled Depth Peel, but the physician needs to keep in mind that it reaches the URD faster and is to be used only after he or she has gained sufficient experience.

SELECTION OF PEEL DEPTH

When choosing the appropriate depth of peel penetration, the physician must consider the clinical condition being treated as well as the patient's skin type, color, and thickness. For epidermal conditions such as actinic keratosis, superficial dyschromia, acne, and rough or sallow skin, one may choose other exfoliative (less potent) chemical peels instead of the ZO Controlled Depth Peel. These include the ZO Invisapeel, the ZO Retinol Stimulation Peel, and the ZO 3-Step Peel. These provide either light exfoliation of the stratum corneum (the former) or heavy exfoliation down to the mid-epidermis (the latter). It is important to note that exfoliation does not thin the skin but may actually thicken the epidermis. These exfoliative peels are unique in that they provide the additional benefit of stimulation and mildly improve wrinkles, scars, large pores, and skin laxity. They can be repeated every 2 to 4 weeks.

As discussed previously, the ZO Controlled Depth Peel can achieve varying levels of penetration: to the PD, the IRD, and the URD. For conditions involving both the epidermis and the dermis, the ZO Controlled Depth Peel to the PD is the most suitable choice because it will improve dermal melasma, actinic keratosis, stretchable wrinkles and scars, general skin laxity, early solar elastosis, and enlarged pores. Peeling to the PD tightens the skin without thinning it or changing its color. This peel can be repeated every 6 to 8 weeks, as needed, especially when treating severe dermal melasma and sun damage. Patients do

TABLE 10.4   Clinical Conditions Treatable with Chemical Peels

Clinical Condition	Procedure
Acne, comedones, flat warts	Exfoliative peels
Epidermal and dermal hyperpigmentation, uneven patches of hypo/hyperpigmentation	ZO Controlled Depth Peel to the papillary dermis (PD)
Actinic keratosis, other premalignant lesions	ZO Controlled Depth Peel to the PD
Large pores	ZO Controlled Depth Peel to the PD (for tightening)
Skin laxity	ZO Controlled Depth Peel to the PD (for moderate tightening)
Fine and medium-to-deep stretchable wrinkles (which disappear with light skin stretching)	ZO Controlled Depth Peel to the immediate reticular dermis (IRD) (for maximal tightening)
ZO Designed Controlled Depth Peel to different depths, including the upper reticular dermis (URD) (for maximal tightening and leveling)	ZO Controlled Depth Peel to the PD or IRD (for tightening)
Stretchable scars	ZO Controlled Depth Peel to the IRD
	ZO Designed Controlled Depth Peel to different depths, including the URD (for tightening and leveling)

not need to discontinue isotretinoin (Accutane) use before a ZO Controlled Depth Peel so long as the peel does not penetrate deeper than the PD.

A ZO Controlled Depth Peel to the IRD provides the greatest amount of skin tightening while reaching the maximal safety depth for most skin types. The ZO Designed Controlled Depth Peel involves performing a peel to the PD and/or IRD, followed by application of additional solution to select areas. This will increase the penetration depth focally to the URD to provide texture improvement with unstretchable wrinkles and scars. The ZO Designed Controlled Depth Peel is used for both tightening and leveling purposes.

Before performing a ZO Controlled Depth Peel, physicians must be adequately trained in performing the peel and in perioperative skin management. The patient's skin should also be conditioned through the appropriate Skin Health Restoration program (see Chapter 2). The skin conditions that particular chemical peels can improve (including various types of the ZO Controlled Depth Peel) are shown in Table 10.4.

PREPARING THE ZO CONTROLLED DEPTH PEEL SOLUTION

ZO Controlled Depth Peel ingredients and their functions are shown in Table 10.5. When developing the ZO Controlled Depth Peel, the color blue was found to be the best choice for revealing the presence of other associated colors that serve as guides in the peeling process, such as the white frost and the pink sign.

TABLE 10.5   The ZO Controlled Depth Peel Ingredients and Their Function

Ingredient	Function
1. TCA	Coagulative agent
2. Blue base*	
a. FD&C Blue #1	Color guide that helps ensure even application of the acid (even blue = even application) and allows for depth signs to be recognized
b. Glycerin	Natural oil that permits easy gliding of the solution, which results in smoother application of the solution
c. Cofactors	Allow bonding of the trichloroacetic acid (TCA) with the blue base for slow release of TCA (slower penetration)
d. Botanical anti-inflammatory agents	Suppress TCA-induced irritation

*The new modified blue peel base (in contrast with Dr. Obagi's previous blue peel base) has a lighter blue color, washes off easily, and contains anti-inflammatory agents.

The ZO Controlled Depth Peel base is packaged within a bottle that has a pump dispenser to dispense the modified blue base. Pipettes and sponges (gauze may be used instead) are also supplied within the same kit. Figure 10.3 shows the components of the ZO Controlled Depth Peel. Before application on a patient, the physician must freshly combine a precise volume of 30% TCA solution with the supplied blue base and mix it together (Figures 10.4 to 10.6). The necessary 30% TCA solution should be obtained from a dependable source. Any remaining unused portion of the mixed preparation should be discarded because gradual evaporation may increase concentration of the TCA within the mixed solution.

In addition to having ready the freshly mixed solution of desired TCA concentration (30% TCA of varying volumes and blue base), the physician should have readily accessible a bottle of normal saline for flushing in the unfortunate case of acid accidentally entering the patient's eyes. Cotton-tipped swabs should also be handy to apply the solution to icepick scars and eyelids.

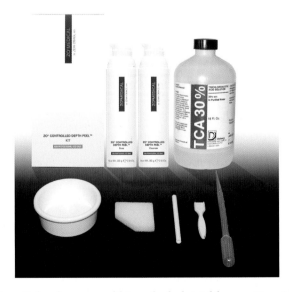

FIGURE 10.3   Essentials: cleanser, rubbing alcohol, trichloroacetic acid 30%, blue base, cup, sponge, transfer pipette, cotton-tipped applicators and brush stick, and spatula.

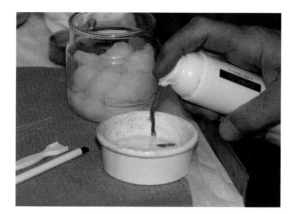

FIGURE 10.4   Adding 6 pumps of blue base to the clear 30% trichloroacetic acid (TCA) solution in the bowl ensures both the proper concentration and slower trichloroacetic acid penetration when it is applied on the skin. To prepare the 20% coat system: 4 mL 30% TCA plus 2 mL (6 pumps) blue base = 6 mL of the 20% concentration. To prepare the 26% to 28% coat system: 8 mL 30% TCA plus 2 mL (6 pumps) blue base = 10 mL of the 26% concentration; 10 mL 30% TCA plus 2 mL (6 pumps) blue base = 12 mL of the 28% concentration.

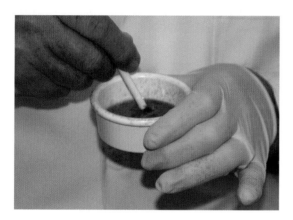

FIGURE 10.5   Mixing the blue base in the bowl that contains 4 to 8 mL of the clear 30% trichloroacetic acid (TCA) solution. In addition to having ready the freshly mixed solution of desired TCA concentration (30% TCA of varying volumes and blue base), the physician should have readily accessible a bottle of normal saline for flushing in the unfortunate case of acid accidentally entering the patient's eyes. Cotton-tipped swabs should also be handy to apply the solution to icepick scars and eyelids.

GENERAL INSTRUCTIONS

Sedation

To control a patient's pain and discomfort, physicians can choose from various methods. Topical anesthetics such as EMLA cream (lidocaine 2.5% and prilocaine 2.5%) are not recommended for use with chemical peels. These agents alter skin hydration and may result in an uneven penetration of the TCA solution. The other three options (local anesthesia, conscious sedation, and general sedation) are acceptable methods for use with chemical peels. Anesthesia is important only before and during the chemical peel; after the procedure, the patient's skin heals painlessly. Regardless of the method the physician chooses, he or she must adhere to local laws in terms of in-office administration of sedation. Furthermore, for safety purposes, patients undergoing conscious sedation should have someone accompany her and drive her home.

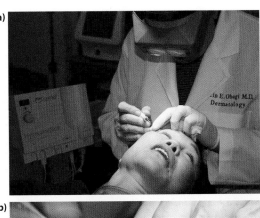

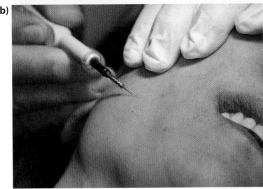

FIGURE 10.6 (a, b) Before administration of the ZO Controlled Depth Peel, the physician can use gentle hyfrecation (electrodessication) to superficially remove certain benign lesions (seborrheic keratoses, flat warts, dermatosis papulosa nigra, acrochorda [skin tags], and junctional nevi) to ensure even and proper penetration of the trichloroacetic acid solution.

Applying the Peel Solution

Patients should arrive the day of the procedure without makeup or jewelry. Hair should be held back with a ponytail holder or a headband. Before administration of the ZO Controlled Depth Peel, the physician can remove certain benign lesions using gentle hyfrecation (electrodessication) to ensure even and proper penetration of the TCA solution (see Figure 10.6).

The patient's face is degreased with alcohol or acetone before the peel solution is applied (alcohol is preferred because it is less irritating). When the face is dry, dip, but do not saturate, a corner of the gauze or sponge (provided in the ZO Controlled Depth Peel kit) into the prepared solution. Begin to apply the solution with short, gentle strokes in all directions, using light pressure. Apply two to five strokes to an area, and then move to another area with a steady speed and rhythm (Figures 10.7 and 10.8). Many physicians prefer to begin with the chin, proceeding to the perioral area, nose, cheeks, and then the forehead. The upper and lower eyelids and other areas can be refined with cotton-tipped swabs. Whether one proceeds in a clockwise or counterclockwise direction, it is important not to return to an already treated area until the solution has been evenly applied to the entire face while respecting the 1 to 2 minutes it takes for neutralization of the applied acid (the period of relative resistance is explained later).

Treating the Perioral Area

Using the same application technique, treat the perioral skin circumferentially all the way down to the mental region. The maximal depth for this area

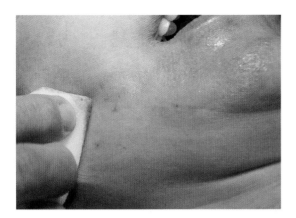

FIGURE 10.7 Applying the ZO Controlled Depth Peel solution (trichloroacetic acid plus blue base) to the face in a controlled, even fashion. Notice the thin and even application of the solution, accomplished by using mainly one corner of the sponge.

is the IRD. Avoid reaching unnecessarily deep levels in this area because scarring can easily occur. This is especially important in the upper lip area where the dermis is thin and little subcutaneous fat rests between the dermis and the underlying muscle. For further correction in this region, it is preferable to repeat the peel (or use another method, such as the CO_2 fractional laser for unstretchable wrinkles) sometime after the peel or 6 to 8 weeks later, rather than attempting deeper correction through a single peel.

To prevent sharp demarcation lines between the neck and the mandibular region, use the feathering technique along the chin and jaw line. To achieve this, apply the solution 1 to 2 inches beyond the main facial treatment site with progressively lighter pressure and progressively shorter acid contact intervals. When the solution has made contact with the skin at these feathering sites, immediately wipe it with a dry tissue. This prevents unintentional deep penetration of the TCA preparation in these peripheral sites. Feathering should achieve a gradually decreasing peel depth, progressing from the IRD to the PD to a deep exfoliation, and ending with a light exfoliation 1 to 2 inches away from the main treatment area (Figure 10.9).

When performing a chemical peel, the maximal safety depth must be observed and respected. With the ZO Controlled Depth Peel, the physician should peel no deeper than the PD or IRD. If the patient requires a deeper peel, a Designed

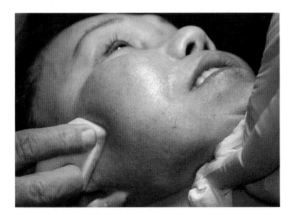

FIGURE 10.8 No free solution is rolling or dripping anywhere as the solution is being applied. The nondominant hand can be used to control any unintentional application of excess solution by removal with a tissue.

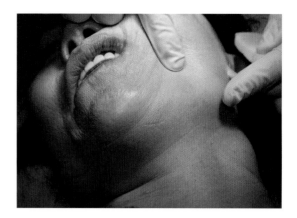

FIGURE 10.9 Proper feathering on the border between the mandibular line and the upper neck is shown here; this is essential to avoid the appearance of a sharp demarcation line.

ZO Control Depth Peel with a 26% to 28% solution (penetrating to a maximal depth of the URD in select sites) may be considered.

Treating the Eyelids

Treating the eyelids helps to eliminate wrinkles and tighten the skin for a better overall cosmetic result. The eyelids should be carefully painted with solution in the same manner as the rest of the face. When coating the upper eyelids, apply the solution in a downward and sideways manner while the patient's eyes remain closed (Figure 10.10). This technique will prevent unwanted opening of the eye. The solution should be applied with only minimal pressure, and it should not drip or run onto already treated skin. Moreover, it should never be allowed to enter the patient's eyes.

When coating the lower lids, the physician must remember to keep the patient's eyes open by lifting and holding the upper lid against the eyebrow bone with his or her thumb. A medical assistant can aid with this maneuver. Apply the solution with horizontal strokes (Figure 10.11). The application should extend beyond the lateral canthi and inward toward the medial canthus. The solution should reach as far superior as the eyelashes and extend inferiorly to the infraorbital rim. At the end of the procedure, the eyelid application should be refined with a cotton swab applicator dipped in solution (Figures 10.12 and 10.13).

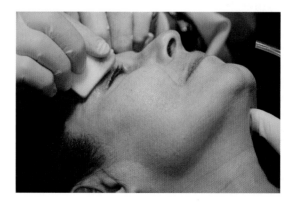

FIGURE 10.10 Application of the ZO Controlled Depth Peel solution to the upper eyelid. Notice the eyes are closed. The sponge is not saturated and not dripping. Application is done sideways and downward.

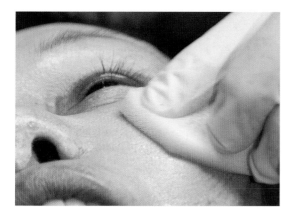

Figure 10.11 Application of the ZO Controlled Depth Peel solution to the lower eyelid. Note that the acid is applied with the eye *open* to ensure optimal visualization and control of acid application. This prevents any free acid from accidentally entering the patient's eyes. If the patient's eyes are closed during this step, acid that might have spread between the eyelids may not be noticed until later. On the lower eyelid, the solution is applied laterally and upward.

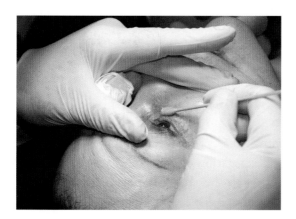

Figure 10.12 When treating the periocular area with the ZO Controlled Depth Peel solution, notice that the eye is open and the lid skin is stretched to prevent any free acids from collecting at the bottom of any fold; stretching the skin ensures even application and fast drying of any solution on the surface.

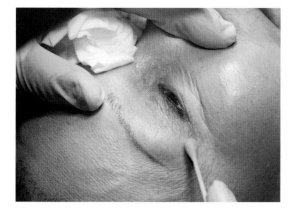

Figure 10.13 Fine-tuning application of the ZO Controlled Depth Peel solution in the periocular areas using a cotton-tipped applicator. This allows the physician to apply the acid solution to areas that were not easily reached with the sponge.

ENDPOINTS AND CLINICAL SIGNS OF A ZO CONTROLLED DEPTH PEEL

Endpoints refer to visible skin changes that indicate the depth of penetration of the TCA solution. Monitoring for specific endpoints allows the physician to stop adding further solution volume after the desired treatment level is reached. Conversely, the physician may continue adding more solution until the peel reaches the chosen depth. This approach produces consistent results and reduces the risk for complications because distinct endpoints correspond to specific ZO Controlled Depth Peel depths (Table 10.6). In contrast, current TCA peels that simply use plain or augmented TCA do not have such clear endpoints. Their results are therefore unpredictable and produce a higher risk for complications.

Despite the publication of a study documenting the correlation of reproducible skin changes to the depth of acid penetration (depth signs), some physicians doubt the existence of these clinically based signs.[3] Recognition of the development of these depth signs requires careful clinical observation and experience. The ZO method of monitoring solution penetration depth is based on the appearance of these signs and allows the physician to perform a safer, more controlled chemical peel.

THE FROST SIGN AND THE PINK SIGN

During a ZO Controlled Depth Peel, TCA will cause a frost to appear on the skin as a result of coagulation of epidermal and dermal proteins. If the acid penetration is limited to the epidermal layer, the skin shows an even blue appearance. An initial speckled, scattered frost may or may not be present at the epidermal level (Figures 10.14 and 10.15). Following the application of more solution volume and deeper penetration, this cloud-like frost will begin

---

TABLE 10.6 Clinical Endpoints at Different Depths of the ZO Controlled Depth Peel

Peel Type and Depth	Color	Frost	Pink Background	Epidermal Sliding
ZO Controlled Depth Peel to the papillary dermis (PD)	Even blue	Thin, transparent, organized white sheet	Present	Present
ZO Controlled Depth Peel to the immediate reticular dermis (IRD)	Even blue	Solid, organized white sheet	Just faded	Just faded
ZO Designed Controlled Depth Peel to the PD, IRD, or upper reticular dermis (URD) (URD focally involved)*	Even blue	Solid frost, white with grayish tone	PD: present IRD: absent URD: absent	PD: present IRD: absent URD: absent
ZO Designed Controlled Depth Peel medium depth to PD, IRD, and URD (URD more extensively involved)†	Even blue	White frost with grayish tone	PD: present IRD: absent URD: absent	PD: present IRD: absent URD: absent

*In the ZO Designed Controlled Depth Peel, the URD is reached in small focal areas of the face.
†In the medium-depth ZO Designed Controlled Depth Peel, the URD is reached to involve larger local areas.

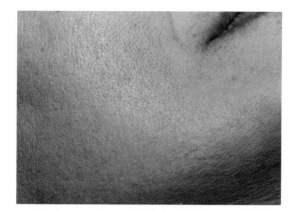

FIGURE 10.14 Early frost formation (speckles) on the treated skin at the epidermal level. Notice that this frost has not yet become confluent to form an "organized" sheet of frost.

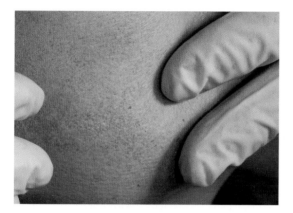

FIGURE 10.15 Denser speckles during early frost formation.

to organize, and a more confluent white sheet will appear. This will occur faster in thin skin than in thick skin.

When the peel reaches the PD, the frost looks like a thin, transparent, organized, white sheet with a pink background (Figure 10.16). This "pink sign" is visible only at certain stages of the peel. When TCA has begun to penetrate the PD, the frost will show the pink background. This is due to the intact blood vessels and continuous blood flow within the PD capillary loops. Frosting of the PD should last for 5 minutes (before total defrosting), which

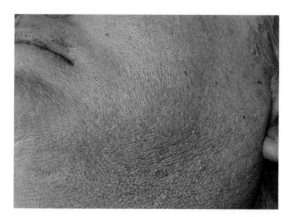

FIGURE 10.16 The treated area now appears to have an organized, sheet-like frost that has an underlying pink background. This appearance is characteristic of a ZO Controlled Depth Peel that has penetrated to the level of the papillary dermis.

confirms that the peel has adequately reached the PD. If the frost starts to fade in less than 5 minutes, more TCA solution should be applied to restore the white frost. This frost should then last an additional 1 to 2 minutes. The peel has reached the IRD when the frost resembles a solid white sheet without any pink background. (When the pink signs start to fade, the IRD and the desired depth have been reached.) The pink sign disappears because of the occlusion or vasospasm within the capillary loops of the papillary dermis, and blood flow in these papillary dermal vessels has stopped. Figure 10.17 shows the progressive levels of vascular reactions during TCA application. If the IRD is the depth desired, no further solution should be applied at this point. If one of the designed URD depths is desired, additional solution can be applied in chosen areas.

Further application of the acid solution will transform the white frost to a grayish color, which indicates that the peel has reached the URD. The moment this grayish tone appears, the physician must stop applying the peel solution. The URD is the maximal depth advisable for a ZO Controlled Depth Peel. In skilled hands and in certain areas of the patient's face, the URD may be reached. Medium to thick skin is ideal for the ZO Designed Controlled Depth Peel, but thin skin is not. Figure 10.18 shows a patient demonstrating all levels of frost simultaneously during a ZO Designed Controlled Depth Peel.

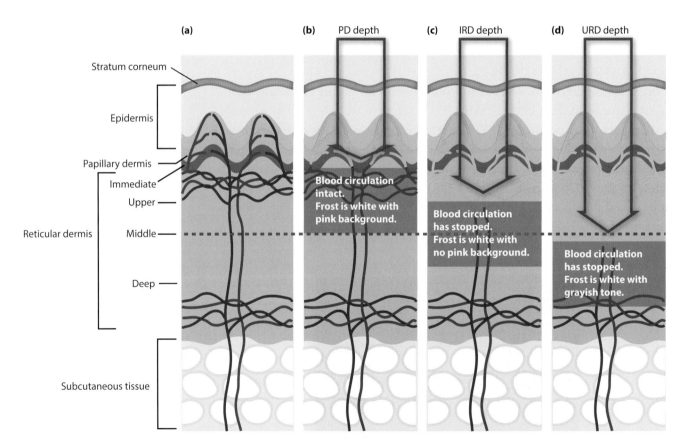

FIGURE 10.17 Progressive levels of vascular reactions during application of the ZO Controlled Depth Peel. When trichloroacetic acid (TCA) has penetrated to the level of the papillary dermis, blood circulation is intact, and the frost is white with a pink background. When TCA has penetrated to the level of the immediate reticular dermis, blood circulation has stopped, and the frost is white with no pink background. When TCA has penetrated to the upper reticular dermis, blood circulation has stopped, and the frost is white with a grayish tone.

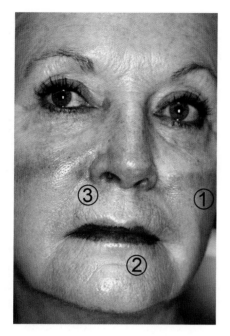

FIGURE 10.18   A patient showing varying depths of penetration and frosting during a ZO Designed Controlled Depth Peel. Note that there are no sharp demarcation lines between the three levels. After this photo was taken, the patient's face was peeled to the appropriate papillary dermis, immediate reticular dermis, and upper reticular dermis levels. (1) White sheet of frost with a pink background at the level of the papillary dermis. (2) White sheet of frost with no pink background at the level of the immediate reticular dermis. (3) Frost with a hint of gray at the level of the upper reticular dermis.

EPIDERMAL SLIDING

Applying TCA to the skin initially causes protein coagulation and precipitation in the epidermis, disruption of anchoring fibrils, initial vasodilation, edema, and a turgid epidermis. These changes allow the epidermis to be moved more freely on the uninvolved dermis (TCA has not yet reached the dermis). If the skin is pinched or pushed, a wrinkling effect occurs in the epidermis and is referred to as the "epidermal sliding sign" (Figures 10.19 to 10.24). This manifestation indicates that the TCA has reached but not completely coagulated the PD. The frost still shows a pink background, however, because the blood flow within the PD capillary loops remains intact.

When the acid has precipitated all components of the PD, the epidermis becomes "fixed" to the dermis as one protein block and is no longer moveable.

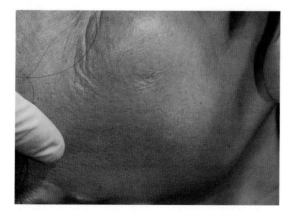

FIGURE 10.19   The epidermal sliding phenomenon on the cheeks and temple. Notice the confluent, sheet-like frost and underlying pink appearance of the treated skin.

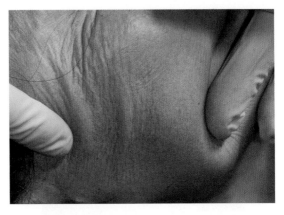

FIGURE 10.20   Epidermal sliding on the cheeks.

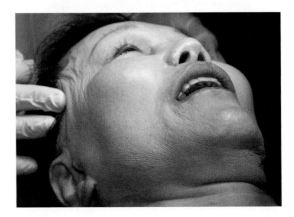

FIGURE 10.21   Epidermal sliding on the temples.

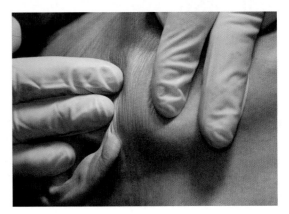

FIGURE 10.22   Epidermal sliding on the upper cheek indicating penetration to the papillary dermis.

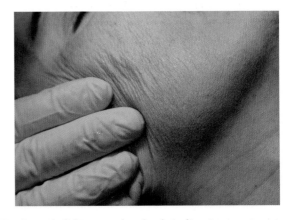

FIGURE 10.23   Epidermal sliding on the cheek indicating penetration to the papillary dermis.

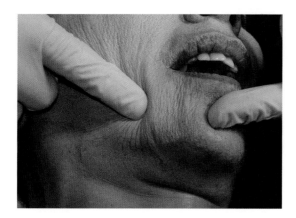

FIGURE 10.24   Epidermal sliding on the lower cheek, indicating penetration to the papillary dermis.

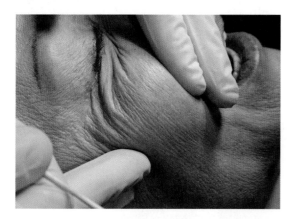

FIGURE 10.25   Epidermal sliding has disappeared on the upper cheeks, indicating that the ZO Controlled Depth Peel has penetrated beyond the papillary dermis to the level of the immediate reticular dermis. Notice the frost without pink in the upper cheek and the presence of epidermal sliding and frost with pink in the lower cheek.

When the epidermal sliding sign disappears, the peel has completely penetrated the PD and has now reached the IRD. The frost here no longer displays a pink background because the capillary loops in the PD have been occluded or constricted by vasospasm, as was shown in Figure 10.18. Figure 10.25 shows the disappearance of epidermal sliding when the peel has reached the level of the IRD.

ENDPOINTS AT COMPLETION OF THE ZO CONTROLLED DEPTH PEEL

With experience, the physician will easily be able to identify the signs at different acid penetration depths (Table 10.7). Of note, the ZO Designed Controlled

TABLE 10.7 Endpoints for a ZO Controlled Depth Peel	
Penetration	*Endpoint*
Papillary dermis	• Frost with a pink background • Epidermal sliding
Immediate reticular dermis	• Frost with minimal to no pink background • No epidermal sliding

Box 10.10

Ideal Depth for the ZO Controlled Depth Peel

- The immediate reticular dermis is the ideal safe depth in all skin types.
- At this depth, the frost appears white (because the pink background has faded), and epidermal sliding has just disappeared.

Depth Peel is ideal for darker skin types because such skin makes it difficult to see the grayish tone of URD penetration. The IRD is the ideal depth of safety in all skin types (Box 10.10). Figure 10.26 shows a properly completed ZO Controlled Depth Peel to the level of the PD, whereas Figure 10.27 shows a properly completed ZO Controlled Depth Peel to the level of the IRD. Figure 10.28 shows a patient demonstrating all of the clinical endpoints during a ZO Controlled Depth Peel.

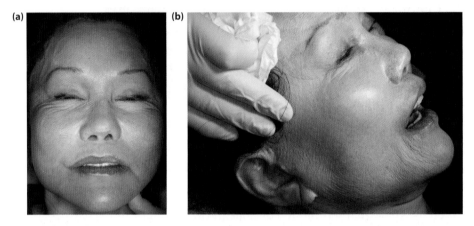

Figure 10.26   (a) Completed ZO Controlled Depth Peel to the level of the papillary dermis. Notice the even bluish-white, sheet-like frost overlying a confluent pink background. (b) Right side view of completed ZO Controlled Depth Peel to the level of the papillary dermis. Notice the even blue color and even frost around the eye.

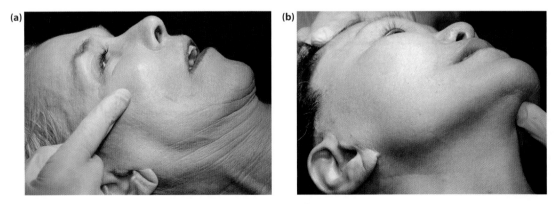

Figure 10.27   (a) Completed ZO Controlled Depth Peel to the immediate reticular dermis. Notice the confluent white, sheet-like frost without an underlying pink background on the face (with the exception of the upper and lower eyelids, which were treated to the papillary dermis level). (b) Completed ZO Controlled Depth Peel to the level of the immediate reticular dermis showing even white frost, which is confluent into a sheet-like appearance *without* an underlying pink background.

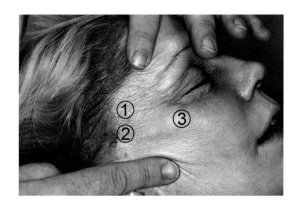

FIGURE 10.28   A patient showing clinical endpoints during a ZO Controlled Depth Peel. (1) Sheet of white frost with pink background. (2) Epidermal sliding (fine wrinkles). (3) White, sheet-like frost with no pink background. If pressure were to be applied, no epidermal sliding would be observed here.

SUPPORTIVE CLINICAL SIGNS TO CONFIRM DEPTH

Supportive clinical signs associated with the specific depth of penetration of a ZO Controlled Depth Peel include 1) defrosting time, 2) skin firmness, and 3) healing time (Table 10.8). The depth of skin injury has an especially high correlation with the expected healing time; the former can help predict the latter.

Frosting signifies the coagulation of epidermal and dermal proteins. After this has occurred, the process of dispersing the precipitated proteins, termed defrosting, begins. Defrosting time depends on skin thickness; the thicker the skin, the longer it takes to defrost. Dermal frost should last 3 to 5 minutes in peels to the IRD level in thick skin and 3 minutes in thin skin.

Following each peel, the practitioner should pinch the skin to feel for firmness to validate the achieved depth. The more proteins coagulated by the action of TCA, the firmer the skin will feel on pinching. In peels that reach the IRD and the URD, one can easily detect an increased level of skin firmness. However, when they reach only the PD, this sign becomes less clear. Firmness is especially pronounced with the ZO Designed Controlled Depth Peel, especially in thick skin.

Healing time is the time required by the skin to complete its re-epithelialization. Because this sign correlates well with the depth of skin injury in all skin types, one can accurately predict healing time if one carefully follows

TABLE 10.8   Supportive Clinical Signs at Different Depths of the ZO Controlled Depth Peel

| Peel Depth | Defrosting Time (min)* | | Firmness | Healing Time (days) |
	Thin Skin	Thick Skin		
Papillary dermis	2-3	4	Light	7 to 8
Immediate reticular dermis	3-4	5-6	Moderate	8 to 10
Upper reticular dermis	5-6	5-8	Strong (leather-like)	10-12

*The difference in defrosting time is due to a range of skin thicknesses: very thick, thick, medium, medium-thin, thin, and so forth. However, 3 to 5 minutes is an acceptable average.

the ZO Controlled Depth Peel endpoints. After the procedure, observing a patient's healing time gives the physician a retrospective indication of the depth achieved by the peel. The observed healing time should be documented in the patient's record.

PATIENT SELECTION AND COUNSELING

As with any dermatologic procedure, physicians can help to ensure the success of the ZO Controlled Depth Peel by selecting appropriate patients and teaching them preprocedure and post-procedure care and explaining expected results. Before undergoing a ZO Controlled Depth Peel, patients should be aware of all features of the peels (Box 10.11).

THE PRE-PEEL OFFICE CONSULTATION

Along with explaining the objectives of ZO Controlled Depth Peel to the patient (leveling vs. tightening), the physician must also address several logistic and

---

Box 10.11

Patient Information

FEATURES OF THE ZO CONTROLLED DEPTH PEEL

1. When properly performed, the ZO Controlled Depth Peel is a well-controlled procedure that can reach specific depths to achieve both medical and aesthetic results.
2. The peel's main objective is to tighten the skin (improve laxity, eliminate stretchable scars and wrinkles).
3. The ZO Controlled Depth Peel offers a high degree of safety and is suitable for all skin types.
4. Even when carefully allowed to penetrate to the depth of the IRD, the ZO Controlled Depth Peel will not thin the skin or cause permanent hypopigmentation or hyperpigmentation.
5. For thin skin, one ZO Controlled Depth Peel down to the depth of the IRD will provide maximal tightening. Thick skin will require two to three treatments with the ZO Controlled Depth Peel to produce equivalent results.
6. For maximum improvement, patients may need more than one ZO Controlled Depth Peel or other procedure.
7. If the peel is to be repeated, the time intervals between peels must be no shorter than 6 weeks for PD peel, 8 to 10 weeks for IRD peel, and 4 to 5 months for URD peel.

medicolegal matters in preparation for the peel. Patient dependability must be ascertained and the importance of program compliance stressed. Clear verbal and written explanation should be given about the preprocedure skin-conditioning regimen, with *at least* 6 weeks (one full keratinocyte maturation cycle) of consistent and thorough program use. The physician must also ensure that the patient has realistic expectations regarding the final result of the peel and is not pregnant or lactating.

The physician should further identify, treat, and control all inflammatory conditions (e.g., acne, folliculitis, active infections) and provide prophylactic treatment to prevent herpes simplex virus (HSV) eruptions before performing a ZO Controlled Depth Peel. If the patient has a history of HSV cold sores, oral antiviral medication should be started to prevent recurrence. Typical antiviral prophylaxis is begun the day before the procedure and continued for 10 days after the procedure. Either acyclovir (400 mg, three times daily) or valaciclovir (500 mg, twice daily) can be used.

At least 1 week before performing the peel, the detailed consent forms should be reviewed with the patient. The physician must ensure that the patient understands the expected recovery time, anticipated reactions (postinflammatory hyperpigmentation [PIH], milia, acne), potential complications (hypertrophic scars, keloids, hypopigmentation, infection), and alternatives to having the ZO Controlled Depth Peel procedure. The patient must also be advised that he or she may need more than one ZO Controlled Depth Peel (or other additional procedures) to achieve an optimal cosmetic result. Pre-peel counseling should also include a thorough discussion regarding the various post-procedure healing stages; instructional videos and photos can be shown to further clarify these to the patient, if available.

The planned method of sedation should also be explained to the patient in detail. If nerve block or conscious sedation is anticipated, patients must be told that they will need someone to drive them to and from the procedure appointment. An anesthesiologist is usually employed to administer nerve blocks and conscious sedation to patients undergoing a ZO Controlled Depth Peel. After the procedure has been completed, patients generally feel no pain.

Patients should have high-quality preprocedure photographs taken without makeup, and these should be kept on file in the office. On the day of the procedure, the patient should be sent home with all of the required post-procedure supplies and a follow-up visit scheduled.

HEALING AND RECOVERY EXPECTATIONS

Patients go through distinct healing stages after a ZO Controlled Depth Peel, and they should know what to expect during each stage (Boxes 10.12 to 10.14). Such stages apply to all resurfacing procedures.

For the ZO Controlled Depth Peel to the PD, the initial healing period lasts 8 days, compared with 10 days for a ZO Controlled Depth Peel to the IRD, and 10 to 12 days for a ZO Designed Controlled Depth Peel (which penetrates to the URD in certain areas).

The first stage of healing has been completed when the skin has re-epithelialized. At this point, the skin is able to tolerate topical treatment with tretinoin

Box 10.12

Day of Procedure and Initial Healing Period

1. Blue color disappears in 1 to 3 days.
2. Total healing time is 7 to 12 days (varies according to depth of peel penetration).
3. Generalized edema and a subsequently darker appearance of skin tone will occur at the treatment site. Prepare patients for this so that they are not alarmed.
4. Home care instructions should begin according to Table 10.9.

Box 10.13

Recovery Period

- Duration: 3 to 6 weeks. Skin may look normal, but most often it will appear red, blotchy, and uneven in color tone after deeper procedures.
- Postinflammatory hyperpigmentation may be present; acne and rosacea may flare.
- When the skin becomes tolerant, patients may restart their full skin-conditioning regimen.
- If indicated, low-dose isotretinoin (20 mg/day) may be added at this time to treat and control certain problems (e.g., acne, rosacea).

Box 10.14

Normalization with Continued Improvement

- Duration: 2 to 3 months. Skin appears relatively normal (scant erythema is possible and/or postinflammatory hyperpigmentation).
- The patient either continues with the preprocedure skin-conditioning regimen or switches to a long-term maintenance regimen when ready.
- If indicated, isotretinoin may be started, continued, or stopped.

and hydroquinone. Patients may resume their preprocedure skin-conditioning regimen, as tolerated. It is essential to restart this topical program (with the exception of mechanical exfoliating agents) as soon as re-epithelialization has occurred because it stabilizes skin color (reduces the risk for PIH), reduces redness, and restores the skin's normal tolerance (barrier function).

The second healing stage is marked by changes within the epidermis and dermis, including redness, uneven color, PIH and collagen production and alignment, and neovascularization. The second healing stage lasts

TABLE 10.9 Post-procedure Home Care Instructions

| Activity | Post-procedure Day | | After Complete Healing |
	Days 1-4	Day 5 Healing	
Cleanse face with nonabrasive cleanser twice daily	X	X	Return to using ZO Medical in the recovery stage
Antiseptic compresses every 2-4 hours while awake	X	X	
Thin layer of petrolatum-based lubricant (after each compress)	X		

approximately 2 to 6 weeks. Accordingly, one must not judge a peel's results until this stage has been completed.

Several elements can delay healing. These include patient-related factors such as picking, excoriation, and cracking of the epidermis due to stretching of the facial skin and improper postpeel management (excessive dryness or moisture). Other conditions that can hinder healing include minor complications such as irritation or infection, which may be avoided through use of wet antiseptic compresses and other home care steps.

POST-PROCEDURE HOME CARE INSTRUCTIONS

Following the ZO Controlled Depth Peel procedure, the patient should be instructed to cleanse the treatment site twice daily with a mild, nonabrasive cleanser (Table 10.9). Cleansing must be gentle in nature, and vigorous rubbing of the skin should be avoided. Antiseptic compresses should be applied four times per day (every 2 to 3 hours while the patient is awake). Antiseptics most commonly used for this include acetic acid 5%, aluminum acetate 0.14% (ZO Medical Surfatrol, one packet mixed with 16 ounces of bottled water), or white vinegar (1 part white vinegar mixed with 9 parts of bottled water). These solutions are applied with 4 × 4 inch gauze pads. Patients should pat skin firmly with the soaked gauze (apply perpendicular pressure with the gauze), without rubbing, for approximately 1 to 2 minutes. Patting with pressure allows serous fluid to be absorbed onto the gauze.

For the first 3 to 5 days following the ZO Controlled Depth Peel, the patient should apply a *thin* layer of a petrolatum-based lubricant (ZO Medical Pomatrol Soothing Ointment) to all treatment areas after application of antiseptic compresses. This hastens healing and prevents premature dryness and scabbing. Applying too thick a layer of this lubricant can cause premature skin peeling and increase the likelihood of post-procedure acne.

Beginning on post-procedure day 5, the patient should discontinue use of the petrolatum-based lubricant (ZO Medical Pomatrol Soothing Ointment) and instead start using a nongreasy (nonocclusive), mild moisturizer (ZO Medical Regencell Epidermal Renewal Creme) after each antiseptic compress. Patients should be encouraged to use this moisturizer frequently throughout the day to prevent premature skin dryness and crust formation. After a thin layer has been applied, it should be gently massaged into the skin until it is fully absorbed. A specially formulated healing kit is also available from ZO Skin Health, Inc. It provides the required three healing elements: step 1—3- to 5-day semiocclusive ointment; step 2—day 5 of healing with a nonocclusive, hydrating and calming lotion; and step 3—antiseptic, anticrusting, calming powder for compresses.

Patients should be cautioned about picking or manually peeling the skin. Clean scissors may be used to cut any loose or hanging skin. When cleansing, water should be splashed gently onto the face, and water pressure from the showerhead should not be allowed to directly contact the treatment area. Excessive facial expressions and stretching of facial skin should be avoided. Loose hair should always be pulled back to avoid contact with the treatment site. Patients should be encouraged to sleep on their back (not on their side or stomach) to avoid rubbing their face on the pillow. Elevating the head with two or more pillows for the first few nights following the procedure is encouraged because it will lessen edema.

PATIENT RESULTS

Figure 10.29 shows a patients who underwent a ZO Controlled Depth Peel to the PD, Figures 10.30 through 10.32 show patients who underwent the peel to the IRD, and Figure 10.33 shows a patient who had a PD level peel and later, after developing HQ resistance, had an IRD level peel. Figures 10.34 through 10.36 show patients who underwent a ZO Design Controlled

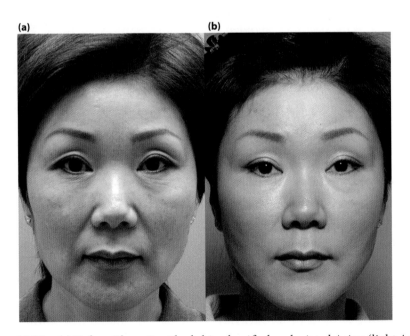

(a)   (b)

FIGURE 10.29 (a) Before. The patient had skin classified as deviated Asian (light Asian), thick, and oily. She was diagnosed as having postinflammatory hyperpigmentation and fine rhytides. (b) One year later. The patient had 6 weeks of an aggressive hydroquinone (HQ)-based Skin Health Restoration program followed by a ZO Controlled Depth Peel to the papillary dermis. After the peel, she continued with the HQ-based protocol for an additional 12 weeks. A non-HQ-based Skin Health Restoration regimen was then used for maintenance.

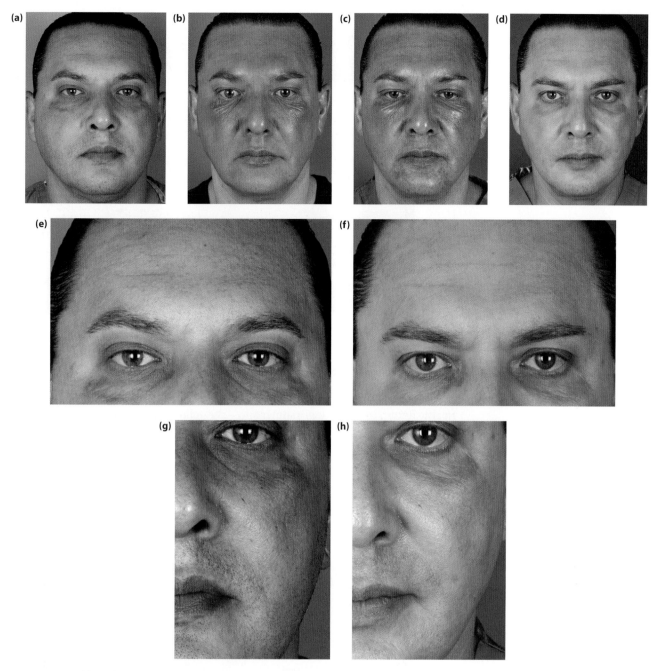

Figure 10.30 (a) Before. The patient had skin classified as deviated white (medium white), thick, and oily. He was diagnosed as having rosacea, sebaceous gland hyperplasia, and associated erythema. Six weeks of skin conditioning was followed by a ZO Controlled Depth Peel to the immediate reticular dermis. (b) The patient on day 1 following a ZO Controlled Depth Peel. (c) The patient on day 5 following a ZO Controlled Depth Peel. (d) One month after the peel. The patient had resumed hydroquinone-based skin conditioning and started isotretinoin, 20 mg/day. (e) Forehead before. The patient had significant gland hyperplasia on the forehead. (f) Forehead after. Many of the sebaceous glands were hyfrecated lightly before the ZO Controlled Depth Peel to the immediate reticular dermis. He was then treated with Skin Health Restoration along with isotretinoin, 20 mg/day for 3 months after healing, which led to the disappearance of most of the hypertrophic sebaceous glands. (g) Cheeks before. The patient had wrinkles, skin laxity, and erythema from rosacea. (h) Cheeks after. The patient's skin is tighter, and erythema has disappeared after using Skin Health Restoration along with isotretinoin following healing from the peel.

Depth Peel, Figures 10.37 and 10.38 show patients who practiced Skin Health Restoration for 20 years and periodically underwent a ZO Controlled Depth Peel. Figures 10.39 through 10.42 show patients who underwent an IRD-level ZO Controlled Depth Peel or a ZO Designed Controlled Depth Peel for leveling and/or tightening.

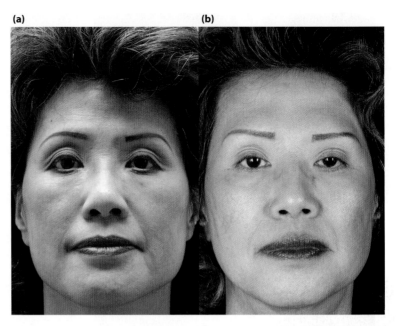

FIGURE 10.31 (a) Before. The patient had skin classified as deviated Asian (light Asian), thick, and oily. She was diagnosed with early signs of aging consisting of rhytides and laxity. (b) One year later. The patient had 6 weeks of an aggressive hydroquinone (HQ)-based Skin Health Restoration program followed by a ZO Controlled Depth Peel to the immediate reticular dermis. After the peel, she underwent 12 weeks of HQ-based Skin Health Restoration. During maintenance, she followed a non-HQ-based skin health regimen.

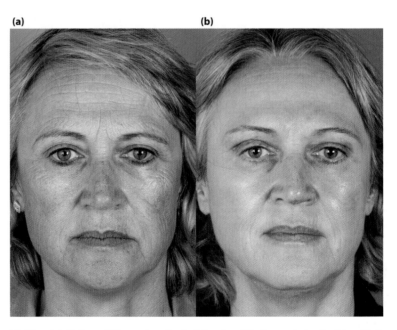

FIGURE 10.32 (a) Before. The patient had skin classified as original white (light white), medium thick, and nonoily. She was diagnosed as having photodamage, rhytides, and laxity. (b) Six months later. The patient had 6 weeks of aggressive hydroquinone (HQ)-based Skin Health Restoration, followed by a ZO Controlled Depth Peel to the immediate reticular dermis. After the peel, she continued with the same ZOMD HQ-based program for 5 months. During maintenance, she followed a non-HQ-based Skin Health Restoration regimen.

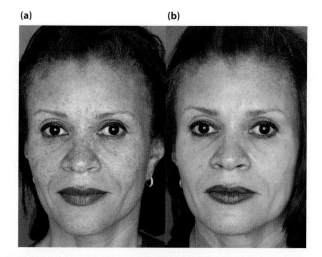

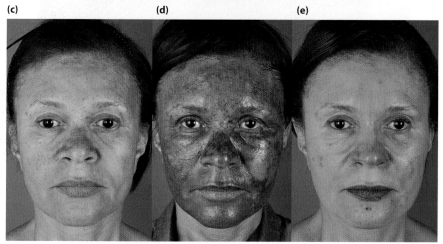

FIGURE 10.33 (a) Before. The patient had skin classified as complex, medium thick, and oily. Complex skin is of mixed racial origin and could be considered to be highly deviated. She was diagnosed with melasma, postinflammatory hyperpigmentation, photodamage, and freckles. (b) Five months later. The patient received 6 weeks of aggressive hydroquinone (HQ)-based Skin Health Restoration, a ZO Controlled Depth Peel to the papillary dermis, and 12 weeks of moderate non-HQ-based Skin Health Restoration. (c) Ten years later. The same patient was using HQ without supervision (obtained from an Internet supplier). She was diagnosed as having melasma, freckles, and HQ resistance. (d) The patient directly after a ZO Controlled Depth Peel. She had 12 weeks of non-hydroquinone (HQ)-based Skin Health Restoration with aggressive epidermal and melanocyte stabilization to eliminate HQ resistance. Following non-HQ-based restoration, she had 6 weeks of aggressive HQ-based Skin Health Restoration. This was then followed by a ZO Controlled Depth Peel to the immediate reticular dermis. (e) Ten days after a ZO Controlled Depth Peel. The patient's skin shows complete healing. She returned to an aggressive HQ-based Skin Health Restoration regimen for three keratinocyte maturation cycles (18 weeks), followed by non-HQ-based maintenance.

ZO CONTROLLED DEPTH PEEL COMBINED WITH OTHER PROCEDURES

As detailed in Chapter 5, combining two or more procedures with different mechanisms of action during the same surgical session can maximize results, minimize invasiveness, and optimize safety. For example, unnecessary depth in areas where there might be higher risk for textural changes or other

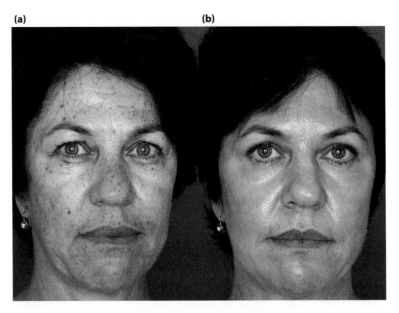

FIGURE 10.34   (a) Before. The patient had skin classified as original white color, thick, and oily. She was diagnosed as having rosacea and photodamage. (b) One year later. The patient had 5 months of Skin Health Restoration and a ZO Designed Controlled Depth Peel (6 weeks after starting the program) during the treatment.

complications can be avoided. A ZO Controlled Depth Peel to the PD and IRD on the entire face, followed immediately by the CO_2 fractional laser to the URD in certain areas, provides better results than either procedure alone. It increases safety because it avoids penetrating to unnecessarily deep levels (e.g., the URD) to achieve the desired tightness while limiting the depth only to areas where leveling is desired. Other combinations include 1) a facelift to remove excessive skin and/or muscle combined with a nonsurgical skin tightening procedure to the entire face by means of a ZO Controlled Depth Peel, 2)

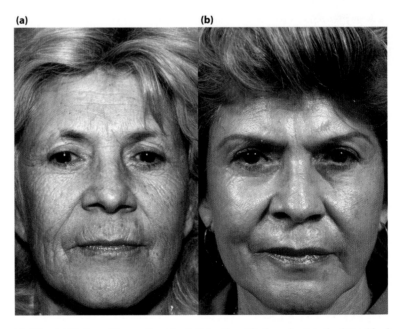

FIGURE 10.35   (a) Before. The patient had skin classified as deviated white (dark white), thick, and nonoily. She was diagnosed as having photodamage and solar elastosis. (b) One year later. She underwent 6 weeks of aggressive hydroquinone (HQ)-based Skin Health Restoration, followed by a medium-depth ZO Designed Controlled Depth Peel 12 weeks after starting the treatment. After the peel, she continued the HQ-based Skin Health Restoration program for 3 more months.

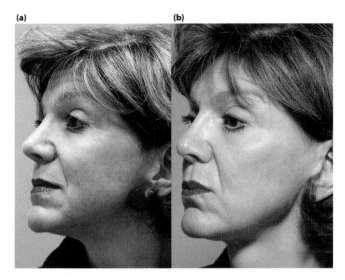

FIGURE 10.36 (a) Before. The patient's skin was an original white color (light white), medium thick, and normally oily. She was diagnosed as having laxity and rhytides. (b) One year later. The patient underwent aggressive hydroquinone (HQ)-based Skin Health Restoration for 6 weeks followed by a ZO Designed Controlled Depth Peel. After healing, she continued with an HQ-based Skin Health Restoration program for 3 months, followed by non-HQ-based maintenance.

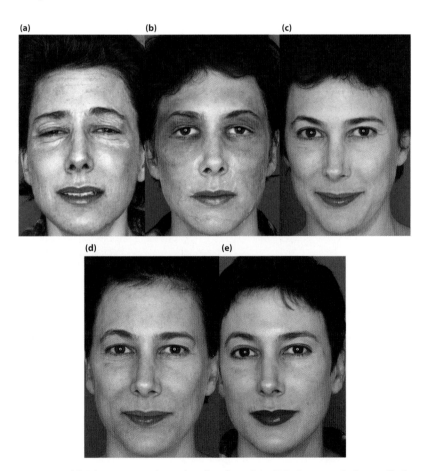

FIGURE 10.37 (a) The patient directly after her first ZO Designed Controlled Depth Peel. (b) The patient 8 days after a ZO Designed Controlled Depth Peel. (c) The patient 1 year later. (d) The patient at age 36 years. The skin of this patient was a deviated white color, normal white, medium thick, and oily. She was diagnosed as having rosacea, early laxity, and rhytides. (e) Twenty years later after undergoing five treatments with the ZO Controlled Depth Peel (three of Dr. Obagi's previous Blue Peels and two of the ZO Controlled Depth Peels) to the papillary dermis, immediate reticular dermis, and upper reticular dermis each time.

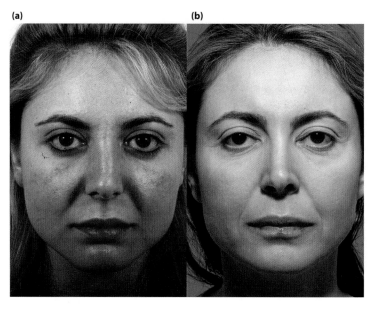

FIGURE 10.38   (a) The patient in 1992. The patient's skin is normal white, medium thick, and medium oily. She was diagnosed with rosacea, large pores, postinflammatory hyperpigmentation, and mild laxity. (b) The patient in 2012. For 20 years, she was treated with multiple courses of hydroquinone (HQ)-based Skin Health Restoration for 5 months at a time. To maintain tightness, she underwent two of Dr. Obagi's previous Blue Peels, followed by two treatments with the ZO Controlled Depth Peel to the immediate reticular dermis (one peel every 4 to 5 years). After certain peels, she started isotretinoin, 20 mg/day for 3 to 5 months. Maintenance was not HQ based.

a vascular or pigment laser treatment combined with a ZO Controlled Depth Peel to the PD simultaneously improves skin texture, restores even color tone, and corrects stretchable wrinkles and scars, and 3) electrodessication and gentle hyfrecation to treat dermatosis papulosa nigra, condyloma acuminata, syringomas, and actinic keratoses combined with a ZO Controlled Depth Peel to the PD or IRD (as shown in Figures 10.43 to 10.45).

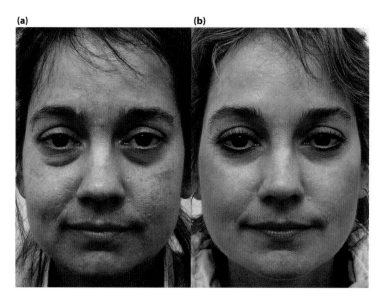

FIGURE 10.39   (a) Before. The patient had skin classified as normal white, medium thick, and oily. She was diagnosed as having laxity, acne scars, and lower eyelid hollowness. Her conditions indicated the need for a tightening procedure. (b) One year later. She had 5 months of hydroquinone (HQ)-based Skin Health Restoration during which a ZO Controlled Depth Peel to the immediate reticular dermis was performed. Notice the tightness, texture improvement, and disappearance of the lower eyelid hollowness.

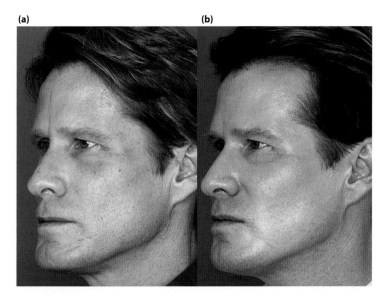

FIGURE 10.40 (a) Before. The patient had skin classified as normal white, medium thick, and oily. He was diagnosed as having rosacea, stretchable acne scars, and sebaceous gland hyperplasia. His conditions indicated the need for a tightening procedure. (b) One year later. He had 6 weeks of non-hydroquinone (HQ)-based Skin Health Restoration followed by a medium-depth ZO Designed Controlled Depth Peel. He then had 3 months of non-HQ-based Skin Health Restoration and isotretinoin, 20 mg/day.

PEELING NONFACIAL SKIN

The skin of nonfacial areas, such as the décolletage, arms, and hands, tends to be poor in sebaceous glands and other adnexal structures. Within the same location, it may be tight and/or loose. For example, the skin on the hands is tight and cannot be pinched in the area of the fingers, but on the dorsum, it is loose. Over the neck area, the skin is tight posterolaterally and loose anteriorly.

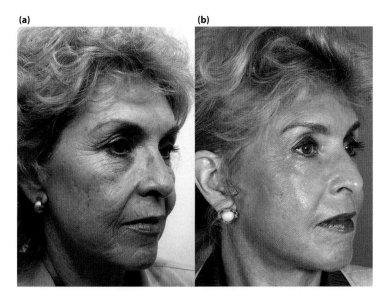

FIGURE 10.41 (a) Before. The patient had skin classified as normal white, medium thick, and nonoily. She was diagnosed as having photodamage, laxity, wrinkles, and acne scars. Her conditions indicated the need for a tightening and leveling procedure. (b) One year later. The patient had 5 months of hydroquinone (HQ)-based Skin Health Restoration and a medium-depth ZO Designed Controlled Depth Peel after 6 weeks of Skin Health Restoration (skin conditioning).

(a)   **(b)**

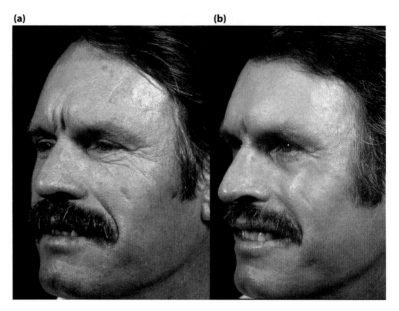

FIGURE 10.42 (a) Before. The patient had skin classified as normal white, thick, and oily. He was diagnosed as having laxity, wrinkles, and a scar on his left cheek. His conditions indicated the need for a tightening and leveling procedure. (b) One year later. The patient had 6 weeks of hydroquinone (HQ)-based Skin Health Restoration followed by a medium-depth ZO Designed Controlled Depth Peel and then 12 weeks of HQ-based Skin Health Restoration.

This is due to the direct attachment of this skin to the underlying muscle with little subcutaneous fat.

In areas where nonfacial skin is loose (can be easily pinched) and where the stratum corneum is thin, frost appears faster compared with areas where the skin is firmly attached (knuckles, toes) or where the stratum corneum is thick. The latter may show only a cloud of speckled frost or no frost at all, despite equal and adequate application of acid solution. In nonfacial skin, the physician should focus on achieving an even blue color and not an even frost.

When painting nonfacial skin with a colorless TCA solution, nonfrosted areas frequently confuse physicians. They believe that these regions have been neglected and that no acid was applied. They therefore paint additional solution to induce a frost. This confusion can lead to unnecessary deep penetration and possible scarring. This does not occur with the ZO Controlled Depth Peel

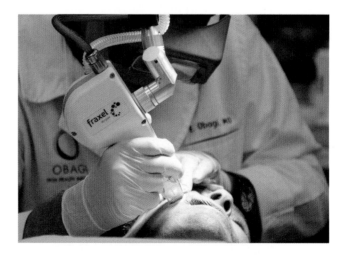

FIGURE 10.43 Dr. Zein Obagi performing a CO_2 fractional laser treatment immediately following the ZO Controlled Depth Peel.

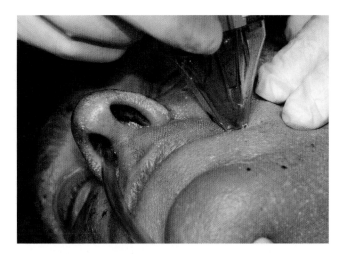

FIGURE 10.44   A CO_2 fractional laser treatment on the unstretchable wrinkles in the perioral area.

because of the presence of the blue color, which easily differentiates painted from nonpainted skin.

PERFORMING A NONFACIAL PEEL

Use the 20% coat system when peeling nonfacial skin and do not exceed the PD in depth. Select a 5% body surface area and apply the coat gradually with even application. Skipped areas are easily made visible by the blue dye in the base. After a coat has been applied, wait 2 minutes for the acid to be neutralized and then paint another. Be sure to maintain an even blue color, similar in intensity, while the frost is slowly progressing. Do not attempt to obtain an even frost. In most cases, one coat of the 20% solution will be enough to reach the PD. Hydrated and pinchable areas will show a sheet of white frost with

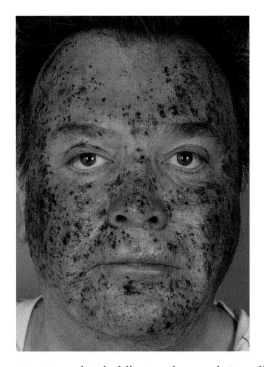

FIGURE 10.45   The patient immediately following the completion of both procedures.

Box 10.15

Peeling Nonfacial Skin

- Use the 20% coat system.
- Select an area to peel that is 5% of the body's surface. If that area is smaller than 5%, decrease the amount of acid solution in the coat proportionately.
- Peel no deeper than the papillary dermis.
- Apply the solution equally and aim for an even blue. After an area shows a sheet of white frost with a pink background, stop the peel. Never attempt to achieve an even frost.
- The areas that frost should display frost with a pink background and epidermal sliding.

epidermal sliding (the dorsum of the hand), whereas firmer, thicker skin (the dorsum of the fingers) may not show any frost or epidermal sliding.

When peeling an area smaller than 5% of the body's surface (as with spot peels), one of two methods may be employed. With the first approach, determine the percentage surface area of the skin to be peeled and then calculate the amount of acid solution needed for one coat (e.g., a 5% surface area will require 4 mL, a 2.5% area 2 mL, and a 1% area 0.8 mL). Then apply the appropriate amount of solution to the chosen area.

With the second method, clinical endpoints are the guide. The physician should apply the solution evenly, wait 2 minutes, and then reapply it again. It is important that an even blue is maintained throughout. After organized, sheet-like frost with a pink background appears within the frosted areas, further application should stop. This is the desired endpoint in nonfacial skin, and application should stop even if other areas are not evenly frosted. Feathering should then be performed between the frosted and nonfrosted areas to prevent any demarcation lines.

Peeling of nonfacial skin is summarized in Box 10.15.

REFERENCES

1. Brody HJ. *Chemical Peeling and Resurfacing.* 2nd ed. St. Louis: CV Mosby; 1997:108-136.

2. Obagi ZE, Sawaf MM, Johnson JB, et al. The controlled depth trichloroacetic acid peel: methodology, outcome, and complication rate. *Int J Aesthetic Restor Surg.* 1996;4:81-94.

3. Johnson JB, Ichinose H, Obagi ZE, Laub DR. Obagi's modified trichloroacetic acid (TCA)-controlled variable depth peel: a study of clinical signs correlating with histological findings. *Ann Plast Surg.* 1996;36:225-237.

SKIN RESURFACING PROCEDURES

Identification and Management of Anticipated Reactions and Potential Complications

Skin reactions, side effects, and serious complications are an invariable part of a dermatologist's career. In fact, the saying, "if you did not have any complications during your medical career, you did not practice medicine," is an undeniable truth. To practice medicine within approved medical standards, a physician must be alert to the possible risks of any procedure or agent used to treat the patient. Furthermore, physicians must be able to maintain a high index of suspicion for potential adverse events, being careful to identify any problems in their early stages and treat them promptly. Dermatologists, plastic surgeons, and other skin professionals are trained to identify abnormal or problematic results and act quickly to improve the outcome, and our patients expect nothing less of us. This chapter is intended to provide the reader with information that may lead to earlier and more effective intervention in the treatment of immediate reactions, anticipated during the recovery stage, as well as in true complications following rejuvenation procedures.

REACTIONS RELATED TO RESURFACING PROCEDURES

Reactions occurring after skin rejuvenation procedures can be divided into the following three types: 1) immediate reactions (occurring 1 to 14 days after the procedure); 2) recovery period reactions (2 to 6 weeks after the procedure); and 3) delayed reactions (3 to 10 weeks after the procedure) (Table 11.1). The first two of these three types of post-procedure reactions can be further subdivided into anticipated versus unanticipated reactions, the latter considered true complications. The third type, delayed reactions, are always considered unanticipated. As such, any reaction occurring after recovery is considered a true complication. With improper treatment, recovery stage complications can carry over into the delayed period.

Before any procedure, the physician needs to counsel the patient on the expected postoperative course. The potential post-procedure adverse events should also be discussed and included on the consent form signed by the patient. When patients are not sufficiently informed about what to expect following a procedure (especially the anticipated reactions), they may become concerned and dissatisfied with the treatment and the physician. It is always good practice to overprepare and underpromise patients so that their expectations are ultimately met or surpassed, and trust in the physician is maintained.

IMMEDIATE ANTICIPATED REACTIONS

Edema

The severity or extent of post-procedure edema is relatively proportional to the procedure's depth of penetration. Specifically, edema is mild following procedures that reach the papillary dermis (PD) and stronger after procedures reaching the immediate reticular dermis (IRD). Edema appears within 24 hours, peaks by the third day, and disappears by the fifth day. The extent of edema varies between patients. Generally, it is more extensive in thin and lax skin and after deeper procedures. In rare cases, it can extend to the neck and upper chest. Because the periocular area of the human skull lacks bone to suppress expansion, edema may be overly prominent around the eyes and, occasionally, the patient's eyes may seal shut. The edema generally does not cause laryngeal symptoms or any other systemic reaction or pain.

Edema does not have to be treated. However, if the physician desires to minimize post-procedure edema, 10 mg of dexamethasone (Decadron) can be administered intravenously during the procedure and a methylprednisolone (Medrol) dose pack applied for 5 days following the procedure on a tapering schedule (6 mg orally first day, 5 mg the next day, etc.). Alternatively, oral prednisone can be used for 7 days, starting with 60 mg the morning after the procedure, tapered daily to 50 mg, 40 mg, 30 mg, 20 mg, 10 mg, and ending with 5 mg. Edema cannot be completely prevented, even with intravenous and oral steroids, but the swelling can be reduced and the patient made more comfortable. Cold compresses, started early and applied gently over the eyes, may help reduce the eyelid swelling.

TABLE 11.1 Possible Reactions (Anticipated and Unanticipated) after Ablative Rejuvenation Procedures*

Immediate (Post-procedure days 1-14)		Recovery† (Post-procedure weeks 2-6)		Delayed (Post-procedure weeks 3-10)	
Anticipated	Unanticipated	Anticipated	Unanticipated	Anticipated	Unanticipated
Edema	Painful vesicles: herpes simplex virus (HSV) eruption	Confluent erythema and mild edema	Painful vesicles: HSV reactivation	Minimal/resolving diffuse confluent erythema	Hypertrophic scarring/keloids
Confluent erythema	Bacterial or yeast infection (If honey-colored exudate: bacterial. If numerous small pustules overlying confluent persistent erythema: yeast)	Postinflammatory hyperpigmentation (PIH)	Bright red erythema with overlying small pustules (yeast/candida)	Minimal/resolving diffuse edema	Scars: hypertrophic and atrophic (occasionally, in severe cases, leading to ectropion formation)
Darkening or dark mask	Allergic reactions	Acne, rosacea flare-up	Persistent erosions or ulcerations (possible secondary aerobic or anaerobic bacterial infection including possible slowly growing atypical mycobacteria)	Delayed-onset PIH (if noncompliance with a proper post-procedure skin regimen)	Hypopigmentation/depigmentation
Oozing	Irritation	Milia	Unexplained delayed re-epithelialization/healing (culture negative)		Sharp demarcation lines
Scabbing (serosanguineous)	Maceration	Demarcation lines	Allergic contact dermatitis to a postoperatively applied topical agent		Sloughing of skin
Pruritus	Ulcerations	Sensitivity			

*Ablative rejuvenation procedures include both fractionated and nonfractionated modalities (fractionated CO$_2$ laser treatment and chemical peels, including the ZO Controlled Depth Peel, respectively).

†With improper treatment, recovery stage complications can extend to the delayed period.

Erythema

A CO_2 laser resurfacing procedure (fully ablative as well as fractionated ablative) and dermabrasion remove some or all surface layers of the skin and expose the dermis. The dermis is exposed during chemical peels that penetrate sufficiently deep. This produces intense confluent redness (erythema) immediately after the procedure that disappears in 7 to 10 days but is followed by less intense erythema (confluent or patchy) that may last a few months. After chemical peels, erythema may last a few weeks following light peels, or 1 to 2 months following deeper peels. Figure 11.1 shows a patient with erythema and sharp demarcation lines following a trichloroacetic acid (TCA) peel to the IRD.

Darkening of the Skin

In contrast to CO_2 laser resurfacing and dermabrasion, in which the immediate post-procedural field has a bloody appearance, TCA peels allow the treated skin on the surface to act as a natural dressing that gradually separates and peels off. After chemical peeling with TCA, the treated surface layers of the skin become darker, like a mask, which later separates and begins to peel away. Following a TCA chemical peel, separation and peeling begins by the third day, accelerates by the fifth or sixth day, and is completed in an average of 7 to 10 days, revealing pinkish and smooth skin. Patients must be advised to allow the skin to peel naturally and not to manipulate or pick the skin or otherwise attempt to remove the peeling skin prematurely.

Oozing

Serous exudates will immediately begin to ooze from the skin after a procedure that reached the IRD or deeper and will persist for 3 to 4 days. To prevent secondary infection and the formation of thick scabs and crusts, oozing fluid must be removed through gentle washing or direct pressure applied (in a

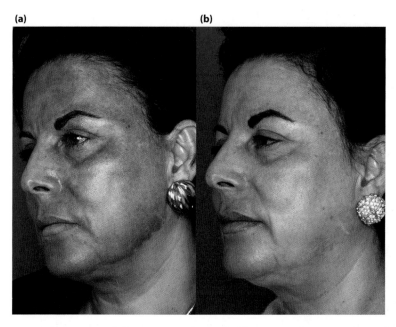

(a) (b)

FIGURE 11.1 (a) A patient following CO_2 fractional laser resurfacing without skin conditioning before and after the procedure. Notice the postinflammatory hyperpigmentation. (b) The patient after 6 weeks of aggressive hydroquinone-based Skin Health Restoration. Notice the improved skin texture and even color tone.

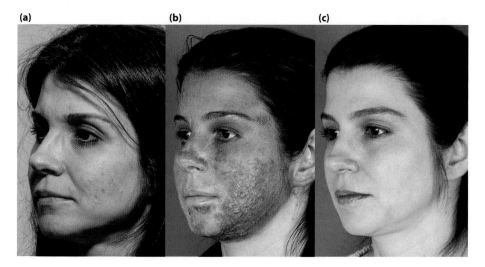

FIGURE 11.2 Scabbing and crusting. (a) A patient with stretchable acne scars. (b) The patient's left cheek shows poor management of a medium-depth peel. Notice the scabbing and crusting. (c) Three months after the peel. The patient has complete healing with use of aggressive, hydroquinone-based Skin Health Restoration.

"patting" manner) with an antiseptic solution, such as ZO Medical Surfatrol, Domeboro, or vinegar-water soaks. If the exudate is not removed and allowed to accumulate, scabs will form increasing the potential for secondary infection.

Scabbing

To decrease the risk for infection, scab thinning or melting should be routinely performed (multiple times throughout the day, as needed) after a chemical peel or any other resurfacing procedure penetrating to the dermis. Specifically, scabs should be melted away by gentle pressing with gauze saturated in an antiseptic solution using ZO Medical Surfatrol at least two to three times per day until complete resolution of the scabs. Scabs should never be forcefully removed by the patient or the physician. Figure 11.2 shows an acne patient with scabbing and crusting following a medium-depth TCA peel.

IMMEDIATE UNANTICIPATED REACTIONS

Herpes Simplex Virus Infection

In patients with a positive history of herpes simplex labialis or even genital herpes, every precaution needs to be taken to prevent the activation of the herpes virus and its appearance on the treated skin area after a procedure. Prophylactic oral antiviral treatment should be initiated the evening before any rejuvenation procedure. A herpes simplex prophylaxis regimen tailored to the patient's history is shown in Table 11.2.

Herpes simplex virus (HSV-1 and HSV-2) spreads rapidly on de-epithelialized, wet skin, especially during the first 7 days following a procedure. Patients can often predict the onset of an HSV flare about 24 hours before the actual eruption by prodrome-related symptoms that include itching, tingling, tenderness, or aching in a previously affected area. This is followed by the formation of vesicles, consisting of serous fluid that contains the infectious virus. Vesicles typically dry out (turn into a dry crust) and heal in approximately 7 to 10 days

TABLE 11.2	Herpes Simplex Prophylaxis Tailored to Patient History		
	Low-Risk Patients	**Medium-Risk Patients**	**High-Risk Patients**
Number of Occurrences/Year	1 or fewer per year	2-3 per year	>3 per year
Prophylaxis	Famciclovir (Famvir) 300 mg twice daily, or acyclovir (Zovirax), 400 mg three times daily, or valacyclovir (Valtrex), 500 mg twice daily started the day before the procedure and continued for 10 days	Same agents as for low-risk group, but started 1 week before the procedure	Same agents as for low-risk group, but started 3 months before the procedure Perform the procedure while the patient is on the treatment

following onset. The labial eruption is usually only slightly painful and, unless it is a manifestation of a primary viral eruption, is not associated with systemic symptoms.

In contrast, a disseminated infection, which is distinguished by vesicular lesions erupting over the entire treatment area, is painful, can occur rapidly, and has a greater potential for leaving scars. Patients must be instructed to notify the physician immediately and return to the office for examination if prodromal symptoms, signaling the onset of an outbreak, occur or if they experience any unusual or increasing pain in the days following the chemical peel or laser treatment. Treatment of herpes simplex infection is shown in Table 11.3. Figure 11.3 shows a patient with disseminated HSV that occurred 5 days after a chemical peel.

Secondary Infection: Bacterial, Viral, or Yeast

A bacterial infection occurring in the treatment areas after the procedure is rare if the patient follows proper home care instructions. However, one should maintain a high index of suspicion of a secondary bacterial infection in patients with a depressed immune system (e.g., those with diabetes), those who demonstrate poor hygiene, and those who are poorly compliant. Pain is the hallmark of a post-procedural infection. Infected areas typically have tender, macerated erosions or ulcerations with a purulent exudate. Concomitant systemic symptoms such as a fever and chills may develop.

When a bacterial or viral infection is suspected, the physician should first obtain a culture for aerobic and anaerobic bacterial and, in certain cases, viral organisms. Following culture, the patient should be started on a broad-spectrum

TABLE 11.3	Treatment of Herpes Simplex Infection
Treatment	**Procedure**
General	Allow skin to dry. Avoid ointments and moisturizers in the affected area.
Compresses	Apply 2% to 5% acetic acid with change of gauze after each contact with skin.
Antiviral ointment	Apply 5% Zovirax ointment or 1% Denavir (penciclovir) cream four to five times daily to lesions only. Discontinue after all lesions have cleared.
Severe cases	May require hospitalization for intravenous antiviral administration.

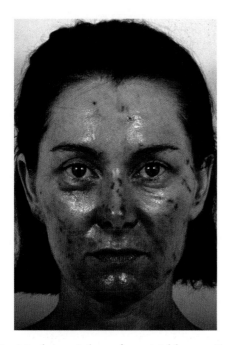

FIGURE 11.3 The patient is shown 8 days after a trichloroacetic acid peel to the papillary dermis. Notice the disseminated vesicles and erythematous lesions. The patient was not given antiviral prophylaxis before or during the procedure. She was given 1 gram of valacyclovir (Valtrex) twice daily for 7 days and topical acyclovir (Zovirax) ointment following the procedure. She cleared well without scarring.

oral antibiotic, such as cephalexin, ciprofloxacin, or cefadroxil. The infected area should be allowed to dry up by avoiding further lubrication (e.g., application of petrolatum-based products) and the patient encouraged to immediately increase the frequency of administration of antiseptic compresses, ZO Medical Surfatrol, three or four times per day. Also, the patient should be instructed to apply topical antibiotic cream (*not ointment*), for example, mupirocin 2% (Bactroban) cream, twice daily to the affected area. Bacterial infections usually respond quickly to treatment. The two most common bacterial causes of skin infections after resurfacing procedures are *Staphylococcus aureus* and (*Streptococcus pyogenes*).

Fungal and yeast infections are rare but can occur, especially in women with a previous history of vaginal yeast infections. Patients with persistent confluent erythema (and occasional overlying small white pustules) that does not respond to oral antibiotics should be suspected of having a possible secondary yeast infection (*Candida albicans* being the most common). Patients with post-procedure sites that appear clinically consistent with a secondary yeast infection should be treated with oral fluconazole tablets for 2 weeks (200 mg the first day and 100 mg for the remainder of the course). Compresses, as described previously, are also advised. A rare possibility in patients during re-epithelialization following deep chemical peel or ablative laser treatment that can cause impaired healing is atypical mycobacteria; these patients are typically not responsive to a course of cephalosporins or tetracyclines. Atypical mycobacteria are slow growing, and tissue cultures are the best method for diagnosis. Although very rare, atypical mycobacteria should be considered in any patient with impaired healing despite standard treatment measures following a resurfacing procedure. After the infection has cleared, lubrication can be resumed. Figure 11.4 shows a patient with infection 8 days after a ZO Controlled Depth Peel. Figure 11.5 shows a patient with infection 8 days after

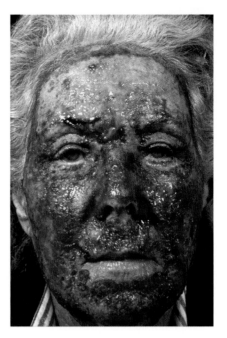

FIGURE 11.4 Eight days after a medium-depth trichloroacetic acid peel. The patient was treated with proper systemic antibiotics (based on culture) and topically with antiseptic compresses and topical antibiotic ointment.

a medium-depth ZO Controlled Depth Peel. Figure 11.6 shows a patient 10 days after a TCA peel.

Allergic Contact Dermatitis

Allergic reactions are rare during the immediate post-procedure period and can be cleared quickly with proper treatment. These reactions are signaled by the appearance of swelling, itching, and erythema in the treated areas and the surrounding skin. The simplest topical agents not containing antimicrobial agents, such as Aquaphor, Vaseline, or petrolatum, are preferred because some topical antibiotics are highly allergic. The most common triggers of allergic

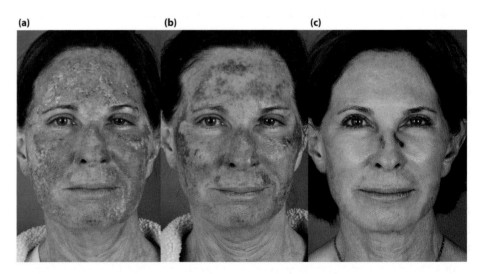

FIGURE 11.5 (a) A patient with photodamage and actinic keratoses. (b) The patient showing delayed healing and infection 7 days after a ZO Controlled Depth Peel to the immediate reticular dermis. She was treated with topical and systemic antibiotics and antiseptic compresses. (c) The patient 3 months after the peel. Notice the keloid on her left lower cheek.

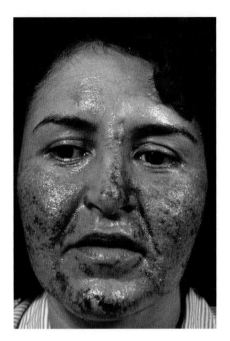

FIGURE 11.6   A patient with an infection 10 days after a trichloroacetic acid peel. Notice the purulent patches on the cheeks indicating infection. She was treated with topical and systemic antibiotics and antiseptic compresses.

contact dermatitis (ACD) in our clinic include neomycin and polymyxin (in certain over-the-counter topical products) and other uncertain home remedies that the patient tried before the clinic visit. Treatment of ACD following a chemical peel or laser procedure can include a Medrol dose pack or another systemic steroid, oral antihistamines, and allowing the skin to dry up for 24 hours. After the reaction has cleared, lubrication with a bland lubricant can be resumed.

Irritant Contact Dermatitis

Irritation of the skin surface after a procedure is common and is usually caused by excessive skin manipulation, such as rubbing, overzealous washing, or scratching before the skin has re-epithelialized (during the first 7 days). After a chemical peel, irritant contact dermatitis (ICD) can also be induced by excessive moisturizing, which ultimately leads to premature skin separation. When comparing the clinical characteristics of ICD and ACD, it is important to know that ICD involves only the treated area, whereas ACD spreads out to affect the surrounding skin. Symptoms consist of burning, redness, and discomfort. Treatment involves gentle handling of skin, use of antiseptic compresses, and allowing the skin to remain dry for 24 hours. Then, home care can be resumed, with the goal of keeping the skin from becoming too dry or too moist.

Premature Skin Separation

Premature skin separation can occur after chemical peels because skin in treated areas remains after the application of acid. In most cases, this treated skin separates slowly and progressively from the underlying skin as skin re-epithelializes. This gradual skin separation is advantageous in that treated skin that was exposed to the peel acts as a natural dressing, providing comfort and allowing re-epithelialization to proceed slowly and naturally. However, if the treated skin is lifted off before completion of re-epithelialization, a raw,

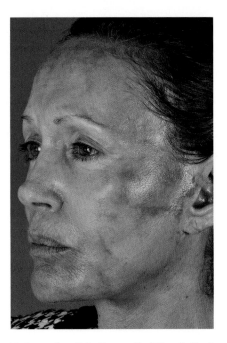

FIGURE 11.7 A patient 10 days after ZO Controlled Depth Peel to the immediate reticular dermis. She peeled away her skin surface 4 days after the peel. Excessive exposure to water during showering caused premature skin separation of the peeled area. Notice the postinflammatory hyperpigmentation and variations in areas of healing.

denuded, sensitive surface is exposed. This can follow excessively vigorous washing of highly moisturized skin if water has been allowed to run on the skin for a long time during a shower (Figure 11.7). It can also follow if the patient picked at the skin and caused excoriations (Figures 11.8 and 11.9). Premature skin separation is associated with significant pain and extreme tightness. Immediate treatment consists of having the patient apply a heavy amount of a bland ointment to the affected areas. In severe cases, patients may need to be prescribed oral pain medication. Although patients may be frightened by premature skin separation, it is ultimately not harmful to the

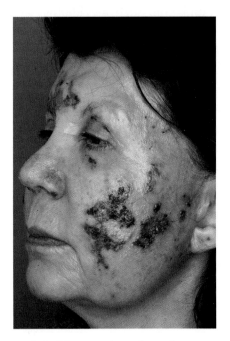

FIGURE 11.8 A patient with scabbing and cracking due to excoriations 8 days after a trichloroacetic acid peel.

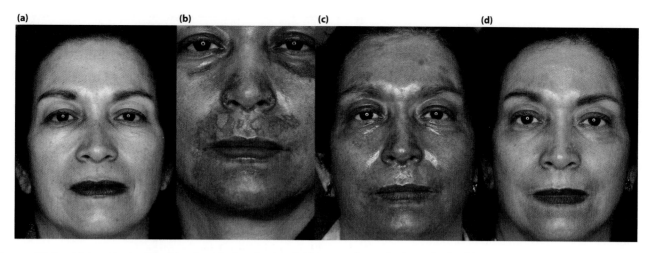

Figure 11.9 (a) A patient with skin classified as deviated white, medium thick, and oily. (b) The patient 10 days after a trichloroacetic acid peel to the immediate reticular dermis. The patient excoriated her face by aggressive washing and picking. (c) The patient 10 days after 5 days of application of fluorinated steroids and aggressive Skin Health Restoration. (d) The patient 1 year later. Notice the improved skin texture and the absence of scarring in the excoriated areas.

skin and does not affect the outcome (with the exception of a possible delay in healing of a few more days). However, premature separation does make skin increasingly susceptible to infection.

RECOVERY STAGE: ANTICIPATED REACTIONS

Erythema

After healing, erythema (redness) can be uniform (confluent) or uneven and blotchy, with deeper red areas usually signaling areas of deeper penetration within the entire treatment field. Erythema is more intense and tends to persist longer following procedures that penetrate deeper than the IRD. This is especially notable in patients with light-colored skin, as well as in patients (regardless of skin type) following administration of ablative procedures, such as the CO_2 fractional laser. Confluent erythema is common, especially in those with white and deviated dark skin types, and is not a true complication. Erythema is usually mild and disappears over the course of 1 week following a ZO Controlled Depth TCA Peel that penetrates to the IRD. Persistent postprocedural erythema is rare after a ZO Controlled Depth Peel that extends no deeper than the PD. However, erythema may persist for approximately 4 to 6 weeks following a ZO Designed Controlled Depth Peel because these have focal areas that are treated as deep as the upper reticular dermis (URD). Similarly, erythema may persist for 3 to 4 months following any deep chemical peel (such as 26% to 28% TCA allowed to penetrate to the URD) or CO_2 fractional laser treatment in patients with very light white or light white skin. The duration and intensity of erythema ranked according to occurrence after certain procedures are shown in Box 11.1. One caveat related to post-procedural erythema is that whenever there is a focal area of intense erythema with an overlying rough texture or an underlying slowly progressive increase in skin thickness, the physician must consider that a hypertrophic scar or keloid may be developing.

Some patients may find that the redness increases when bending, exercising, or drinking alcohol. This is usually a vascular phenomenon (vasodilation), which diminishes in both incidence and intensity over time without

281

Box 11.1

Likelihood of Post-procedural Erythema According to Treatment Type

CO_2 fractional laser $\geq$ dermabrasion > phenol chemical peel > ZO Designed Controlled Depth Peel > standard ZO Controlled Depth Peel > exfoliative chemical peels

treatment. Use of alpha-hydroxy acid (AHA) products in concentrations higher than 4% should be avoided for 3 weeks after deeper chemical peels as well as CO_2 fractional laser because these agents strip the stratum corneum, which can worsen and prolong the erythema.

Uneven redness (blotchiness) is more likely to occur after combined procedures, for example, a 26% to 28% TCA ZO Controlled Depth Peel to the entire face immediately followed by CO_2 fractional laser treatment to the perioral and periocular areas because these achieve variable depths. Erythema may be longer lasting in fair or thin skin and in individuals who previously have had CO_2 laser (fractionated as well as fully ablative, non-fractionated), a phenol chemical peel, or dermabrasion. Fissuring, cracking, picking, or rubbing of scabs after a procedure can produce more intense, localized erythema. Patients with severe solar elastosis may exhibit intense, blotchy erythema mixed with less erythematous or normal-appearing areas (marbleization). This is due to variable penetration without proper feathering between deep and less deep levels or to an uneven response to the procedure. The latter can occur if skin is not adequately pretreated with a strong topical regimen in the weeks preceding the chemical or laser treatment. A summary of erythema after certain procedures and in different skin types is shown in Table 11.4. Box 11.2 shows the temporary nature of postprocedure erythema.

Treatment of Erythema

When the severity of erythema is mild, it can be left untreated, and it will resolve spontaneously. If treatment is desired for mild erythema, nonfluorinated hydrocortisone (0.05% to 1%) cream can be used for 1 week and then repeated, as needed, two to three times in an on-and-off cycle. Stimulation with topical tretinoin cream is preferred; it can increase the intensity of

TABLE 11.4	Erythema after Different Procedures and Skin Types	
Skin Type	*Procedure*	*Erythema*
White and deviated dark skin	Chemical peels to the papillary dermis (PD) or deeper and ablative laser treatments	Usually uniform; lasts for 3 to 4 weeks
Very light white or light white skin		Lasts 3 to 4 months (especially following CO_2 laser treatment and deep chemical peels)
Very light white to dark skin	ZO Controlled Depth Peel to the IRD	Usually mild and disappears after 1 week
	ZO Designed Controlled Depth Peel to the PD	Rare
	Combined procedures	Uneven redness (blotchiness) more likely

Box 11.2

In certain cases, post-procedure erythema may be prolonged, but it eventually disappears and is never permanent.

erythema initially but should shorten its overall duration. Sunscreen and moisturizer should be used if there is dryness. For severe erythema and significant, uneven redness, treatment with a fluorinated topical steroid (e.g., clobetasol) for 1 week, stopping for 1 week, and repeating the on-off schedule two to three times may help while the patient is using tretinoin. Occasionally, in patients who have severely photodamaged skin and irregular redness (marbleization) that is unresponsive to the previously mentioned creams, it may be necessary to perform a chemical peel (to the PD or deeper) or a home retinol peel to even out the blotchiness. In these cases of persistent blotchy erythema, one should not repeat fractionated CO_2 laser surgery in hopes of treating the erythema because the skin may not tolerate the effects of additional thermal damage. In severe cases, topical vitamin C, oral beta-carotene, and gingko biloba supplements may provide some benefit. Exposure to infrared wavelengths may also help.

Postinflammatory Hyperpigmentation

Uneven pigmentation, including areas of postinflammatory hyperpigmentation (PIH), is the result of temporary melanocytic hyperactivity following skin injury from any procedure that extends to the PD or below. PIH is usually limited to the epidermis, but the dermis may be involved on rare occasions. The incidence of PIH increases with deeper procedures and in patients with the deviated type of skin color. Sun exposure without sunscreen or sun-protective clothing soon after the procedure can exacerbate PIH. The potential for PIH also increases after treatment complications, including irritant and allergic contact dermatitis, and secondary infection during the healing stage.

PIH can persist for 2 to 3 weeks after light procedures and for 4 to 6 months after deeper procedures. However, with aggressive early topical treatment (bleaching and blending), it can resolve completely in 2 to 6 weeks (Box 11.3).

Box 11.3

Duration and Resolution of Postinflammatory Hyperpigmentation

■ Postinflammatory hyperpigmentation (PIH) can persist 2 to 3 weeks after light procedures and 4 to 6 months after deeper procedures. However, with aggressive early topical treatment (bleaching and blending), it can resolve completely in 2 to 6 weeks.

■ Use of the skin conditioning principles before and after the procedure helps to reduce both the incidence and severity of PIH.

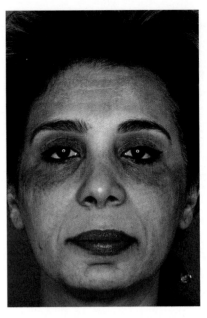

FIGURE 11.10 A patient with skin classified as deviated white (dark), medium thick, and nonoily following periorbital CO_2 fractional laser treatment without previous skin conditioning. Notice the postinflammatory hyperpigmentation.

Use of the skin conditioning principles before and after the procedure also helps to reduce both the incidence and severity of PIH. Repeated ZO Controlled Depth Peels (at intervals of at least 4 to 6 weeks in between peels) to blend skin color and any demarcation lines can be performed if topical treatment does not restore an even skin tone. Excessive skin oiliness can reduce the effectiveness of topical agents used for skin conditioning. In stubborn cases, postprocedural sebum reduction, for example, with the use of oral isotretinoin for at least 2 to 3 weeks, may be necessary. Figures 11.10, 11.11, and 11.12 show patients with PIH following CO_2 fractional laser treatment without previous skin conditioning. Figure 11.13 shows a patient with severe PIH following a peel with an unknown agent. With poor treatment, PIH that appeared at the

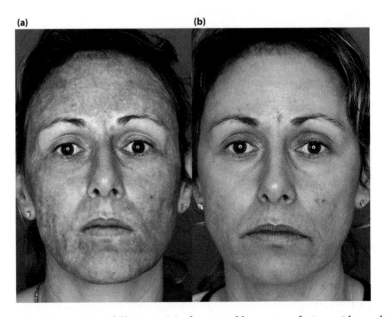

FIGURE 11.11 (a) A patient following CO_2 fractional laser resurfacing without skin conditioning before and after the procedure. Notice the postinflammatory hyperpigmentation. (b) The patient after six weeks of aggressive HQ-based Skin Health Restoration. Notice improved skin texture and even color tone.

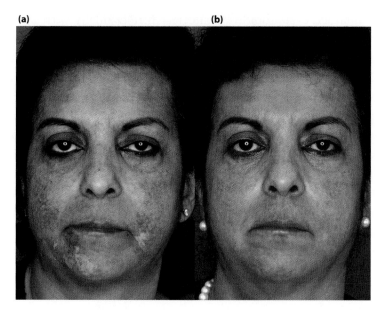

FIGURE 11.12 (a) A patient following CO_2 resurfacing without previous skin conditioning. Notice the postinflammatory hyperpigmentation and depigmentation. (b) The patient 6 months following aggressive hydroquinone-based Skin Health Restoration. Notice the restoration of normal skin color tone and repigmentation of the depigmented areas.

recovery stage can persist to the delayed stage. Persistent PIH is considered to be an unanticipated reaction and a true complication.

Acne or Rosacea Flares

Patients with oily or thick skin and those who are acne prone may experience a flare of cystic or comedogenic acne, usually 2 to 4 weeks after the procedure. However, in rare cases, it may begin as early as 4 to 5 days after the procedure.

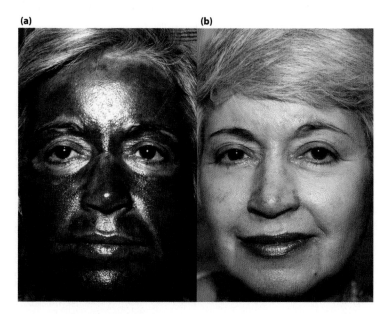

FIGURE 11.13 (a) A patient 6 months after a peel with an unknown agent. Notice the severe postinflammatory hyperpigmentation and the normal skin color around the eyes. (b) The patient 6 months after aggressive hydroquinone-based Skin Health Restoration during which a monthly ZO Controlled Depth Peel to the papillary dermis was performed for a total of three peels. Notice the restoration of normal skin appearance.

Large, inflamed cysts should be injected intralesionally with 2 to 2.5 mg/mL of triamcinolone acetonide (Kenalog). Topical ointment or moisturizer may be applied lightly when needed for comfort, but the skin should be kept somewhat dry in the healing stage. Acne flares can be minimized or prevented by skin conditioning before and immediately after healing and, if necessary, by using topical or systemic antibiotics in acne-prone individuals. Patients with a history of active acne can be given a 10-day course of twice-daily oral antibiotics, such as a tetracycline, macrolide, or third-generation cephalosporin, starting the evening before the procedure. If necessary, a 4- to 5-month course of isotretinoin (Accutane) can be prescribed for patients who are to have a peel not extending deeper than the PD. If the acne is severe, oral isotretinoin can also be started immediately or soon after the procedure. Peels to the IRD level have been performed in patients taking oral isotretinoin *before* the procedure without any ill effects. However, for procedures penetrating deeper than the level of the IRD, isotretinoin should be discontinued for at least 6 to 8 months before the procedure.

Milia

Milia are likely the result of excessive re-epithelialization or sebum production that caused pore closure and accumulation of sebum and keratin. Milia are more common following procedures that penetrate to depths deeper than the IRD. Treatment consists of mechanical removal with a #11 blade or comedone extractor, light hyfrecation with an epilating needle, and the daily use of topical tretinoin to prevent recurrence. If not treated, milia can persist for 3 to 4 months or longer and can become quite problematic.

Demarcation Lines

Demarcation lines are the result of inadequate feathering between treated and untreated areas during a procedure, especially in those that penetrate deeper than the IRD. Prevention of demarcation lines can be achieved by performing a combination treatment such as fractionated CO_2 laser resurfacing of the face, followed by the administration of a ZO Controlled Depth Peel to resurface the neck. Post-procedural demarcation lines can be treated by performing a second procedure (exfoliation or a light peel) to even out any abrupt changes between treated and untreated areas. One or more ZO Controlled Depth Peels that penetrate to the PD may be needed for adequate correction; standard ZO Controlled Depth Peels can be repeated every 4 to 6 weeks, as needed. During these "corrective" peels, special attention should be given to the process of feathering. The peel should reach the IRD on the dark margin of the demarcation line and penetrate to progressively shallower depths as it extends to encompass normal skin up to 3 to 4 inches away from the line. Demarcation lines can also be treated by aggressive skin conditioning consisting of twice daily topical bleaching, blending, and stimulation, which extends to encompass normal skin 3 to 4 inches beyond the initial treatment areas. A patient with demarcation lines following a TCA peel to the IRD was shown in Figure 11.1.

Enlarged Pores

With advancing age, enlarged pores appear because of a relative loss of perifollicular elastin in the papillary and upper reticular dermis. In individuals with thick skin, preexisting enlarged pores, sebaceous gland hypertrophy or hyperplasia, acne, or other underlying causes of excessive oiliness, pores may appear enlarged 3 or 4 weeks after re-epithelialization following a procedure that extended deeper than the IRD. This is usually a transient phenomenon because the pores return to their normal size 6 to 10 weeks after new elastin and collagen have been formed. In contrast, following certain deeply penetrating procedures, such as a phenol peel, dermabrasion, CO_2 laser resurfacing (nonfractionated or fractionated, in which settings are overly aggressive with respect to the density of microcolumns of destruction), or a medium-depth ZO Designed Controlled Depth Peel, a mild degree of fibrosis surrounding the hair follicle within the PD can prevent restoration of elastic tissue in that area and lead to the appearance of enlarged pores.

Whenever there is wide involvement of the URD, there is potential for subsequent loss of elastin and overproduction of thick, fibrotic-like collagen. Unfortunately, there is no currently available treatment that can fully correct enlarged pores. However, a few keratinocyte maturation cycles of skin conditioning with aggressive stimulation may increase the production of elastin in the PD, thus softening the fibrotic areas enough to induce the desired pore tightening. In cases of extensive areas of enlarged pores, a ZO Controlled Depth Peel to the level of the PD can be helpful because of the enhanced production of elastin in the PD after this peel. This chemical peel can be repeated every 4 to 6 weeks, for a total of two to three times, as needed. Reassessment every 4 to 6 weeks following a chemical peel should be performed to determine whether additional peels are necessary. For enlarged pores resulting from sebaceous gland hypertrophy or hyperplasia and excessive skin oiliness, a 3- to 5-month course of oral isotretinoin (Accutane) can be effective when added to the skin conditioning or Skin Health Restoration program.

RECOVERY STAGE: UNANTICIPATED REACTIONS

Marbleization
Marbleization is a term that describes an uneven post-treatment pigmentary response that may occur after a chemical peel or ablative laser procedure that penetrates unevenly over the treatment area. It can also occur if feathering intended to blend variable depths of penetration was unevenly applied. Marbleization has been observed following ZO Designed Controlled Depth Peel, dermabrasion, and fractionated CO_2 laser surgery performed on skin with deep, fibrotic scars or on severely photodamaged skin with extensive solar elastosis. Certain areas of damaged or poorly hydrated skin do not frost equally (compared with adjacent areas of undamaged, adequately hydrated skin) following a TCA peel. A similar phenomenon can be seen following ablative (CO_2) laser treatment, when the depth of penetration is uneven, even after extra passes. After healing, certain areas that appear as if they were not treated may be admixed with areas that responded well to treatment, with the latter appearing red and smooth. The poorly responding areas may represent very dense, damaged elastin or severely fibrotic tissue that did not adequately respond to the acid or ablative laser treatment. In most cases, aggressive stimulation by daily or twice-daily application of topical tretinoin tends to

reduce the differences in appearance within 3 to 4 months. However, in severe cases of marbleization, one or more future chemical peels or laser treatments may be needed to achieve optimal cosmesis. The occurrence of marbleization can be minimized by ensuring that patients comply with a longer and more aggressive preprocedure skin conditioning regimen.

Persistent Skin Sensitivity

After undergoing a procedure reaching the URD or deeper, patients with thin, dry, fragile skin or in areas with sparse adnexal structures (e.g., the upper chest) may develop intolerance to external factors, including applied topical agents. This state of extreme sensitivity can persist for weeks to months and is often accompanied by severe erythema. Excessively deeply penetrating treatments may yield postoperatively persistent skin sensitivity. Also, multiple other underlying cutaneous factors can be at fault, including poor circulation, defective keratinization, an inadequate number and density of adnexal structures, and defective barrier function. In thin skin, the maximal depth of treatment penetration should be the PD; only rarely in thin skin should the treatment penetrate to the depth of the IRD. Patients with thin skin are treated by gradually building skin tolerance and improving the skin's barrier function through a program that includes 2 to 3 months of daily stimulation with topical tretinoin (Box 11.4; see Chapter 2). Topical steroids should generally not be used in these cases because they can thin the epidermis, increase skin fragility, and further weaken the barrier function. However, topical steroids can occasionally be used—for a limited amount of time—to reduce the severity of a patient's anticipated reaction to tretinoin.

Persistent Erythema

Erythema is quite common after procedures penetrating to depths below the IRD, including those that penetrate to the URD. Persistent erythema, defined as persisting for 6 to 12 months after a procedure, is more pronounced and prolonged in patients with thin, dry, or severely sun-damaged skin. The cause is not known, but it is likely that a defect in keratinization that leads to a weak barrier function (as discussed in the previous section) is at fault. Persistent erythema is difficult to treat, and long-term steroid treatment should be avoided. In certain situations, correcting the keratinization defect and building up skin tolerance gradually using the principles of correction and stimulation has been successful.

Box 11.4

Treating Persistent Skin Sensitivity

Persistent skin sensitivity can be treated by gradually building skin tolerance and improving the skin's barrier function through a 2- to 3-month program of stimulation.

Treatment of persistent erythema can be described as "treating fire with fire." Tretinoin or retinol is used in gradually increasing concentrations, amounts, and frequency of application to which the patient's skin initially responds with more severe erythema and sensitivity. Treatment for 1 to 2 days with a mild topical steroid to reduce skin inflammation while strengthening the barrier function is permitted but with decreasing frequency. This should continue until natural skin tolerance has been restored, which may take 5 to 6 months. Transient hypersensitivity, on the other hand, is common in all skin types after a procedure. It is characterized by 1 to 2 weeks of poor tolerance to topically applied agents, sun exposure, or changing ambient temperatures. Transient hypersensitivity may occur with or without erythema and is treated in the same manner.

DELAYED UNANTICIPATED REACTIONS (TRUE COMPLICATIONS)

Unlike immediate post-treatment reactions and those that appear relatively early during healing and are temporary and resolve spontaneously, delayed, unanticipated reactions are true complications that appear later and may be permanent. The more common complications in this category are hypertrophic reactions, keloids, hypopigmentation, depigmentation, and ectropion.

Hypertrophic Reactions

Hypertrophic "reactions" are distinct from hypertrophic scars or keloids. They are erythematous, firm, indurated plaques that can be flat or raised, appear in a linear or cobblestone-like distribution, or are grouped into plaques and may be pruritic. Hypertrophic areas are usually well demarcated and have limited growth. The most susceptible areas are the upper lip, cheeks, and lower eyelids, especially in areas treated with a chemical peel or ablative laser procedure penetrating to a depth below the IRD. Areas with long-standing crusts or cracks, sites that the patient has picked or peeled and areas of prior secondary infection are also at risk. Hypertrophic reactions can usually be detected 2 to 3 weeks after re-epithelialization. Concomitant erythema may or may not be present. Pinching the involved skin reveals a thicker texture than that of surrounding skin. Under magnification, hypertrophic areas appear as rough, pearly patches with fine, raised threads or papules.

Hypertrophic reactions can sometimes resolve slowly without treatment, but resolution can be hastened through intralesional or topically applied corticosteroids. A potent steroid cream, such as clobetasol, should be liberally applied twice daily and massaged into the affected areas as soon as the reaction has been identified. Flurandrenolide-impregnated tape, applied at bedtime, releases a steady dose of steroid that can help in rapid resolution. Intralesional injection of steroid (e.g., triamcinolone acetonide at a concentration of 10 mg/mL) into the stroma of the thickened areas is helpful. Every effort should be made to avoid injecting the steroid into normal skin because this can cause atrophy. A combined treatment approach with flash lamp pulsed dye (FLPD) laser treatments and intralesional steroid injections may also be effective. The

> ### Box 11.5
>
> ### Hypertrophic Reactions
>
> - Hypertrophic reactions can sometimes resolve slowly without treatment, but resolution can occur faster with use of injected or topical corticosteroids.
> - With proper treatment, hypertrophic reactions usually disappear quickly without residual scarring.

laser treatment should be performed 2 weeks apart from the steroid injection because heat generated by the laser inactivates the steroid. Intralesional steroid administration helps calm and shrink the hypertrophic reaction, which makes subsequent laser treatments more effective. With proper treatment, hypertrophic reactions usually disappear quickly without residual scarring (Box 11.5). Figure 11.14 shows a hypertrophic reaction following CO_2 fractional laser treatment without previous skin conditioning.

Keloids

Keloids (hypertrophic scars) should be suspected in areas showing localized thickening and persistent erythema after a procedure (Box 11.6). The affected areas thicken quickly to produce a tumor-like growth that extends beyond the margins of injury to include areas of normal skin. Erythema, deformity, and retraction of surrounding skin are often seen, and symptoms of itching and pain are common. Keloids are more likely to form after a medium-deep to deep procedure in the upper lip area, jawline, shoulders, back, and chest, and in individuals with a prior history of atypical healing or keloid scar formation elsewhere. A keloid rarely forms after a PD- or IRD-level peel.

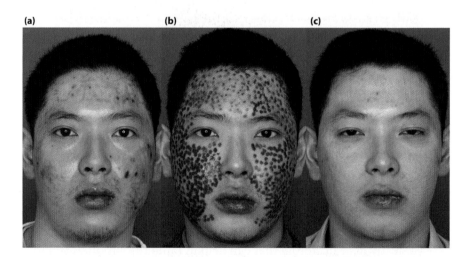

(a)   **(b)**   **(c)**

FIGURE 11.14 (a) A patient with hypertrophic reactions 6 months after CO_2 fractional laser treatment without previous skin conditioning. (b) Appearance after treatment with the flash lamp pulsed dye (FLPD) laser. (c) One year later. The patient had aggressive, non-hydroquinone-based Skin Health Restoration with epidermal stabilization and stimulation. The patient had four FLPD treatments and two ZO Retinol Stimulation Peels. Notice the skin's normal texture and appearance.

Box 11.6

Persistent Erythema Indicates Keloids

Any localized, persistent erythema should be considered an early sign of a keloid scar unless proved otherwise.

The rate of keloid formation is much higher in black and Asian (5% to 10%) patients than in white patients with light skin (1% to 2%). Infections, cracking, or scabbed areas that the patient has picked during the healing phase are also at increased risk for keloid formation. Figure 11.15 shows a patient with a hypertrophic reaction and keloid following a CO_2 fractional laser treatment without previous skin conditioning. Figure 11.16 shows a patient with a hypertrophic reaction and keloid following a medium-depth TCA peel without previous skin conditioning. Figure 11.17 shows a patient with keloids following a medium-depth TCA peel.

Treatment of keloids should be aggressive and begin as soon as possible after detection. Intralesional injection of a steroid (triamcinolone acetonide at a concentration of 10 mg/mL) into the stroma of the thickened areas is the primary initial therapy; injections are typically repeated every 3 to 4 weeks, as needed. In the early stages, keloids should be covered with silicone gel sheeting as much as possible. If keloid growth is not curbed following the first triamcinolone acetonide (Kenalog) injection, one should switch to intralesional injections of triamcinolone hexacetonide (Aristopan), 20 mg/mL, diluted to 10 mg/mL or, in severe cases, undiluted. Care must be taken when injecting triamcinolone hexacetonide because it is a very potent steroid that can also cause skin atrophy. Injection of 0.5 to 1 mL into a lesion every 4 to 6 weeks is

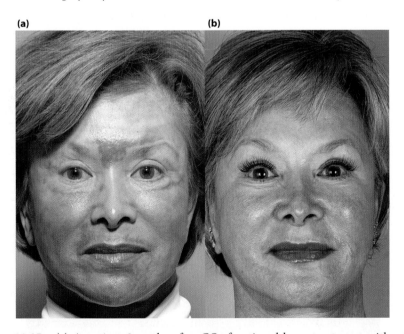

(a) **(b)**

FIGURE 11.15 (a) A patient 3 weeks after CO_2 fractional laser treatment without previous skin conditioning. Notice the hypertrophic reaction on the cheeks and an early keloid in the glabellar region. (b) The patient after 8 weeks of aggressive non-hydroquinone-based Skin Health Restoration, two flash lamp pulsed dye laser treatments, and intralesional steroid injections.

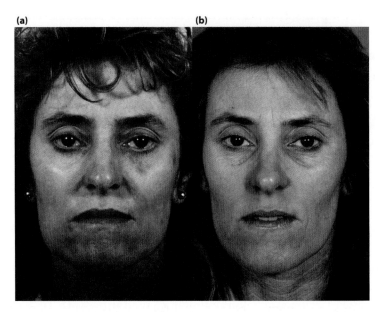

FIGURE 11.16 (a) A patient showing a hypertrophic reaction and early keloid formation 3 weeks after a medium-depth TCA peel without previous skin conditioning. (b) The patient 5 months after aggressive hydroquinone-based Skin Health Restoration during which three flash lamp pulsed dye laser treatments were performed and intralesional steroid was injected. Notice the restoration of normal skin appearance.

the maximum. Alternating injections of triamcinolone acetonide with triamcinolone hexacetonide is helpful in the case of large keloids.

For early-growing keloids, recombinant interferon alfa-2b (Intron A), a water-soluble protein that exerts its activity by binding to specific receptors on the cell surface, is an alternative treatment. The intracellular events that follow binding include enzyme induction, suppression of cell proliferation, suppression of collagen production, decrease of immunomodulating activities, and inhibition of virus replication in virus-infected cells. A dose of 1 million

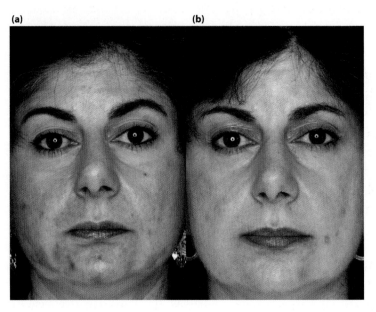

FIGURE 11.17 (a) A patient with keloids following a medium-depth trichloroacetic acid peel. (b) The patient following Skin Health Restoration, four sessions of flash lamp pulsed dye laser treatment, and five sessions of intralesional injection of steroids. Notice the total clearance of keloids.

international units (IU) is injected intralesionally in one treatment, repeated three times weekly, not to exceed a total of 5 million IU per week. Both Intron and intralesional steroids can be used to treat the same keloids, with the steroid injected once every 3 to 6 weeks and Intron three times each week. However, Intron should not be injected 3 days before or 3 days after steroid injections because the delay between treatments permits the steroid to settle within the keloid before the Intron is administered; if the two are administered less than 3 days apart, the Intron will "flush out" the steroid from the area where it was placed. Compression and manual massage of keloids have been shown to be independent factors that help prevent progression and hasten resolution of keloids. This treatment is based on the assumption that occlusion suppresses the action of fibroblasts, but the exact mechanism has not been defined. Thus, flurandrenolide-impregnated tape is a useful home treatment for keloids because it administers pressure as well as slowly releasing steroids directly into keloids. Treatment with the FLDP laser once every 4 to 6 weeks until resolution is helpful in shrinking the keloid, eliminating the redness, and improving the surface texture.

Scars

Scarring (full-thickness destruction or slough) is rare, occurring only after deep, poorly controlled procedures, such as deep chemical peels, dermabrasion, or CO_2 laser resurfacing. Scarring can also occur following these deep procedures when they are performed on a skin flap at the same time that a facelift is performed. This is because deep, ablative procedures on a skin flap may compromise the blood supply to the tissue with resulting full-thickness necrosis (no collateral blood supply is available in these cases to prevent tissue necrosis). Scars can also occur after a severe infection during the healing stage. Some sloughing scars that appear as small indentations or shallow lines can be corrected after a few months by repeated resurfacing, a "spot treatment" with TCA (typically 30% to 40% concentration), or a repeat TCA peel to the full area previously treated (typically 20% to 30% TCA concentration). Figure 11.18 shows a hypertrophic reaction and skin slough following a facelift procedure.

Hypopigmentation and Depigmentation

Hypopigmentation is caused by a dysfunction or a reduced number of functioning melanocytes. The likelihood of occurrence is correlated with the depth of the procedure and with the underlying thickness or fragility of the patient's skin. For example, areas of hypopigmentation are relatively common following deeply penetrating treatments such as phenol peels, medium to deep TCA peels, ablative CO_2 laser resurfacing, and dermabrasion. Patients with severe photodamage, thin or fragile skin, or skin that has previously been treated with dermabrasion or phenol peels are more susceptible.

After medium-depth TCA peels, hypopigmentation improves with time before becoming permanent. Hypopigmentation can sometimes be treated successfully by early aggressive stimulation with tretinoin for 3 to 4 months or recurrent administration of psoralen plus ultraviolet A light (PUVA) to regenerate melanocytes (Box 11.7). If these fail, blending and feathering into untreated areas with a PD-level peel, such as the ZO Controlled Depth Peel, may be effective.

FIGURE 11.18 The patient had necrosis and skin slough following a facelift that resulted in scarring. Notice fibrosis and depigmentation in the necrotic area after healing.

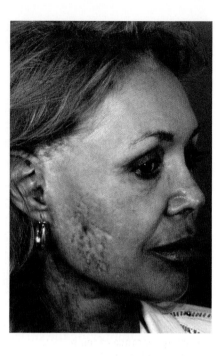

Box 11.7

Hypopigmentation can sometimes be treated successfully by early aggressive stimulation with tretinoin for 3 to 4 months or psoralen plus ultraviolet A light (PUVA).

Depigmentation (the complete loss of skin color) is caused by a total destruction of underlying melanocytes. Very white, sharply demarcated macules or patches, resembling islands surrounded by normally colored skin, appear following deep procedures performed in thin skin, skin poor in adnexal structures, or severely photodamaged skin. Areas of depigmentation may also appear after resolution of focal secondary infection, complicating such

FIGURE 11.19 A patient with skin classified as complex (from India) showing depigmentation and uneven color tone 1 year after CO_2 laser resurfacing.

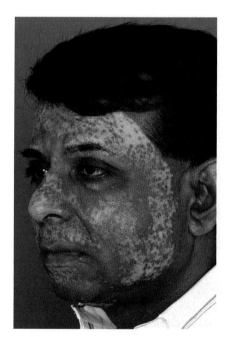

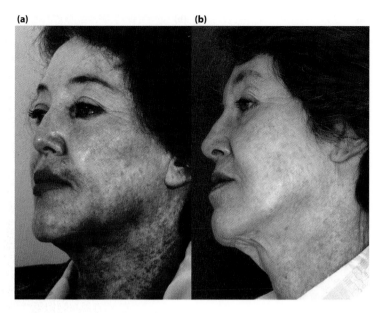

Figure 11.20 (a) A patient 6 months after a phenol peel. Notice the depigmentation, uneven appearance of telangiectasia, and erythema. (b) The patient after non-hydroquinone-based Skin Health Restoration followed by three flash lamp pulsed dye laser treatments and a ZO Retinol Stimulation Peel. Notice skin improvement (texture) and the permanent hypopigmentation.

procedures. Treatments to correct depigmentation are usually futile. However, attempts can be made with epidermal grafts or epidermal and dermal punch grafts, along with aggressive stimulation with tretinoin. Hypopigmentation of the darker areas surrounding the white skin in order to produce more even coloration can also be helpful but should be only considered a last resort. If loss of color is extensive in distribution, monobenzone 20% (Benoquin) cream can be used to depigment the residual dark areas of skin. However, treating depigmented patches by inducing the loss of pigment in surrounding areas of skin (making the former appear less noticeable) is a cumbersome process, has potentially toxic side effects, and takes a long time to work. Figure 11.19 shows a patient with complex skin type showing depigmentation 1 year after CO_2

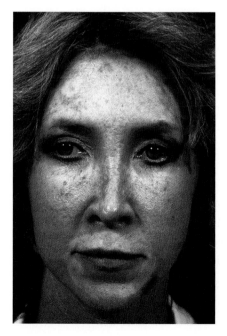

Figure 11.21 A patient showing permanent perioral depigmentation after a localized phenol peel.

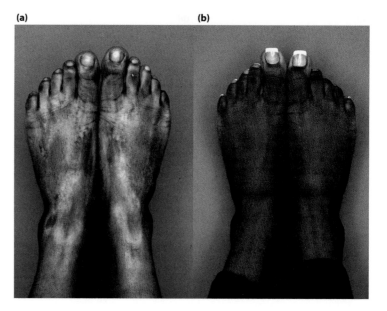

(a) **(b)**

FIGURE 11.22   (a) A patient's feet 10 years after first- and second-degree burns that were treated with hydroquinone (HQ) and a variety of topical agents. Notice the hypopigmentation and areas of near depigmentation. The patient's skin was classified as original black. (b) One year after treatment. The patient underwent non-HQ-based Skin Health Restoration for epidermal and melanocyte stabilization, stimulation, and blending. Intralesional steroid was injected into fibrotic areas, and three exfoliative TCA peels were performed. Notice the improved texture, even color, and attractive nails.

Box 11.8

Performing the Lid Snap Test

- With your fingers, press the skin 4 inches below the lower lid and move it upward with a gentle pull in ½-inch increments.
- The point at which the lid margin is pulled down should be noted as the point at which an IRD peel should end and a PD-level peel begin.

---

laser resurfacing. Figures 11.20 and Figure 11.21 show patients with depigmentation following a phenol peel. Figure 11.22 shows a patient with hypopigmentation on his feet following first- and second-degree burns.

Ectropion

Ectropion (eversion of the eyelid margin) is more likely to occur after procedures penetrating deeper than the PD performed on lower eyelids that are already lax (weak snap test). Unintentionally deeper chemical peels or CO_2 laser resurfacing can cause full-thickness injury to the thin and lax skin of the eyelids, resulting in ectropion or scleral show. True ectropion should be distinguished from false ectropion in that the latter may appear secondary to retraction of the lower eyelid during the edematous period after the peel or during the early tightness period after CO_2 laser resurfacing. To prevent ectropion, the lid snap test should be performed on every patient to tailor the depth of the procedure in the eyelid area (Box 11.8). True ectropion can be corrected surgically with skin grafts.

CHAPTER 12

LASER AND ENERGY SOURCES IN SKIN HEALTH AND REJUVENATION

E. Victor Ross, MD

LASER DEVICES AND THEIR APPLICATIONS

The role of energy sources in skin health and rejuvenation has expanded greatly over the past 20 years. From the early argon and CO_2 lasers to present-day fractional lasers and radiofrequency equipment, the ever-enlarging array of devices allows for many applications. On the other hand, that same large list has made the selection of the best equipment for particular skin maladies an ongoing challenge. In this chapter, we review lasers and other energy sources from first principles and develop a logical proposal for optimal device selection.

DEVELOPMENT OF LASERS IN DERMATOLOGY

The first laser (ruby) was used for pigmented lesions. Between 1980 and 1990, only argon, Nd:YAG, and CO_2 lasers were added to the dermatology field. The first laser "designed" for a specific skin condition was the pulsed dye laser (PDL).[1-5] The development of this laser and its parameters for port wine stain (PWS) was based on a logical selection of pulse width and wavelength such that very spatially localized heating was achieved. In those early days of lasers in dermatology, the primary applications were not cosmetic but medical in nature. If one reviews the literature before 1996, almost every treated condition was a benign tumor or vascular anomaly.

By the middle of the 1990s, three developments expanded the role of lasers in cutaneous medicine. One was the introduction of CO_2 laser resurfacing, another was the introduction of nonpurpuric settings for vessel reduction, and a third was Q-switched lasers for removal of tattoos and pigmented lesions. However, two procedures transformed the laser dermatology arena more than any other development, at least from a commercial perspective. One was laser hair reduction, now the most popular laser procedure in the world, and the second was the application of the intense pulsed light (IPL) for full-face and off-the-face rejuvenation. These two procedures themselves were novel enough, but the delivery of these procedures by nonphysicians broadened the type of practices providing them and likewise the number of patients who underwent laser procedures.

LASERS FOR PIGMENT REDUCTION

Modern lasers and other therapeutic light sources are developed to maximize target selectivity and minimize collateral damage. Based on the absorption of specific chromophores, namely blood, melanin, and water, one can achieve very high localized temperatures.[5] The greatest selectivity occurs with hemoglobin and melanin because their distribution in the skin is discrete. Water, on the other hand, is ubiquitous in the skin so that high temperature confinement is established by either using 1) a shorter pulse, 2) a very small spot (fractional lasers; vide infra), or 3) a wavelength where absorption is so strong that thermal damage is minimal adjacent to the laser impact. Based on an understanding of the relative absorption of the three major chromophores in the skin (Box 12.1), one can devise logical strategies to treat a number of skin conditions (Figure 12.1).

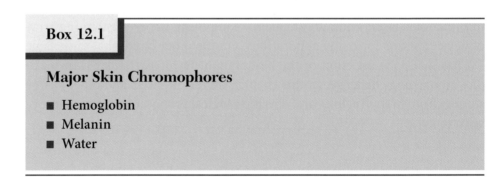

Box 12.1

Major Skin Chromophores

■ Hemoglobin
■ Melanin
■ Water

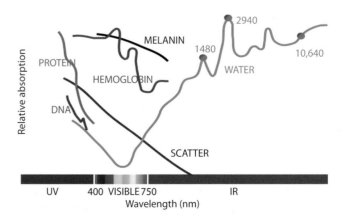

FIGURE 12.1   Spectrum of the three major skin chromophores.

TABLE 12.1   Popular Laser Settings for the Treatment of Telangiectasia

	Pulse Width (ms)	Fluence (J/cm²)	Spot Size (mm)	Cooling
Pulsed dye laser (nonpurpuric settings)	6-40	6-12	5-10	Cryogen spray or cold air
Large-spot KTP laser	8-20	6-12	8-12	Sapphire contact
Intense pulsed light	10-30	Variable	Up to 10 × 30 mm on face	Sapphire contact

The most rewarding applications for laser technology are those in which the ratio of absorption of the target versus normal skin enjoys the greatest value. One of these is the vasculature, where until the 1980s, one was confined to treatment with nonselective tools such as electrosurgery for telangiectasia and where there were essentially no effective options for broader vascular pathologies such as rosacea and port wine stain (PWS) (although the CO_2 laser was applied with varying results for PWS).[6] With typical vascular laser applications, the ratio of absorption of the blood vessel versus surrounding skin is more than 100:1. For skin rejuvenation, the most common vascular maladies are rosacea, telangiectasia, keratosis pilaris rubra faceii, flushing (which some consider a variant of rosacea), and poikiloderma (of the neck). The three most commonly applied tools are the KTP (potassium titanyl phosphate) laser (more rigorously called a frequency doubled, long-pulsed Nd:YAG laser), the PDL, and the IPL. All three devices have been applied with relatively equal effects, depending on settings. For telangiectasia, we have listed the most popular settings with particular equipment in Table 12.1.

The endpoint in successful vessel reduction is either 1) persistent bluing of the vessel or 2) constriction of the vessel so that it is almost invisible. For larger vessels, a longer wavelength laser might be required, such as the alexandrite laser, 810-nm laser, or 1,064-nm laser. An alternative is a multiple wavelength IPL coupled with a longer pulse (>50 ms) in which a spectral shift allows for deeper penetration than with shorter pulses (5 to 20 ms). Periorbital blue veins respond particularly well to longer wavelength lasers, where the 1,064-nm laser can be applied with a 2- to 3-mm spot, 20- to 40-ms pulse width, fluence of 120 to 180 J/cm², and surface cooling to achieve predictable closure. Metal internal corneal eye shields should accompany the use of the laser in this region, where the retina can be damaged by the deeply penetrating infrared light.[7,8] For smaller, finer vessels in fair-skinned patients, visible (VIS) light devices can achieve vessel closure (Figure 12.2). For darker skinned patients, the 1,064-nm laser often provides the greatest ratio of vascular damage to epidermal damage. A conundrum is the tanned or dark patient with "fine vessel" disease, such as poikiloderma, where shorter wavelengths might be required for vessel closure but where those wavelengths are also likely to damage the epidermis. In these cases, we have found the PDL to be preferable to other interventions, primarily because of the cooling efficacy of the dynamic cooling device (DCD, cryogen spray cooling.).[9]

In addition to vascular lesions and redness, VIS light devices can also target pigment dyschromias, where, depending on the wavelength and pulse duration, melanin within melanosomes can be selectively heated. To illustrate the use of VIS light in rejuvenation, we examine treatment in the patient in

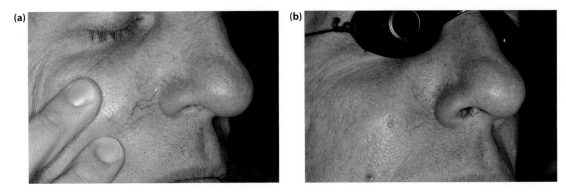

FIGURE 12.2 Right mid-cheek vessel before 532-nm laser (a) and just after treatment with a 4-mm spot KTP device at 12 J/cm², 15-ms pulse width, and contact cooling (b).

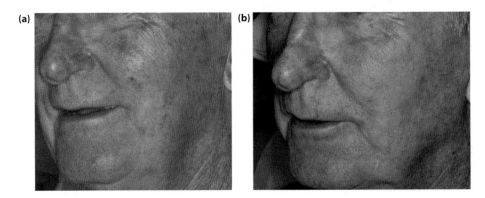

FIGURE 12.3 (a) Pretreatment cheek showing lentigines and telangiectasia. (b) Three months after treatment with an intense pulsed light (Icon, Palomar Medical Technologies, Max G handpiece, 32 J/cm², 10 ms).

Figure 12.3. This patient shows excessive pigment and vessels. There are multiple possible treatment strategies. In one scenario, a pulsed-light device is applied to the entire face. The settings are adjusted so that one pass achieves reduction in brown and red dyschromias. Numbing cream is typically applied to the face about 1 hour before the procedure. Settings are device dependent, but generally the lowest settings that achieve "immediate" pigment darkening or vessel stenosis are applied. Test spots can be applied just before application of numbing cream in a representative area of the face and reviewed just before treatment (on removal of the numbing cream about 1 hour later). Although 1 hour is inadequate to determine the full extent of the reaction, this interval is sufficient to avoid gross overtreatment or undertreatment, and with experience, one can use this technique to improve outcomes. Test spots, evaluated only 5 to 10 minutes after the procedure, are almost impossible to interpret and in many cases can result in overtreatment or undertreatment. The safest patients to treat are those with a lighter skin type where there is maximal contrast between red and brown dyschromias and background skin. As the background skin color increases or lentigines become lighter, the sweet-spot fluence, where selective heating of the target is achieved, becomes smaller. In acutely tanned skin, the injured dermis and epidermis should not be treated. Treatment should be deferred until most of the sunburn erythema has resolved. Although treatment of chronically tanned skin in regions with year-round sun is suboptimal, treatment avoidance of all tanned skin is impractical. With experience, such skin can be treated as long as the operator is careful to reduce fluence to avoid overheating of background skin (Box 12.2).

Box 12.2

Treatment with Visible Light Devices

- VIS light devices can be used to treat:
  - Vascular lesions and redness
  - Pigment dyschromias
- In pigment dyschromias
  - Melanin within melanosomes can be selectively heated
  - As the background skin color increases and/or lentigines become lighter, the sweet-spot fluence, where selective heating of the target is achieved, becomes smaller
- The safest patients to treat are those with maximal contrast between red and brown dyschromias and their background skin

With a large spot KTP laser or IPL, one pass of the device can reduce red and brown spots. In the presence of contact cooling, overheating of the background skin is preventable. The PDL can also be applied for red and brown dyschromias; however, in the most common configuration, in which a cryogen cooling device is incorporated into the system, epidermal pigmented lesions are often overcooled, and two passes must be applied (one with and one without the cooling device). Alternatively, the PDL can be equipped with contact cooling or refrigerated air. These cooling accessories have a lower cooling protection factor (CPF) and are less likely to overcool the targeted epidermal pigmented lesions than their lower CPF counterparts. The long pulsed alexandrite laser and 810-nm diode lasers have also been used for pigment dyschromias.[10]

For discrete lesion treatment, the Q-switched ruby, alexandrite, and 532-nm lasers achieve excellent clearance of most lesions (Box 12.3). The confinement of heat to the melanosomes offers a quick recovery with almost no damage to surrounding skin. Even with pulse stacking, collateral damage is minimal, and side effects such as scarring are unlikely in the absence of infection. Hand lentigines respond predictably well to this approach. Also, low-contrast lesions, where the degree of pigment in the lesions compared with the surrounding skin is small, are a good indication for this technology. Alternatives to Q-switched lasers for low-contrast lesions include "masking" down larger spots to a smaller spot where the lesion size and spot sizes are similar (Figure 12.4). Special adaptors can also be used to decrease the spot

Box 12.3

Lasers for Discrete Lesion Treatment

The Q-switched ruby, alexandrite, and 532-nm lasers achieve excellent clearance of most discrete pigmented lesions.

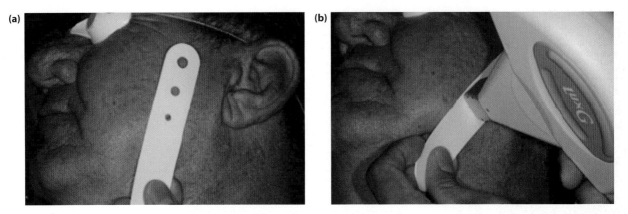

Figure 12.4 (a) A Teflon mask used to protect normal skin. A small lentigo is present within the smallest "hole." (b) The intense pulsed light handpiece is applied over the area. The mask protects the background slightly tanned skin. (From Soon SL, Victor Ross E. Letter: use of a perforated plastic shield for precise application of intense pulsed light. *Dermatol Surg.* 2008;8:1149-1150.)

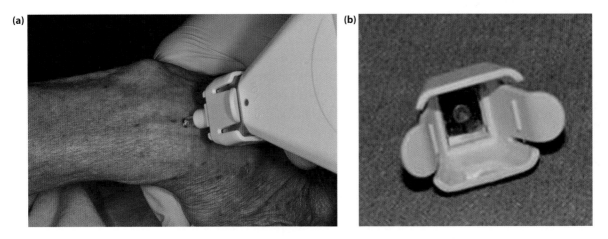

Figure 12.5 An adaptor truncates the 10- × 15-mm sapphire window down to 4 mm.

size. In this manner, higher fluence can be applied to the lesion without damaging the background skin (Figure 12.5). Ablative CO_2 and erbium YAG lasers can be applied as well.

Often the patient presentation includes widespread actinic keratoses (AKs) in addition to dyschromias (Figure 12.6.). In this scenario, reduction of the AKs is an important component in rejuvenation. If one treats the facial dyschromias and neglects AKs, a red splotchiness will persist where the AKs are observed, and the patient will not achieve optimal results. Adding topical aminolevulinic acid with photodynamic therapy (ALA/PDT) is a good option for this presentation. We apply the ALA 1.5 hours before light treatment. Initially we use IPL, KTP, or PDL to reduce red and brown dyschromias, followed immediately by 3 to 8 minutes of blue light. We have ceased use of numbing cream in this protocol because the cream enhances the PDT effect in an unpredictable way (most likely by accelerating the penetration of ALA). In the absence of cream, we offer facial nerve blocks.

Idiopathic guttate hypomelanosis is another challenging condition. These white lesions, which are commonplace on the arms and legs, most likely represent small lightly pigmented seborrheic keratoses. Liquid nitrogen, ablative lasers, and most recently, fractional ablative lasers have been applied with some success.[11,12] We have found that the best way to improve this condition is

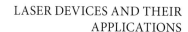

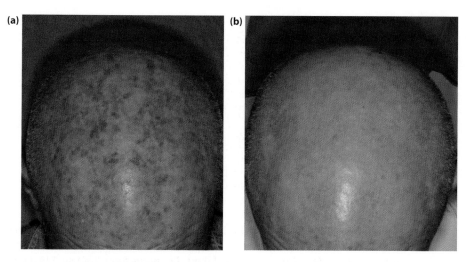

FIGURE 12.6 (a) Patient with widespread actinic keratoses and lentigines. (b) One month after treatment with aminolevulinic acid with photodynamic therapy combined with Q-switched alexandrite laser.

to simply reduce the dyschromia around the lesions and improve the overall homogeneity of skin coloration on the arms and legs.

One common conundrum after laser treatment of pigmented lesions is recurrence and worsening of pigment in the area (postinflammatory hyperpigmentation [PIH]). Patients should be counseled that both of these sequelae are possible. Lighter skinned patients are less likely to experience early lesion recurrence and PIH. Studies have shown that for skin types IV and V, longer pulsed (non-Q-switched) technologies are less likely to cause PIH.[13] On the other hand, Q-switched lasers are more likely to achieve complete clearance. Substances that can suppress PIH include topical corticosteroids, hydroquinone, and retinoids. Sun avoidance is also critical in prevention.

LASERS FOR HAIR REMOVAL

As with pigment reduction, hair removal with light relies on pigment contrast between the hair follicle and the epidermis (Box 12.4). Melanin is the initial target, and heat diffusion from melanin in the hair matrix and possibly the shaft is required for hair follicle destruction. Complete destruction of the dermal papilla ensures permanent hair removal. Typical endpoints are charring of the hair at the surface and perifollicular edema (PFE). Depending on the pulse duration, fluence, hair thickness, and hair color, varying degrees of PFE are observed. Longer pulses, thinner light hairs, and lower fluence are associated with reduced PFE. In the early years of laser hair reduction, permanent removal was the goal. However, as the field matures, patterns have evolved regarding the likelihood of permanence and the required number of sessions. Many of these patterns depend not only on the thickness and color of hair and laser parameters but also on the specific anatomic region, as well as the age and gender of the patient. Based on a literature review and clinical experience, the bikini area and axilla are the most predictably successful regions for laser hair reduction. Other regions that enjoy good success are legs and arms. Men's backs show mixed results, with many patients requiring maintenance

Box 12.4

Lasers for Hair Removal

- Hair removal with light relies on pigment contrast between the hair follicle and the epidermis.
- Melanin is the initial target.
- Permanent hair removal is no longer the goal. Instead, patterns have evolved regarding the likelihood of permanence and required number of sessions.
- The bikini area and axilla are the most predictably successful regions. Other regions that enjoy good success are legs and arms. Men's backs show mixed results. Women's faces have shown the greatest variability in responses.
- Optimal laser parameters for hair removal selectively target the hair bulb while preserving the epidermis.
- Long pulsed alexandrite, 810-nm diode, and Nd:YAG lasers, as well as the IPL, are the most effective devices for hair removal.
- Paradoxical laser-induced growth stimulation (PLIGS) has become a major issue, especially in female facial areas.

treatments even after as many as six sessions spaced 2 to 3 months apart. Women's faces have shown the greatest variability in responses.

Generally, optimal laser parameters for hair removal selectively target the hair bulb while preserving the epidermis (Figure 12.7). Shorter pulses generate higher peak temperatures but can result in hair shaft vaporization during the pulse such that the latter portion of the pulse energy is not applied to follicle heating. Longer pulses have been shown to generate a larger cylinder of residual thermal damage; however, fluence must be much larger to reach a threshold T (the temperature required for pan follicular cellular death), particularly for lighter, thinner hairs.

A large number of devices have been applied in laser hair removal. The initial ruby laser has been largely replaced by long pulsed alexandrite, 810-nm diode, and Nd:YAG lasers, as well as the IPL. Larger spot sizes have allowed for faster treatment times (determined by cm^2/s). A review of laser hair removal and specific considerations is found in the publication by Ross and colleagues.[14] The focus of laser hair removal has been optimized hair follicle heating, but phenomena such as paradoxical laser-induced growth stimulation (PLIGS) and resistant anatomical regions have redirected consideration to hair biology.

The optimal intervals for laser reduction have been determined based on a mathematical model that considers the hair cycle.[15,16] The model shows that longer intervals are indicated for areas with longer telogen phases. For skin types I to IV, IPL, alexandrite, and 810-nm diode lasers can all be applied with a reasonable safety window, where the fluence to achieve laser hair removal is less than that to cause epidermal damage. For type V or VI skin, the 1,064-nm laser enjoys a much greater safety window. Also, in tanned patients and in areas where

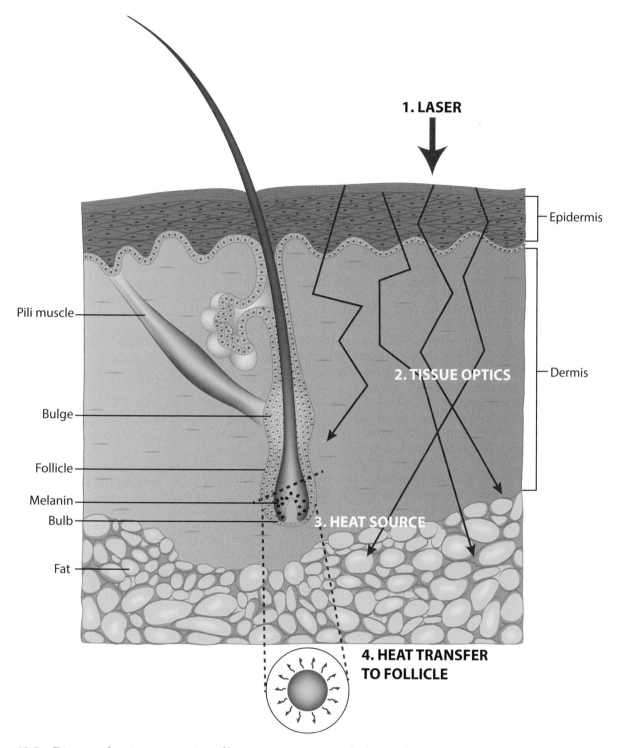

1. LASER

Epidermis

Pili muscle

2. TISSUE OPTICS

Dermis

Bulge

Follicle

Melanin

Bulb

3. HEAT SOURCE

Fat

4. HEAT TRANSFER TO FOLLICLE

FIGURE 12.7 Diagram showing progression of laser tissue interaction for hair reduction. (From Ross EV, Ladin Z, Kreindel M, Dierickx C. Theoretical considerations in laser hair removal. *Dermatol Clin.* 1999;17(2):333-355, viii.)

melanin concentration is greater (pubic region), longer wavelength lasers can be used with less risk for epidermal damage.

Some IPLs feature handpieces with filtering or pulse modulation that shift the emission spectrum toward the infrared. The handpieces can be applied safely in most skin types. Still, if one's practice primarily serves darker skinned patients, the 1,064-nm laser is a good first choice. Because the 1,064-nm laser offers an enviable ratio of hair bulb to epidermal heating, even for lighter skin, one might suggest that the 1,064-nm laser is the ideal first laser for laser

Box 12.5

Characteristics of Lasers Used for Hair Removal

Alexandrite: 755 nm (near infrared) (most effective on pale skin and not safe on very dark skin at effective settings)

Pulsed diode array: 810 nm (near infrared) (for pale to medium skin)

Nd:YAG laser: 1,064 nm (near infrared) (made for treating darker skin types, though effective on all skin types as long as hair is dark)

Intense pulsed light: 810 nm (not a laser, but used for hair removal) (for pale to olive type skin, depending on the type of filter and settings)

hair removal in any practice, even one with mostly lighter skinned patients. However, larger spot Nd:YAG lasers tend to peak at about 70 J/cm², a fluence that would prove inadequate for destruction of lighter hairs (blond through sandy brown). Studies have explored sequential and simultaneous delivery of two wavelengths (755 and 1,064 nm) for laser hair removal for some slightly darker patients with lighter hairs. In these cases, an 80/20 mixture of 1,064 to 755 nm achieved the optimal combination of hair reduction, epidermal protection, and pain tolerance.[17,18] Characteristics of lasers used for hair removal are shown in Box 12.5.

PLIGS has become a major issue, especially in female facial areas (Figure 12.8).[19] Most of these cases have occurred when thinner hairs in the cheek, neck, and sideburn areas were treated. In some cases, even areas adjacent to the treated area have grown more hair, suggesting that subsurface light scattering at lower fluence might paradoxically stimulate hair growth. Almost every laser device has been reported as a culprit. Corrective actions have included cooling the nontargeted adjacent area, using ever-increasing fluence and/or shorter pulse width, using different wavelengths, making a second pass over the area in the same treatment session, and having patients return 1 week after treatment for a second treatment. In the latter scenario, one theory suggests

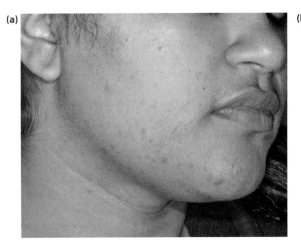
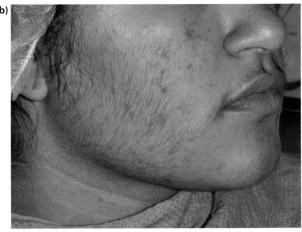

Figure 12.8 Paradoxical laser-induced growth stimulation. Note increased hair after four treatments about 2 months apart. Parameters were 40 J/cm², 3 ms, 1,064 nm, and cryogen spray cooling.

that the initial treatment induces differentiation of the follicle, rendering it more susceptible to laser injury 1 week later. PLIGS does not tend to improve naturally. Although some clinics have abandoned facial hair removal in women altogether, most facilities continue to perform laser hair removal but confine treatment to areas of thicker hair, avoiding the areas and hair types most susceptible to this phenomenon. Studies report some synergy between Vaniqua (Allergan, Inc., Irvine, CA), a prescription hair removal cream, and laser hair removal, and this combination treatment is one option for PLIGS-plagued patients.[20,21] Spironolactone, which antagonizes the male hormone at the skin level to directly stop new hair growth, can also be used in conjunction with laser treatment.

Pain with laser treatment is variable but tends to be proportional to the thickness, color, and density of hair. It follows that treatment of men's beards (normally only treated with PFB) generates the greatest pain. Topical anesthetics usually suffice in pain reduction, although some sensitive patients might require oral analgesics or anxiolytics. For some hair types and regions, the 1,064-nm laser tends to generate more discomfort than 755- and 810-nm lasers. IPL overall tends to generate the least discomfort. An exception to 1,064 lasers being the most painful are scenarios in which the hair is thin and light enough that insufficient heat is generated in the follicles. In general, as long as the hairs are sufficiently thick, longer pulses tend to produce greater pain than shorter pulses.

LASERS FOR SKIN RESURFACING

Until 2006, laser skin resurfacing was carried out in a confluent manner, and the efficacy, risks, and recovery intervals tended to be proportional to the total depth of injury. A number of side effects contributed to the reduction in full-face laser resurfacing cases from 1994 to 2000. Infections, prolonged erythema, pain, and scarring were not uncommon.[22,23] However, a common long-term side effect was hypopigmentation, which tended to occur along the lateral jawline and perioral area (Figure 12.9). Also, neurotoxins and later hyaluronic acid fillers were introduced into the cosmetic arena, allowing laser resurfacing to play only a complementary role in skin rejuvenation. Beginning in 1997, investigators reported the first results of nonablative, nonfractional lasers.[24] The term selective dermal heating was introduced, wherein a laser, using water as a chromophore, was coupled with surface cooling to spare the epidermis and heat a subsurface slab of skin from 200 to 800 μm below the epidermis. Wavelengths from 1,320 to 1,540 nm were applied with these devices. In the end, higher settings resulted in unacceptably high levels of pain and side effects. But when parameters were reduced, wrinkle and acne scar improvements were so marginal that only sophisticated imaging tools could show the changes.[25] Most of these devices are no longer manufactured.

Fractional Lasers
Nonablative Fractional Lasers
By 2006, nonablative fractional rejuvenation (NAFR) was introduced and has continued to enjoy success. NAFR relies on wavelengths that are relatively

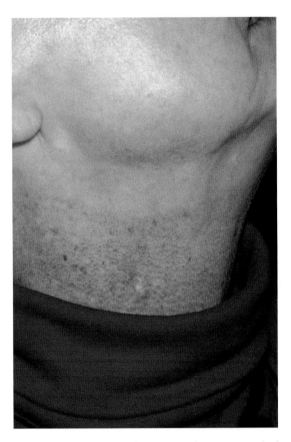

FIGURE 12.9 Patient 1 year after CO_2 confluent resurfacing. Note the hypopigmentation.

weakly absorbed by water.[26-28] Unlike their nonfractional counterparts, small micro-columns of thermal damage are generated with diameters of 100 to 300 μm. Density (or the cross-sectional percentages) tend to range from 10% to 50% per treatment session. The first commercially available fractional laser was the Fraxel Restore (Solta Medical, Hayward, CA). This laser emits 1,550-nm radiation with 120-μm diameter spots at typical pulse energies. The device uses unique scanning technology (intelligent optical tracking system [IOTS]) that randomly places beamlets across the skin as the tip rollers cover the skin surface. Multiple passes are made until a preset density, determined by the treatment level, is achieved. The scanner is able to measure the speed over the skin and adjusts the beamlet rate to accommodate the speed. Although optically the micro-beam size remains constant, with increasing pulse energies, the zone of thermal damage increases. Conventional wisdom dictates that conditions with deeper microscopic changes (acne scars) are best treated with lower densities and higher pulse energies, whereas superficial surface irregularities (pigment dyschromias and fine lines) are optimally treated by lower pulse energies and higher densities. More recent additions to the nonablative fractional armamentarium are the Palomar 1,540-nm laser (Palomar Medical Technologies, Burlington, MA); Mosaic laser (Lutronic, Inc., Fremont, CA); Cynosure Affirm CO_2 laser (Sentient Medical Technologies, Kamas, UT); and the new Lumenis ResurFX (1,565 nm) (Lumenis Ltd., Yokneam, Israel). These lasers use a stamping mode in which a larger beam is separated into beamlets by a diffraction lens.

When applying fractional lasers, visible endpoints are vague, such that the operator must rely on "recipes" for successful rejuvenation. The user must track the number of passes so that critical total surface densities are not exceeded. Bulk cooling, either through frequent application of a contact roller or through refrigerated cold air, is useful for overall skin protection and analgesia. Indications for fractional nonablative lasers are extensive, but the three most common "rejuvenative" indications are fine wrinkling, pigment reduction, and scars. Wrinkle reduction is achieved after a number of treatments, spaced usually about 1 to 3 months apart, when higher depths and densities are applied. In another scenario, lower densities and depths can be applied with either home devices or less powerful clinic-based technologies where the treatments can even be applied on a daily basis.

Ablative Fractional Lasers
Ablative fractional resurfacing (AFR) lasers emit radiation at 2,790 nm, 2,940 nm, or 10,600 nm.[29,30] The relative absorption by water is roughly 1 to 2 orders of magnitude greater than in NAFR. The types of lesions created by AFR devices can be divided into 1) deeper narrower wounds (the most common type) and 2) more superficial broader wound types (500 to 1,500 µm in diameter). In the former case, the depth exceeds the width of the lesion and the geometry is akin to lawn aeration. In the latter case, the fractional geometry mimics a "lily pad on the pond" type of injury.

Rational Use of Fractional Lasers and Common Applications
NAFR is a more practical approach for patients because recovery side effects are typically confined to erythema and swelling. Also, NAFR can be combined with other procedures; for example, in a patient with telangiectasia and lentigines, an IPL, KTP laser, or PDL can be applied just before NAFR. Similarly, neurotoxins and fillers can be used before the procedure. Shortcomings associated with NAFR include 1) poor reduction in perioral rhytides; 2) only partial improvement in excessive pigmentation; 3) possible worsening of melasma, particularly with higher pulse energies and densities; and 4) variable degrees of pain. Also, in some cases, acneiform eruptions occur in the acute follow-up period. Despite conventional wisdom that multiple sessions are required for rejuvenation, many patients are satisfied with only one treatment as long as that treatment is repeated every year. In another approach, three to six treatments are carried out with 1- to 2-month intervals, again with a high likelihood that a repeat series of treatments would be applied every 1 to 2 years.

Often the approach to an individual patient is based on the precise "cosmetic" presentation, the willingness of the patient to accept filler and neurotoxins as part of the "solution," the available lasers in the practice, and the tolerance for downtime. The goal is to play to the respective strengths of the interventions. For example, in a 55-year-old patient with deep perioral wrinkles and multiple lentigines, the physician should first determine the patient's primary concern. If, for example, perioral wrinkles are particularly bothersome, a conventional CO_2 or erbium laser can be applied around the mouth and a fractional ablative laser over the remainder of the face. Neurotoxins and fillers can be applied in the same session. If the patient has little time for recovery, a program of VIS light technologies combined with NAFR can be applied. Box 12.6 provides a summary of the use of fractional lasers.

Box 12.6

Summary of Fractional Lasers

- The Fraxel Restore (Solta Medical), the first nonablative fractional laser (NAFR):
  - Emits 1,550-nm radiation with 120-μm diameter spots at typical pulse energies
  - Uses unique scanning technology that randomly places beamlets across the skin as the tip rollers cover the skin surface
  - Entails multiple passes until a preset density is achieved
- Other nonablative fractional lasers are the Palomar 1,540-nm laser, Lutronic Mosaic laser, Lumenis 1565-nm laser, and Cynosure Affirm CO_2 laser.
- With fractional lasers, conditions with deeper microscopic changes (acne scars) are best treated with lower densities and higher pulse energies. Superficial surface irregularities (pigment dyschromias and fine lines) are optimally treated by lower pulse energies and higher densities.
- The three most common "rejuvenative" indications for NAFR are fine wrinkling, pigment reduction, and scars.
- Nonablative fractional lasers can be combined with other procedures.
- With NAFR, recovery side effects are typically confined to erythema and swelling.
- NAFR shortcomings include poor reduction in perioral rhytides, only partial improvement in excessive pigmentation, and possible worsening of melasma.
- Often the approach to an individual patient is based on:
  - The precise "cosmetic" presentation
  - The willingness of the patient to accept filler and neurotoxins as part of the "solution"
  - The available lasers in the practice
  - The tolerance for downtime
- Fractional ablative:
  - Can achieve good wrinkle reduction around eyes and cheeks after one treatment; the durability of the response is variable
  - Reduces perioral wrinkles but not as well as confluent resurfacing
  - Is less likely to cause hypopigmentation, scarring, and infection than confluent resurfacing
  - Is an excellent tool for scars

NONINVASIVE SKIN-TIGHTENING PROCEDURES

Probably nothing in the skin rejuvenation arena is more controversial and challenging than noninvasive deep skin tightening (Box 12.7). The controversy includes the definition of "tightening" itself as well as establishing objective assessment tools for efficacy. Often the results are three-dimensional such that simply examining a standard photo is inadequate

Box 12.7

Skin Tightening

- Skin tightening is the visible reduction in jowls, neck laxity, and so forth, as opposed to a reduction in fine wrinkles.
- The Thermage device (Solta Medical) is a noninvasive skin-tightening technology that delivers radiofrequency energy through a square cooled tip.
- Multiple passes and lower energy settings called for with recent Thermage algorithms provide consistent tightening and reduced side effects (pain, fat atrophy).
- Resurfacing with the CO_2 laser provides for at least temporary skin tightening, as do deeper applications of the erbium YAG laser.

for assessment. Regarding the definition, we refer to "skin tightening" as a visible reduction in jowls, neck laxity, and so forth, as opposed to a reduction in fine wrinkles. There are several noninvasive skin-tightening technologies. The most common are radiofrequency (RF) devices, followed by halogen lamps (infrared heating), and ultrasound. Noninvasive RF has enjoyed a 10-year market experience, beginning with the Thermage device (Solta Medical), in which RF energy is delivered through a square cooled tip coupled to a fine dielectric membrane that distributes the electrical field somewhat evenly over the skin. Early approaches relied on one pass and a high-energy setting, whereas more recent algorithms call for multiple passes and lower energy settings. In this scenario, tightening has remained consistent and side effects (pain, fat atrophy) have been reduced. Unlike the Thermage device, most other RF devices use a motion technique in which the skin is heated over a certain temperature and time (i.e., 41° C at surface for 3 to 10 minutes). In this scenario, the tip is moved back and forth over the surface until the skin achieves a certain surface temperature or becomes intolerably hot. More than 10 devices use this approach of large-volume, low-level heating. Although most patients report a warm or hot sensation after treatment, with an associated sense of "tightening," few objective studies support a strong role for these devices.

In designing a skin-tightening application or any energy-based application, the operator should consider the basis for the underlying cosmetic concern. For example, in skin tightening, for which the most common complaint is sagging of the lower face, multiple factors contribute to "loose" skin, including volume loss, elastic tissue loss, bony recession, relaxation of the suspensory ligaments associated with the superficial muscular aponeurotic system, and others. It follows that a logical approach to skin tightening should address these factors. Among the technologies applied for skin tightening, some older technologies that heat superficially do provide tightening. A primary example is the CO_2 laser, in which production of collagen in the dermis and possibly resetting of the wound-healing matrix provide for at least temporary skin tightening. Likewise, deeper applications of the erbium YAG laser have achieved some skin tightening. Cutis laxa, in which even very young patients

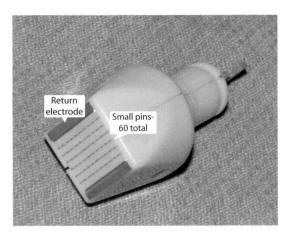

Figure 12.10 Fractional RF device (Fractora). The tip is placed against the skin, and the machine sends radiofrequency current to each of the 60 pins.

show skin sagging, is a good example of the importance of elastic tissue in skin health.

Fractional radiofrequency devices (e.g., Viora, Jersey City, NJ; Fractora, Invasix, Irvine, CA) and other sublative RF fractional devices (eMatrix, ePrime; Syneron and Candela, Irvine, CA) deliver RF energy in a bipolar fashion whereby the return electrodes are typically placed at the perimeter of the square applicator (Figure 12.10). The energy is delivered through small micropins at a certain pitch. Small wounds are created at the skin surface. In this configuration, the superficial energy deposition is best suited for fine wrinkle reduction and acne scar treatment. Another device creates microplasmas on the skin surface to improve scars, striae, and wrinkles (Pixel RF, Alma Lasers, Buffalo Grove, IL).

Halogen lamps have also been applied for skin tightening. The lamps, emitting radiation from about 1.2 to 1.7 μm, are coupled with cooling at the surface and achieve heating about 1 to 2 mm deep in the skin. Like their nonfractional RF counterparts, these devices rely on large volume and relatively small temperature elevations for the desired effect.

Ultrasound devices have been studied for skin tightening. One device, Ulthera (Ulthera, Mesa, AZ), creates 1-mm^3 wounds 2 to 5 mm deep in the skin, depending on the transducer. With each application, a line of coagulative wounds is produced. The number of lines can vary depending on the needs of the patient. In the most recent scenarios, multiple passes are made in some areas with different transducers.

Another device, ePrime, uses an RF design in which five sets of paired electrodes are impaled by a spring action about 2 mm deep in the skin. The electrodes are angled at about 25 degrees from the skin surface. Insulation prevents the superficial portion of the electrode from damaging the epidermis and the very superficial dermis. Studies have shown an increase in elastin production and a volumization effect after treatment. Optimally the procedure is paired with other procedures so that patients observe the immediate as well as the delayed effect of the procedure. This coupling of procedures is a recurrent theme for procedures with very small immediate effects. Often a patient will respond best when engaged by an immediate response (i.e., IPL for red brown spots, neurotoxins, filler) that complements the deeper tightening procedure.

FUTURE DIRECTIONS

Of the major advances in lasers and other energy-based technologies, some landmark changes have been the addition of skin-cooling, platform-based rejuvenation systems, fractional lasers, and deeper heating RF and ultrasound systems. Nonetheless, several common cosmetic ailments have defied laser treatment. Among these are melasma, idiopathic guttate hypomelanosis (discussed earlier), sebaceous hyperplasia, lightly pigmented seborrheic keratoses, white hair, and multicolored tattoos. Future light sources might be designed that can improve these common conditions.

Engineering advances will miniaturize lasers. Diodes will become increasingly commonplace; diode chips will replace some high-powered solid-state lasers. These diode chips enjoy a much higher effectiveness compared with traditional lasers. IPLs will continue to improve with improved lamp filtration, better cooling, and larger spots. A new device, the TRASER (total reflection amplification of spontaneous emission of radiation),[31] which combines some of the attributes of IPL and laser, will likely become commercially available and allow for a large number of monochromatic wavelengths from one device.

Laser complications result primarily from unfamiliarity with the device and a lack of understanding of laser-tissue interactions. Experience with a few devices is preferable to dabbling with many types of light-based technologies. When performing a laser procedure, operators must apply all of their senses to minimize the likelihood of side effects. Endpoints should always prevail over settings. With experience, one's eyes provide excellent feedback insofar as applications addressing surface concerns. However, for deeper heating (RF, Ulthera), one relies on time-tested recipes for safety and efficacy. The introduction of real-time assessments of subsurface temperature should enhance outcomes and increase safety within the field of deeper dermal and fat heating.

Most complications result from overheating the epidermis when treating brown and red dyschromias or in laser hair reduction (Figure 12.11). Underestimation of background epidermal pigment is often a contributor or, even more commonly, underestimation of a tan. Technique can also contribute to complications. For example, poor contact between the skin and handpiece tip, particularly in concave or convex areas, can result in inadequate cooling. Air is a good insulator, so that any air between the skin and the handpiece can result in surface overheating. Another cause for complications is a failure to understand heat transfer, which is one of the foundations of laser-tissue interactions. For example, in making multiple passes of a fractional laser over a shorter time, bulk heating of the skin can occur. Skin heating with short pulsed lasers is immediate, on the same time scale as the laser pulse; however, cooling is slow, on the order of milliseconds and, for larger targets, even seconds. Box 12.8 provides a summary of future directions with lasers.

Much to-do is made of skin typing in establishing laser settings, particularly in laser scenarios for darker skin. By convention, operators are discouraged from treating darker skin types, out of fear of either immediate complications or delayed PIH. However, skin typing was developed to guide practitioners in optimizing ultraviolet treatments for psoriasis, not for laser applications. Although skin typing is related to constitutive pigmentation and epidermal tolerance, real-time melanin assessment is a more valuable tool. To that end,

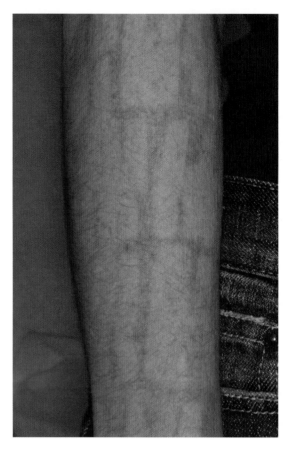

FIGURE 12.11   Note the hypopigmentation after intense pulsed light treatment. This type of side effect will usually resolve over 6 to 12 months.

Box 12.8

Future Directions with Lasers

- Lasers will be miniaturized.
- Diodes lasers and diode chips will replace some high-powered solid-state lasers.
- Intense pulsed light (IPL) will continue to improve with improved lamp filtration, better cooling, and larger spots.
- A new device, the TRASER (total reflection amplification of spontaneous emission of radiation),[31] which combines some of the attributes of IPL and laser, will allow for a large number of monochromatic wavelengths from one device.

---

manufacturers have developed devices for bedside assessment of skin melanin to aid in parameter selection.[32] One of these devices is the Skintel (Palomar Medical Technologies), a built-in skin meter that reports pigment levels from the skin through Bluetooth to the base unit. A recommended range of settings is then displayed for the provider (Figure 12.12).

PIH is a common sequela in treatment of darker skin; however, the risk for PIH should only be considered a relative contraindication to laser surgery. In some cases, the depth of injury needed to improve the skin lesions exceeds the

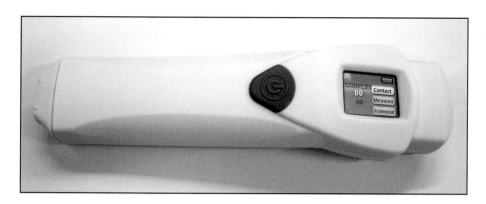

FIGURE 12.12 Pigment meter (Skintel). The tip is applied on skin, and the meter measures the real-time skin color.

depth that causes PIH. A good example is acne scarring, where deeper NAFR or AFR is required for marked improvement. More superficial treatments can achieve scar reduction, but deeper treatments are more likely to achieve success. If a patient shows melasma and acne scarring, the physician should counsel the patient that PIH (and worsening of melasma) might be likely if treatments are carried out aggressively enough to see meaningful scar improvement.

PROBLEMATIC CONDITIONS

Despite the long list of lasers and other energy-based technologies, some skin conditions are still only mildly improved by lasers, and indeed, in some cases less expensive nonlaser technologies are still preferred (Box 12.9). Melasma, for example, is often best treated by retinoids, bleaching creams, and sunblocks.[33] Sebaceous hyperplasia has been treated by a number of lasers, but recurrences are frequent, and the risk for scarring tends to increase with the likelihood of a durable response. Syringomas and other benign adnexal tumors respond to ablative lasers, but given their microscopic location in the dermis, very deep ablation must be carried out to achieve a durable response. Fractional lasers have recently been applied to a number of conditions. In one recent paper, a CO_2 fractional laser was applied to syringomas with a partial response.[34-36] However, the use of fractional lasers in "nonfractional" conditions (e.g., AKs) is still controversial. Dark circles under the eyes are a common patient complaint and, depending on the precise patient presentation, are likely the result of increased vasculature, excessive pigment, a trough-like condition under the eye, and thinner skin that increases light transmission and shows the underlying orbicularis muscle.[37,38] We have found that dark circles due to true hyperpigmentation do respond to noninvasive, Q-switching 1,064-nm lasers. Traditional resurfacing has also proved effective, but often only after PIH resolves months after the treatment. Carefully placed fillers can also diminish dark circles in selected patients.

Red striae can be improved with vascular lasers. Older striae improve after ablative or nonablative fractional treatment. Still, results are somewhat unpredictable, and PIH is common and persistent in some patients with darker skin. Striae alba have been particularly challenging to improve with lasers. More recently, NAFR and AFR, as well as fractional RF technologies, have been applied.

Box 12.9

Laser Treatment of Problematic Conditions

- Patients with melasma and acne scarring may see PIH and worsening of melasma with aggressive laser treatment (that may be needed to achieve meaningful scar improvement).
- Recurrences of sebaceous hyperplasia are frequent after laser treatment.
- Very deep ablations must be carried out to achieve a durable response with syringomas and other benign adnexal tumors.
- The use of fractional lasers in "nonfractional" conditions (e.g., actinic keratoses) is controversial.
- Dark circles under the eyes do respond to noninvasive, Q-switching 1,064-nm lasers.
- Red striae can be improved with vascular lasers, and older striae improve after ablative or nonablative fractional treatment, but results are somewhat unpredictable, and PIH is common and persistent in some patients with darker skin.
- Scar rehabilitation or improvement is a growing application in laser dermatology, but improvement is gradual and incremental.
- Early red acne scars are treated with vascular-specific devices, and PIH is treated with pigmented lasers. More mature scars, if they are of the boxcar type, can be treated by nonablative fractional rejuvenation or ablative fractional laser.
- Light should not normally be a first-line acne treatment, and creative use of topical and oral medications is usually sufficient to treat acne.
- Visible light devices (and more recently alexandrite and Nd:YAG lasers) can be applied for reduction of redness and flushing after the papules and pustules of rosacea have been reduced by oral and topical drugs.[43]
- Laser removal or lightening of true nevocellular nevi is controversial.
- The excimer laser is helpful for pigment restoration in facial skin with vitiligo.

Scar rehabilitation or improvement is a growing application in laser dermatology. Depending on the type of scar, the provider can use a mix of vascular devices and fractional lasers to improve range of motion, color, and texture. In scar assessment, one should look for scar features that differentiate the scar from normal surrounding skin. For example, after a motor vehicle crash, one might observe traumatic tattooing, hyperemia, and later PIH (Figure 12.13). In this scenario, a combination of a dedicated pigment and vascular laser, as well as a fractional laser, can prove helpful. In the consultation, the concept of scar rehabilitation should be discussed with the patient, with an emphasis on gradual incremental scar improvement. Impairments of both form and function should be corrected in an effort at normal skin restoration. Typically, for hypertrophic and keloid scars, intralesional corticosteroids and 5-fluorouracil can be added to the treatment routine.

Acne scar treatment should be based on the morphology of the scars. Goodman has established a comprehensive grading system with a logical

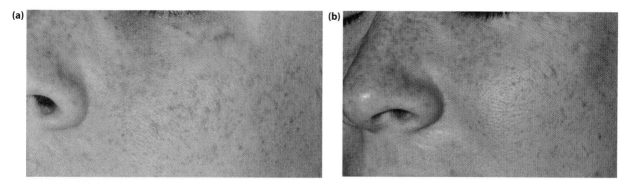

(a)   **(b)**

FIGURE 12.13   (a) Traumatic tattoo before treatment. (b) The patient after one treatment with Q-switched 1,064-nm laser.

treatment program based on scar features.[39,40] Early red scar areas are treated with vascular-specific devices, and PIH is treated with pigmented lasers. More mature scars, if they are of the boxcar type, can be treated by NAFR or AFR. Rolling scars can be treated by filler and subcision and laser. Icepick scars can be treated by the CROSS (chemical reconstruction of skin scars) technique. In our experience, although AFR tends to improve scars more than NAFR on a per session basis, we have found that most patients prefer a series of NAFR treatments.

Light-based treatment of active acne has been touted as a bona fide technique to reduce papules, pustules and redness. In our experience, light should not normally be a first-line acne treatment, and creative use of topical and oral medications is usually sufficient to treat acne. However, a role for light in acne is reasonable under certain patient presentations. For example, for temporary improvement of redness, vascular targets are logical and effective, and IPL, PDL, and KTP are all useful. For acne refractory to treatment with isotretinoin or when that drug is contraindicated (e.g., pregnant patients, depressed patients), ALA/PDT can be very useful. We have found that the greatest effect is seen after treatment regimens as outlined by Sakamoto and colleagues.[41,42] where long incubation times, red light, and higher fluence are applied (about 50 to 200 J/cm^2). Under these conditions, especially when the treatments are carried out two or three times at 2- to 3-month intervals, results similar to those obtained with oral isotretinoin can be achieved. However, under these conditions, often desquamation, discoloration, acne flares, and PIH are observed. Gentler forms of PDT with shorter incubation times, blue light, and shorter irradiation times have shown mixed results.

For rosacea patients, after the papules and pustules have been reduced by oral and topical drugs, visible light devices (and more recently, alexandrite and Nd:YAG lasers) can be applied for reduction of redness and flushing.[43] Often multiple treatments are required, and treatment packages must be repeated every 6 to 12 months. Some patients are particularly resistant to treatment, and antihistamines and topical vasoconstrictive agents must be added to the therapeutic "soup."

Laser removal or lightening of true nevocellular nevi is controversial. However, as long as the nevus shows benign features and the patient is educated regarding the relative risks, certain nevi may be safely removed. Among nevi most often considered for removal are small junctional nevi in darker patients. They can be lightened by a series of Q-switched or long-pulsed alexandrite lasers or, alternatively, a series of a switched YAG lasers. Another possibility is ablation by the CO_2 or erbium YAG laser, where one can use magnification to ablate the nevus layer by layer with multiple passes. The advantage over shave excision is the precision of removal because the operator is not committed to one depth across the entire lesion. Normally we use a 0.2- to 2-mm spot size, and with magnifying loops, we very carefully ablate the lesion until a very slight depression is observed. We have also used the Surgitron (Ellman International, Hicksville, NY) with a fine loop or needle to achieve excellent cosmetic results. If the patient is mainly concerned regarding the color of the nevus versus its exophytic nature, we recommend a formal elliptical excision or no treatment at all.

Vitiligo has been treated with the excimer laser. As a form of targeted ultraviolet therapy, the laser at 308 nm is near the peak action spectrum for repigmentation potential with a relatively lower risk for erythema than 290 nm. We have found the laser helpful for pigment restoration in facial skin (about 80% repigmentation after 20 to 30 treatments delivered twice a week). Off-the- face treatments have proved to be more resistant; however, after 30 to 50 treatments, we have observed considerable repigmentation of the knees, neck, and hands in some patients.

Devising a laser strategy for a particular patient should be based on a good understanding of laser tissue interactions and wound healing. With experience, a logical approach can be designed that accommodates the recovery constraints of the patient. The complementary nature of neurotoxins and fillers to the laser arsenal is a major advance in skin rejuvenation. In most cases, an individualized approach is best for both provider and patient. Undertreating the patient is always better than overtreating, and operator and patient safety should take precedence over other concerns for the successful laser surgeon.

REFERENCES

1. Anderson RR, Parrish JA. Microvasculature can be selectively damaged using dye lasers: a basic theory and experimental evidence in human skin. *Lasers Surg Med.* 1981;1(3):263–276.

2. Apfelberg DB, Maser MR, Lash H, Rivers J. The argon laser for cutaneous lesions. *JAMA.* 1981;245(20):2073–2075.

3. Greenwald J, Rosen S, Anderson RR, et al. Comparative histological studies of the tunable dye (at 577 nm) laser and argon laser: the specific vascular effects of the dye laser. *J Invest Dermatol.* 1981;77(3):305–310.

4. Anderson RR, Jaenicke KF, Parrish JA. Mechanisms of selective vascular changes caused by dye lasers. *Lasers Surg Med.* 1983;3(3):211–215.

5. Anderson RR, Parrish JA. Selective photothermolysis: precise microsurgery by selective absorption of pulsed radiation. *Science.* 1983;220(4596):524–527.

6. Anderson RR. Carbon dioxide lasers: a broader perspective. *Arch Dermatol.* 1987; 123(5):566–567.

7. Eremia S, Li CY. Treatment of face veins with a cryogen spray variable pulse width 1064 nm Nd:YAG laser: a prospective study of 17 patients [comment]. *Dermatol Surg.* 2002;28(3):244–247.

8. Lai SW, Goldman MP. Treatment of facial reticular veins with dynamically cooled, variable spot-sized 1064 nm Nd:YAG laser. *J Cosmet Dermatol.* 2007;6(1):6–8.

9. Chang CJ, Nelson JS. Cryogen spray cooling and higher fluence pulsed dye laser treatment improve port-wine stain clearance while minimizing epidermal damage. *Dermatol Surg.* 1999;25(10):767–772.

10. Trafeli JP, Kwan JM, Meehan KJ, et al. Use of a long-pulse alexandrite laser in the treatment of superficial pigmented lesions. *Dermatol Surg.* 2007;33(12):1477–1482.

11. Goldust M, Mohebbipour A, Mirmohammadi R. Treatment of idiopathic guttate hypomelanosis with fractional carbon dioxide lasers. *J Cosmet Laser Ther. 2012;* May 8 [Epub ahead of print].

12. Kim SK, Park JY, Hann SK, et al. Hypopigmented keratosis: is it a hyperkeratotic variant of idiopathic guttate hypomelanosis? *Clin Exp Dermatol. 2012;* Apr 20 [Epub ahead of print].

13. Kono T, Manstein D, Chan HH, et al. Q-switched ruby versus long-pulsed dye laser delivered with compression for treatment of facial lentigines in Asians. *Lasers Surg Med.* 2006;38(2):94–97.

14. Ross EV, Ladin Z, Kreindel M, Dierickx C. Theoretical considerations in laser hair removal. *Dermatol Clin.* 1999;17(2):333–355, viii.

15. Kolinko V, Littler CM. Mathematical modeling for the prediction and optimization of laser hair removal. *Lasers Surg Med.* 2000;26(2):164–176.

16. Kolinko VG, Littler CM, Cole A. Influence of the anagen:telogen ratio on Q-switched Nd:YAG laser hair removal efficacy. *Lasers Surg Med.* 2000;26(1):33–40.

17. Bernstein EF, Basilavecchio L, Plugis J. Bilateral axilla hair removal comparing a single wavelength alexandrite laser with combined multiplexed alexandrite and Nd:YAG laser treatment from a single laser platform. *J Drugs Dermatol.* 2012;11(2):185–190.

18. Nilforoushzadeh MA, Naieni FF, Siadat AH, Rad L. Comparison between sequential treatment with diode and alexandrite lasers versus alexandrite laser alone in the treatment of hirsutism. *J Drugs Dermatol.* 2011;10(11):1255–1259.

19. Desai S, Mahmoud BH, Bhatia AC, Hamzavi IH. Paradoxical hypertrichosis after laser therapy: a review. *Dermatol Surg.* 2010;36(3):291–298.

20. Hamzavi I, Tan E, Shapiro J, Lui H. A randomized bilateral vehicle-controlled study of eflornithine cream combined with laser treatment versus laser treatment alone for facial hirsutism in women. *J Am Acad Dermatol.* 2007;57(1):54–59.

21. Smith SR, Piacquadio DJ, Beger B, Littler C. Eflornithine cream combined with laser therapy in the management of unwanted facial hair growth in women: a randomized trial. *Dermatol Surg.* 2006;32(10):1237–1243.

22. Ragland HP, McBurney E. Complications of resurfacing. *Semin Cutan Med Surg.* 1996;15(3):200–207.

23. Apfelberg DB. Side effects, sequelae, and complications of carbon dioxide laser resurfacing. *Aesthet Surg J.* 1997;17(6):365–372.

24. Lask G, Lee PK, Seyfzadeh M, et al. Nonablative laser treatment of facial rhytides. In: Anderson RR, ed. *Lasers in Surgery: Advanced Characterization, Therapeutics, and Systems VII.* Vol. 2970. San Jose, CA: Society of Photo-Instrumentation Engineers; 1997:338–349.

25. Kopera D, Smolle J, Kaddu S, Kerl H. Nonablative laser treatment of wrinkles: meeting the objective? Assessment by 25 dermatologists. *Br J Dermatol.* 2004;150(5): 936–939.

26. Rahman Z, Alam M, Dover JS. Fractional laser treatment for pigmentation and texture improvement. *Skin Ther Lett.* 2006;11(9):7–11.

27. Weiss RA, Gold M, Bene N, et al. Prospective clinical evaluation of 1440-nm laser delivered by microarray for treatment of photoaging and scars. *J Drugs Dermatol.* 2006;5(8):740–744.

28. Tierney EP, Kouba DJ, Hanke CW. Review of fractional photothermolysis: treatment indications and efficacy. *Dermatol Surg.* 2009;35(10):1445–1461.

29. Trelles MA, Mordon S, Velez M, et al. Results of fractional ablative facial skin resurfacing with the erbium:yttrium-aluminium-garnet laser 1 week and 2 months after one single treatment in 30 patients. *Lasers Med Sci.* 2009;24(2):186–194.

30. Paasch U, Haedersdal M. Laser systems for ablative fractional resurfacing. *Expert Rev Med Devices.* 2011;8(1):67–83.

31. Zachary CB, Gustavsson M. TRASER: total reflection amplification of spontaneous emission of radiation. *PLoS ONE.* 2012;7(4):e35899.

32. Dolotov LE, Sinichkin YP, Tuchin VV, et al. Design and evaluation of a novel portable erythema-melanin-meter. *Lasers Surg Med.* 2004;34(2):127–135.

33. Sardana K, Chugh S, Garg VK. Which therapy works for melasma in pigmented skin: lasers, peels, or triple combination creams? *Indian J Dermatol Venereol Leprol.* 2013;79(3):420–422.

34. Brightman L, Geronemus R. Commentary: treatment of syringoma using an ablative 10,600-nm carbon dioxide fractional laser. *Dermatol Surg.* 2011;37(4):439–440.

35. Cho SB, Kim HJ, Noh S, et al. Treatment of syringoma using an ablative 10,600-nm carbon dioxide fractional laser: a prospective analysis of 35 patients. *Dermatol Surg.* 2011;37(4):433–438.

36. Akita H, Takasu E, Washimi Y, et al. Syringoma of the face treated with fractional photothermolysis. *J Cosmet Laser Ther.* 2009;11(4):216–219.

37. Xu TH, Yang ZH, Li YH, et al. Treatment of infraorbital dark circles using a low-fluence Q-switched 1,064-nm laser. *Dermatol Surg.* 2011;37(6):797–803.

38. Roh MR, Chung KY. Infraorbital dark circles: definition, causes, and treatment options. *Dermatol Surg.* 2009;35(8):1163–1171.

39. Goodman GJ. Treating scars: addressing surface, volume, and movement to expedite optimal results. Part 2: more-severe grades of scarring. *Dermatol Surg.* 2012;38(8):1310–1321.

40. Goodman GJ. Treating scars: addressing surface, volume, and movement to optimize results: part 1. Mild grades of scarring. *Dermatol Surg.* 2012;38(8):1302–1309.

41. Sakamoto FH, Torezan L, Anderson RR. Photodynamic therapy for acne vulgaris: a critical review from basics to clinical practice: part II. Understanding parameters for acne treatment with photodynamic therapy. *J Am Acad Dermatol.* 2010;63(2):195–211; quiz 211–192.

42. Sakamoto FH, Lopes JD, Anderson RR. Photodynamic therapy for acne vulgaris: a critical review from basics to clinical practice: part I. Acne vulgaris: when and why consider photodynamic therapy? *J Am Acad Dermatol.* 2010;63(2):183-193; quiz 193–184.

43. Neuhaus IM, Zane LT, Tope WD. Comparative efficacy of nonpurpuragenic pulsed dye laser and intense pulsed light for erythematotelangiectatic rosacea. *Dermatol Surg.* 2009;35(6):920–928.

NUTRACEUTICALS AND THEIR ROLE IN SKIN HEALTH RESTORATION

Kevin Nagengast, PharmD

NUTRACEUTICALS

The fact that the skin is the least nutrient supplied yet largest organ of the body compels us to choose nutraceuticals that are well formulated to realize optimal results in skin health. Most components essential for healthy skin are first used elsewhere in the body, as determined by higher priority, such as, the brain, liver, and kidneys. Because the skin receives what is left, it is necessary to supplement the essential nutrients in the highest of quality, in the correct form, carried in an appropriate vehicle, and delivered with sufficient quantity. With many complex interactions possible within and between nutritional supplements, the perfect skin nutraceutical regimen demands a deeper understanding of the intricacies of each essential component. As we approach each nutraceutical with a pragmatic and scientific eye, a review of the current literature is provided. Attention to the details as we review the future of skin health from the inside out is key to achieving total skin health.

Without a clearly developed methodology for carrying botanicals, vitamins, and minerals across the skin's barrier, there can be minimal absorption and effectiveness achieved. Correctly supplementing a standard diet with essential elements for healthy skin can dramatically improve the appearance, elasticity, fullness, and glow of the skin. By addressing each category of supplementation, this section will cover an array of mechanisms to promote positive skin outcomes. The survey of nutraceuticals, as we shall call them, will detail antioxidants, vitamins, cofactors, enzymes, amino acids, and the related botanicals that contain them. Through the correct use of nutraceuticals, a universal approach to the treatment of skin conditions from the inside out, as an adjunct and option for the prescriber, can achieve optimal results. Nutraceuticals are an excellent approach to achieving skin health in addition to the use of topical creams when a patient, for example, may not be a candidate for procedures such as peels, lasers, or surgery because of disease or a compromised immune system.

There are several modalities and guidelines for using oral supplements, such as vitamin C for colds and vitamin D for supplementing lack of exposure to the sun; however, there are limited data on using nutraceuticals to aid in achieving skin health. An overview of the current data will assist the practitioner in selecting the proper nutraceuticals for skin health.

CLINICAL STUDIES AND RESEARCH

It is common practice for clinical studies to evaluate outcomes based on the patient's subjective feedback and an arbitrary scoring system. The advent of newer technology provides tools for the practitioner to document the effectiveness of oral supplementation beyond what can be seen by the naked eye. Such devices use processors to analyze the surface of the skin for discoloration, hydration, ultraviolet radiation (UVR) damage, wrinkles, and more. Objectively assessing skin rejuvenation by emphasizing clinical, functional, and histological aspects will lead to more accurate evaluations. Although technology has allowed for advances in clinical trials to measure the benefits of supplementing with nutraceuticals, there are few trials using these technologies for practitioners to evaluate.

MARKET

According to *Consumer Reports,* 50% of adults in the United States currently use nutraceuticals. The market for skin health supplements is rapidly expanding, creating an opportunity for dermatologists and skin care professionals to add a new tool in the fight against aging. Selecting the correct ingredients can be a cumbersome task of navigating through the limited literature available on ingredients classified as "cosmetic." Because these supplements are complementary, as opposed to a replacement to current prescription and other therapeutic topical regimens, they require patient education and expertise to create a unique oral supplementation protocol to complete the patient's comprehensive maintenance program.

The role of nutraceuticals in skin health is to supplement the current treatments and enhance patient outcomes where traditional therapies fall short. Most patients are willing to add to their skin care routine if additional benefits and correction can be achieved. Although taking pills orally is usually not a patient's first choice, oral supplementation has the unique advantage over topical application of benefiting the whole body. The added benefits of nutraceuticals include the perception of luxury, natural sourcing, being less invasive than procedures, and achieving overall skin health at a faster rate than with other therapies alone. The goals of nutraceuticals for skin health are 1) to prevent and protect the skin from harmful UVR and other environmental and internal stressors; 2) to rejuvenate skin, enhance results, and improve its appearance; 3) to minimize side effects and maximize efficacy; and 4) to create an easy application for compliance to meet the patient needs (Table 13.1).

DOWNSIDE OF NUTRACEUTICALS

Unlike pharmaceutical-grade products, nutraceuticals tend to lack high-quality studies because of the high cost and time required of clinical trials. Products available in the marketplace, including chain stores and other health-related outlets, provide numerous products with little to no information to guide the patient to an appropriate, safe, and effective supplement. Regulatory agencies such as the U.S. Food and Drug Administration (FDA) limit claims made about a nutraceutical product: the product cannot be advertised as having the ability to treat, cure, diagnose, or prevent a disease. However, nutraceuticals may state their effectiveness with phrases such as "improves the appearance of wrinkles" or "enhances skin glow" rather than making a specific medical claim related to disease or skin function.

TESTING THE EFFECTIVENESS OF NUTRACEUTICALS

Manufacturers of nutraceuticals are not required to submit detailed information including chemistry, mechanism of action, pharmacokinetics, toxicity, and interactions to the FDA. The German Commission E is one source available to evaluate the clinical evidence behind the reasonable use of nutraceuticals. However, much of the available nutraceutical detailing is lacking for currently popularized nutraceuticals for skin health. Further, many formulations use "cocktails" or products with numerous ingredients, making a review of all of the active ingredients complicated and tedious. The common practice of "more ingredients are better" can lead patients to duplicating ingredients when more than one combination nutraceutical product is used. It is well documented that products such as antioxidants and skin-lightening products are more effective with multiple ingredients, providing a variety of mechanisms of action. Unfortunately, many companies analyze

TABLE 13.1   Goals and Benefits of Nutraceuticals

Goals	Benefits
To prevent and protect the skin from harmful ultraviolet rays and other environmental and internal stressors	Less invasive than procedures The perception of luxury Natural sourcing
To rejuvenate the skin, enhance results, and improve the appearance of damaged skin	Faster rate of achieved skin health than with topical creams alone
To minimize side effects and maximize efficacy	
To create an easy application for compliance to meet the patient needs	

their safety based on the safety profile of *individual ingredients* rather than the final formulation. This leaves room for interactions within the formulation, generating possible side effects and decreased potency.

The ideal oral skin health supplement creates an immediate result, has a low side-effect profile, is applicable to a variety of skin conditions, and has long-lasting preventative benefits. *Such a product does not currently exist in the nutraceutical marketplace.*

MECHANISMS OF ACTION OF ANTIOXIDANTS

Several mechanisms of action are required to address the various internal and external stresses created by our environment. The first line of defense is creating a protective barrier to UVR by either deflection or the transfer of UV energy into heat. As solar UVR and our body's own metabolic pathways create reactive oxygen species (ROS), constantly depleting our available antioxidants, supplementation becomes essential to replenish and restore our body's supply of antioxidants. For the sake of simplicity, all oxidative agents and oxidative stress will be referred to as ROS. Supplementation of antioxidants can result in 1) protecting and promoting collagen by stimulating production and inhibiting matrix metalloproteinase (MMP), which breaks down collagen; 2) supporting the skin's structural integrity; 3) strengthening the barrier function; 4) reducing the transepidermal water loss (TEWL); 5) increasing cell turnover; and 6) upregulating DNA repair enzymes.

ANTIOXIDANTS

The most common nutraceuticals promoting skin health are antioxidants. Benefits include protection from oxidative and UVR damage, which is responsible for accelerating the aging process and DNA damage. Current thinking in skin health promotes the application of multiple antioxidants, addressing protection through multiple mechanisms of action.

Environmental stressors, including UVR, industrial pollutants, cigarette smoke, and chemical oxidants, and internal stressors, including normal metabolic reactions, create destructive ROS. The supplementation of bioactive antioxidants is aimed at replenishing the endogenous antioxidant pool, reducing pro-inflammatory mediators, and preventing oxidative chain reactions and DNA damage.

Some DNA damage can be prevented by antioxidants because they effectively arrest ROS activity, preventing the chain reaction of oxidation that can lead to misreading and a change in the DNA sequence referred to as a mutation. The direct absorption of UVR causing DNA cross-linking is not prevented by antioxidants because free radicals are not involved in this process. These reactions are extremely dangerous, leading to mutations that are linked to cancers, including squamous and basal cell carcinomas. To lessen the chances of these dangerous DNA mutations, patients can take advantage of physical blockers, including sunscreens, protective clothing, and visors. DNA repair

Box 13.1

Physical sunblocks, together with antioxidants, can provide ultraviolet
radiation protection.

requires multiple steps, including specific repair enzymes to replace damaged,
cross-linked sites. The damage to DNA strands can ultimately lead to 1) new
genes; 2) the release of stress signals, including tumor necrosis factor-α and
interleukins; and 3) the upregulation of MMP-1 in fibroblasts that will result
in collagen degradation. Through multiple mechanisms, the chronic exposure
to UVR and toxins will physically and superficially result in photodamaged,
uneven, aged skin. Antioxidants can effectively support skin health, resulting
in brighter, healthier, and more even-looking skin.

The requirements for UVR protection are fulfilled by using multiple mechanisms of action, including absorption or reflection with physical sunblocks
and antioxidants such as vitamin C, vitamin E, beta-carotene, and selenium
to eliminate ROS (Box 13.1).

Plant evolution has provided for multiple mechanisms to protect from
damaging solar UVR exposure. Popular botanicals in skin health contain
hundreds of different chemical constituents, many possessing antioxidant
properties. The main categories of plant active components having antioxidant properties for oral supplementation are polyphenols and carotenoids.
Polyphenols provide plants with pigmentation and oxidative protection.
Carotenoids have a similar structure to vitamin A, protecting from UVR and
ROS. There are more than 600 carotenoids identified, with 10% of these acting
as precursors to vitamin A, often referred to as having provitamin A activity.
Commonly used carotenoids include astaxanthin, lutein, lycopene, and zeaxanthin. Popular polyphenols are ellagic acid from pomegranate, curcumin
from turmeric, epigallocatechin gallate (EGCG) from green tea, genistein in
soybeans, and silymarin from marigolds.

CURCUMIN

Curcumin is the yellow-orange constituent of turmeric root. Categorized as
a polyphenol antioxidant, it is commonly used as a spice, food coloring, and
food preservative preventing discoloration from oxidation. Structurally similar to resveratrol, curcumin has anti-inflammatory activity and is believed to
prevent the breakdown of ceramides, the major lipid in cell membranes supporting the skin barrier.

ELLAGIC ACID

Ellagic acid is found in many fruits and vegetables, with the highest amount
present in pomegranate and berries. This phytochemical antioxidant is
unfortunately poorly absorbed, rapidly metabolized, and readily eliminated

by the body. Benefits include skin lightening by inhibiting tyrosinase, anti-inflammatory activity, and protection from UVR-induced collagen degradation by blocking MMP.

EPIGALLOCATECHIN-3-GALLATE

EGCG is the main component of green tea and is also found in grape seeds and buckwheat to name a few. EGCG has shown promising applications in skin health with photoprotective properties, anti-inflammatory activity, and ability to stimulate keratinocyte proliferation. Black tea has lower amounts of EGCG than green tea because of the intense processing of the leaves.

GENISTEIN

Genistein, known as an isoflavone of the polyphenol family, is primarily isolated from soybeans. This phytoestrogen has a similar structure to human estrogen but has weak estrogen and antiestrogen effects. Genistein benefits the skin by increasing skin thickness and decreasing facial wrinkling in women. Other benefits include protection from UVR, ROS, lipid peroxidation, and increased collagen gene expression. Genistein is also used to reduce skin discoloration, erythema, and inflammation.

LUTEIN

Lutein, lycopene, and zeaxanthin are all similarly structured carotenoid antioxidants. Classified as food coloring in the United States, they are often used for their bright yellow, orange, or red color. Lutein is well known for its use in age-related macular degeneration (AMD) for its ability to absorb blue light and prevent UVR damage. It is believed to have similar benefits as antioxidants for UVR absorption.

NIACINAMIDE

Niacinamide is converted to niacin *in vivo* and has similar effectiveness to niacin, without causing skin flushing at high doses. Niacin and its derivatives are used for their anti-inflammatory benefits, encouraging skin turnover, and lightening effect on the skin. Niacinamide is thought to contribute to skin lightening by inhibiting the transfer of melanosomes from melanocytes to epidermal keratinocytes.

FRENCH MARITIME PINE BARK

French maritime pine bark of the species *Pinus pinaster* is a newer popularized antioxidant capable of regenerating vitamins C and E to their reduced and active forms. Benefits include improvements in skin elasticity, hydration, and collagen synthesis.

SILYMARIN

Silymarin, commonly sourced from milk thistle, is an antioxidant of the polyphenol group employed to reduce inflammation, protect from UVR, and promote skin healing. Silymarin possesses anticancer attributes for the skin and other cancers.

UBIQUINONE

Ubiquinone, or ubidecarenone, is more popularly referred to as coenzyme Q10 or simply CoQ10. As an antioxidant, CoQ10 is popularized for its benefits in heart failure patients by preventing lipid peroxidation. CoQ10 regenerates reduced vitamin E and is regenerated by alpha-lipoic acid. Ubiquinone has been shown to decrease collagen breakdown by decreasing collagenase, and it enhances healing after laser skin treatments.

ASCORBIC ACID

Ascorbic acid (L-ascorbic and ester-C forms of vitamin C) is a very effective antioxidant, second only to vitamin E in abundance within the skin. Vitamin C is used in numerous skin products with benefits including the reduction of wrinkles, decreased skin inflammation, reversal of damage from UVR exposure, brightened skin, repair of damaged DNA, and stimulation of collagen and elastin synthesis.

VITAMIN E

Vitamin E is the primary antioxidant in the stratum corneum. Actively regenerated by alpha-lipoic acid, glutathione, and ubiquinone, vitamin E is effective at soothing dry skin, preventing UVR damage, and providing anti-inflammatory benefits. Continuous supplementation is required to keep levels elevated within the skin. Combining vitamin E with ascorbic acid has been shown to work synergistically to decrease UVR-induced erythema.

GRAPE SEED EXTRACT

Grape seed extract possesses antioxidant, anti-inflammatory, antihistaminic, and antimutagenic substances. Grape seed's numerous beneficial ingredients include EGCG, alpha-lipoic acid, vitamin E, and oligomeric proanthocyanidins (OPCs) that stabilize collagen and elastin. Oral supplementation has been shown by one study to reduce the risk for squamous cell carcinoma, the second most common skin cancer in the United States.

RESVERATROL

Resveratrol is found in high quantities in grape skin, pomegranate, and some berries. Commonly associated with the benefits of the Mediterranean diet and the "French paradox" phenomenon, resveratrol is readily absorbed and rapidly metabolized. Resveratrol has been shown to inhibit tyrosinase and to have anti-inflammatory benefits and carcinopreventive properties.

BETA-CAROTENE

Beta-carotene is the most important and popularized provitamin A. Two vitamin As are released upon cleaving beta-carotene, promoting benefits such as the growth, repair, regeneration, and differentiation of epithelial cells, including cohesiveness, keratinization, and immunomodulation. Oral bioavailability of beta-carotene is low and dependent on the source, quantity, and fat content in the diet. Overconsumption of foods high in beta-carotene, including carrots, sweet potatoes, and pumpkins, and supplementation may cause carotenodermia, or orange skin, but is highly unlikely to cause hypervitaminosis A.

VITAMIN D

Vitamin D is essential to skin health, creating a dilemma between sun exposure providing for synthesis of vitamin D, weighed against the sun damaging UVR-induced aging and increased cancer risk. The recommendation for employing photoprotective measures may compromise vitamin D sufficiency. Nonetheless, there is not an established safe level of UVR exposure to provide for cutaneous vitamin D synthesis without increasing the risk for skin cancers. Vitamin D is fat soluble, stored in the liver and fat, and not a true vitamin because it is produced cutaneously through UVR. Vitamin D often refers to both vitamin D_2 (ergocalciferol) and vitamin D_3 (cholecalciferol) forms. Vitamins D_2 and D_3 are essentially equivalent because our bodies use them similarly, with the exception of vitamin D_3 possibly having a higher bioavailability than vitamin D_2 at higher doses. Although a precise dose and correlated vitamin D serum level have not been established for optimal skin health, the supplementation of vitamin D for most patients can safely be recommended at daily doses up to the upper limit (UL) of 4,000 IU.

Vitamin D Source
Vitamin D is obtained from epidermal photosynthesis, through dietary means, and from additional supplementation. The human body synthesizes vitamin D from provitamin D_3 (7-dehydrocholesterol) through UVB irradiation. Dietary sources are fatty fish, egg yolks, and supplemented products, including dairy, cereal, and orange juice. The highest amounts of vitamin D are found in fatty fish, especially swordfish, salmon, and tuna (Table 13.2).

Food	IU per Serving
Swordfish, cooked (3 oz)	566
Salmon, cooked (3 oz)	447
Tuna, canned (3 oz)	154
Orange Juice, fortified (1 cup)	137
Milk (1 cup)	115-124
Egg (1 large)	41
Cereal, fortified (1 cup)	40

TABLE 13.2   Dietary Sources of Vitamin D

Data from the U.S. Department of Agriculture, Agricultural Research Service. Website: www.ars.usda.gov.

Vitamin D Deficiencies

Vitamin D deficiency is linked to a number of diseases and conditions affecting the bones, gastrointestinal tract, heart, lungs, kidneys, and thyroid, including diabetes, cancer, and inflammatory conditions. Low vitamin D serum levels may be due to numerous reasons. A deficiency in UVB absorption and vitamin D activation may be the result of high amounts of melanin in the skin, limited effective sun exposure because of climate or occupation, and older age, which is associated with less exposure and less efficient synthesis. UVB irradiation is also blocked by glass, and all but half will penetrate clouds and pollution. Sunscreens and clothing can also block UVB rays from reaching the skin. Strict diets including vegan and lactose avoidance may also limit vitamin D intake (Box 13.2). Because some dietary fat is required for vitamin D absorption, high-dose oral supplementation or intramuscular injection may be necessary for patients with fat malabsorption, including those with gastric bypass or liver disease. Vitamin D is fat soluble and sequestered by subcutaneous fat, so obese patients may have low serum levels owing to limited release of vitamin D into circulation. Activation of vitamin D to its active form 1,25(OH)$_2$D may be limited because of kidney dysfunction, steroid therapy, or inflammatory disease.

Vitamin D Toxicity

The risk for toxicity is highly unlikely from excessive UVR exposure or a diet high in vitamin D foods and is usually due to supplementing vitamin D above the UL of 4,000 IU to 10,000 IU or more daily. One study found vitamin D supplementation of 5,000 IU/day gave rise to serum 25(OH)D levels of 100 to 150 nmol/L. High 25(OH)D levels are considered above 125 nmol/L, and toxic levels are suggested to be above 500 nmol/L. Symptoms of toxicity include arrhythmias, polyuria, and weight loss. As calcium levels increase

Box 13.2

Strict diets, fat malabsorption, and obesity can decrease serum vitamin D levels.

with vitamin D levels, kidney stones and calcification of vascular and soft tissue, including the heart, kidneys and intestine, can occur.

Vitamin D Monitoring Levels

Vitamin D exposure is measured through serum levels of the vitamin D forms 25(OH)D and the bioactive form 1,25(OH)$_2$D (Box 13.3). 25(OH)D has a long half-life of 15 days and is recognized as the best biomarker for exposure to vitamin D. In contrast, the 1,25(OH)$_2$D levels are highly variable with a half-life of less than a day and are affected by changing levels of serum parathyroid hormone (PTH), calcium, and phosphorus. 1,25(OH)$_2$D levels are only significant when vitamin D deficiency is severe. A serum vitamin 25(OH)D level for optimal skin health has yet to be agreed on, although monitoring may be useful to identify patients at risk with potentially low levels and those with high and possibly toxic levels.

Vitamin D Supplementation

The recommended dietary allowances (RDA) for adults is 600 IU/day for those aged 70 years and younger and 800 IU/day for those older than 70 years (Box 13.4). The RDA recommendations are suspected to be too low and do not take into account vitamin D that is synthesized from UVR. Thirty-seven percent of the U.S. population take a daily supplement containing vitamin D. The National Health and Nutrition Examination Survey (NHANES) from 2005 to 2006 showed a mean 25(OH)D level above 50 nmol/L, consistent with intake of vitamin D from diet and supplements equivalent to the RDA amounts. Supplementation of vitamin D has a nonlinear relationship with 25(OH)D levels. Estimates state that with doses less than 600 IU/day, serum 25(OH)D levels will increase 2.3 nmol/L for every 40 IU supplemented daily. Doses greater than 1,000 IU/day are estimated to increase serum 25(OH)D levels by 1 nmol/L for every 40 IU supplemented per day.

Box 13.3

Vitamin D Monitoring Levels

Low level and at risk: <30 nmol/L (12 ng/mL)

- Low bone mineral deposits: osteomalacia in adults, rickets in children
- Secondary hyperparathyroidism

Potentially at risk for inadequacy: 30-50 nmol/L (12-20 ng/mL)

- Osteoporosis through reduced calcium absorption

Adequate levels: ≥50 nmol/L (≥20 ng/mL)
High levels: >125 to 150 nmol/L

- Long-term effects not yet defined

Toxic: >500 nmol/L (>200 ng/mL)

Note: 1 nmol = 0.4 ng/mL.

Box 13.4

Recommended Dietary Allowances for Vitamin D*

- For 1-70 years old: 600 IU/day (15 μg/day)
- > 70 years old 800 IU/day (20 μg/day)

*Note: 1 μg = 40 IU.

The Ultraviolet Radiation Exposure Quandary

The benefits of sun exposure are boasted to increase vitality and release endorphins, raising vitamin D levels, stimulating epidermal melanization, and increasing the tumor suppressor "guardian of the genome" p53 in the skin. The accumulation of p53 in the skin can interrupt the cell cycle of damaged cells to allow for the upregulation of DNA repair and stimulate apoptosis if irreparably damaged. The quandary of sun exposure versus protection lies in determining a "safe" amount of UVR, allowing for the benefits without the negative consequences. UVR and sun exposure are described as the "complete carcinogen" because they are indirectly and directly mutagenic, with nonspecific damage leading to the initiation and promotion of tumors. UVR damage also attributes to skin pigmentation changes, atrophy, wrinkling, epidermal hyperplasia, and cell death.

Skin Cancer

The prevalence of skin cancer is on the rise and is currently the most common cancer, with an estimated 1.5 million cases per year in the United States. UVR exposure is the major cause of the three most common skin cancers: basal cell carcinoma, squamous cell carcinoma, and malignant melanoma. Skin cancers are also responsible for more than half of all malignancies. Those at highest risk are individuals genetically predisposed to UVR sensitivity, individuals with fair skin, and immune-compromised patients. Surgical resection can often leave imperfections such as scars and is not a solution to skin health. UVR protection and vitamin D supplementation are the essential preventative steps a person can take to lower their risk for skin cancer.

Vitamin D and Skin Cancer Studies

Whereas many antioxidants have been shown to decrease DNA damage from ROS, vitamin D is unique in its ability to not only lessen DNA damage but also increase DNA repair of both oxidative damage and dimmer formation. However, in one study, a positive correlation between serum 25(OH)D levels and basal cell carcinoma has created an uncertainty of their interconnection. The same UVR that damages DNA and increases the risk for epidermal malignancy is also responsible for vitamin D synthesis. Vitamin D and vitamin D receptors (VDRs) play an important role in protecting skin from cancer formation by controlling keratinocyte proliferation and differentiation, as well as enhanced cell survival. The question arises of whether the increased survival of UVR-induced DNA-damaged cells could lead to increased risk for cancer.

Cells lacking VDR in mice exposed to UVR were predisposed to epidermal tumor formation, specifically basal cell carcinoma. This study speculates that VDR limits tumor formation and promotes DNA repair. Topically applied 1,25(OH)$_2$D protects from UVR-induced photodamage, increases DNA repair of dimmer formations, increases cell survival, and increases p53 expression. Topically applied vitamin D also regulates VDR proliferation, differentiation, and signaling. Vitamin D facilitates DNA repair following UVR exposure by increasing p53 in keratinocytes and melanocytes and increasing nucleotide excision repair enzymes.

Vitamin D Conclusion

Because vitamin D is available in very few foods, oral supplementation remains advisable for most patients. Without a safe level of UVR exposure established to adequately synthesize vitamin D, the recommendation for photoprotection, especially for fair-skinned individuals, necessitates our continued advocacy. Vitamin D has protective effects against carcinogenic actions of UVR by preventing UVR-induced cell death and DNA damage, increasing the rate of DNA repair, inhibiting UVR-induced immunosuppression, and upregulating endogenous antioxidants. For most patients, it is recommended to increase a diet with foods rich in vitamin D and to incorporate safe supplementation (Box 13.5).

GLUTATHIONE

Glutathione is arguably the most important antioxidant in the body and has the greatest potential for being beneficial in skin health. Glutathione within the skin can regenerate other antioxidants, protect from UVR-induced ROS, detoxify, and provide skin-lightening benefits.

Maintaining generous quantities of glutathione throughout the body and skin is essential for the management and maintenance of optimal skin health. Ubiquitous throughout the body, including the skin, glutathione is known as the master antioxidant, life extender, detoxifier, and mother of all antioxidants. It is cited in more than 100,000 scientific articles, providing insight into its significance as an essential component to life as the most vital intracellular and extracellular antioxidant.

Glutathione is widely known for its detoxification in the liver of many harmful compounds, including medications, carcinogens, and other toxins. Throughout the body, glutathione also 1) protects cells from ROS damage, 2)

Box 13.5

Vitamin D Chart

7-dehydrocholesterol (pre–vitamin D$_3$) → UVR (UVB) → vitamin D$_3$ → liver (25-hydroxylase) → 25(OH)D (calcidiol) → kidney (1α-hydroxylase) → 1,25(OH)$_2$D (calcitriol) (active form)

acts as a cofactor for the activation and regulation of numerous enzymes, 3) complements the immune system, 4) is an effective amino acid transporter, and 5) is involved in DNA, protein, and prostaglandin synthesis. Glutathione is also used as a whitening agent because it inhibits tyrosinase activity. The lack of glutathione is associated with poorer health and a weaker immune system. Low glutathione levels are also associated with elevated oxidative stress, aging, and many diseases.

Bioavailability

Glutathione is a small protein readily digested when consumed orally without appropriate protection from digestive enzymes. For glutathione to reach its target in the skin, it first must survive the gastrointestinal tract, be absorbed across the intestinal barrier, remain active through first-pass metabolism by the liver, and continue on through the circulation to reach the skin. Unfortunately, weak cellular absorption is observed owing to its large structure and lack of sufficient transport mechanisms.

Supplementation

To enhance the benefits of glutathione, multiple mechanisms are necessary to maintain elevated levels in the body, including providing sufficient essential precursors, cofactors, regenerators, and lifestyle modifications such as diet and exercise.

Glutathione concentrations are increased when essential precursors, in particular cysteine-containing compounds such as *N*-acetylcysteine and cystine, are ingested. Folate, selenium, vitamin B_6, and vitamin B_{12} are also essential cofactors required for the production and regeneration of glutathione. Alpha-lipoic acid and vitamins C and E can also regenerate oxidized glutathione. To effectively increase levels, measures must be taken to decrease various stress conditions that deplete glutathione. Supplementing the diet with dietary glycine, silymarin, and sulfur-rich foods, such as garlic, onions, broccoli, and kale, is also beneficial. Studies suggest that regular exercise may also improve glutathione levels.

ENZYMES AND COFACTORS

SELENIUM

Selenium is an essential trace element, acting through enzymes as an antioxidant, providing UVR protection, and stimulating elastin formation. Further studies are necessary to evaluate selenium's potential and appropriate dose for tumor suppression and skin health.

ALPHA-LIPOIC ACID

Alpha-lipoic acid supplementation benefits include antioxidant properties, chelation of heavy metals, and possible anti-inflammatory benefits.

Alpha-lipoic acid is only 50% absorbed orally, has a short half-life, and is quickly reduced to dihydrolipoic acid (DHLA). As an active metabolite, DHLA is capable of regenerating the antioxidants glutathione, vitamin C, vitamin E, and ubiquinone. Alpha-lipoic acid's application in skin health includes antioxidant properties, increased collagen synthesis, and lightening dyspigmentation.

ZINC

Calamine, a natural topical containing the active ingredient zinc oxide, has been in use for centuries to sooth inflammation. Zinc in its ionic form (Zn^{2+}) has important attributes to skin health not only for its ability to reduce irritation but also for its ability to absorb and reflect UVR and to accelerate wound healing through re-epithelialization and improved elasticity, as well as its anti-inflammatory properties. Numerous enzymes require zinc for activity, including those necessary for the synthesis of the retinol-binding protein and the vitamin A transport protein. Without adequate zinc, symptoms of vitamin A deficiency, including severe dermatitis, can appear, regardless of the presence of vitamin A.

The RDA of zinc is 15 mg/day for adults. Oral consumption of zinc, although established in wound healing, requires further research in skin health. As a natural sun block, zinc taken orally can absorb and reflect radiation within the skin, potentially generating free radicals within the dermis, eliciting an inflammatory response. Despite the rarity of a deficiency, zinc's importance as a cofactor necessitates our attention and encouragement for patients to receive an adequate intake for healthy skin.

AMINO ACIDS AND PEPTIDE SUPPLEMENTS

PEPTIDES

Peptides are amino acid chains providing many functions, including cellular regulation and communication between cells. Peptides also affect neurotransmitter release, act as carriers for cofactors, and are involved in many complex enzymatic steps in the skin, including the production of collagen. Long peptides with a large molecular size can create an obstacle to effectively penetrating the skin for topical application, often requiring a sophisticated carrier system to provide sufficient quantities for therapeutic results. Smaller peptides containing only a few amino acids are much more likely to traverse the skin barrier than larger, complex peptides known as proteins. Oral supplements of peptides are unlikely to bestow benefits in their intact form because they are readily digested by proteases on oral ingestion, releasing their individual amino acid components for absorption. Amino acid and protein supplements are frequently consumed in weight-loss and muscle-building nutritional regimens, replenishing the essential building blocks for protein and enzyme synthesis, and possibly providing other benefits, including increased energy, a lean body, and muscle support. A few proposed oral supplements include collagen, elastin, and spirulina, which may provide benefits in skin health as protein and ultimately amino acid supplements.

Collagen plays an integral role in providing strength and flexibility to the skin as the most abundant and significant component of connective tissues. Known as collagen I in the skin, it is created largely by fibroblast, mainly of the amino acids proline, glycine, and alanine. Identified as a skin constituent that becomes more rigid and declines in functioning with aging, optimizing collagen's vigor is often a target for skin rejuvenation therapies. By breaking down the collagen to what is commonly referred to as hydrolyzed collagen, an increase in the absorption of the essential amino acids is provided.

Elastin is the elastic polypeptide in connective tissue providing the ability of skin to stretch and return to its original shape. Because oral supplementation of elastin is likely to be broken down before reaching the skin, benefits are conceivably due to providing essential amino acids.

Spirulina, a blue-green algae, is an ancient food that contains all of the essential amino acids, as well as antioxidants and vitamins. Spirulina is 60% protein by weight, making it a great oral protein supplement option for skin health.

Although supplemented peptides are likely to be broken down to their essential amino acids, the pendulum can be swayed to lean toward higher use of these amino acids through greater availability. More research is required, including enhanced technologies for providing the skin with these essential amino acids and peptides for oral consumption.

GROWTH FACTORS

Numerous growth factors are involved in complex and synergistic combinations to stimulate collagen, elastin, and glycosaminoglycans. They are also involved in regulating epithelial proliferation, differentiation, and other cellular functions. Transforming growth factor-α is involved in the regulation of systemic inflammation, including the pro-inflammatory condition psoriasis. One nutraceutical, curcumin, has been shown to decrease transforming growth factor-α in vivo, which may be used to decrease skin inflammation.

HYALURONIC ACID

Hyaluronic acid has viscoelastic and lubricating properties that make it useful in osteoarthritis, cosmetic fillers, and topicals for its humectant properties benefiting atopic dermatitis, eczema, wounds, and ulcers. Hyaluronic acid will increase retinoic acid use and keratinocyte proliferation, supporting skin hydration. The quantity of hyaluronic acid in the skin decreases with age, UVR exposure, and ROS exposure. Constantly degraded and synthesized, hyaluronic acid production can be stimulated by retinol and inhibited by hydrocortisone. Oral supplements of hyaluronic acid without a protective delivery system are likely to be readily metabolized before absorption.

SPECIFIC INDICATIONS

SKIN LIGHTENING

Patients with dyspigmentation from photoaging, hyperpigmentation from melasma, and postinflammatory hyperpigmentation are best treated with products that help balance overactive melanin production and uneven distribution. To address this situation, most active ingredients for skin-lightening inhibit tyrosinase, the rate-limiting enzyme in the biosynthesis of melanin.

Glabridin, obtained from licorice, is the most commonly used tyrosinase inhibitor in nutraceutical products. Another popular tyrosinase inhibitor is ascorbic acid, which interacts with the copper ion binding on tyrosinase. Arbutin, a derivative of hydroquinone from the bearberry fruit, paper mulberry from the mulberry tree roots, aloesin from aloe vera, resveratrol from grapes, and ellagic acid from berries are also tyrosinase inhibitors. Vitamin A derivatives are commonly used for lightening of skin. The effectiveness of vitamin A analogs in reducing skin pigmentation are likely due to their ability to inhibit tyrosinase, accelerate epidermal turnover, and interfere with melanosome transfer to keratinocytes.

Nutraceuticals that lighten and even pigmentation may also work through other mechanisms of action in addition to inhibiting tyrosinase. For example, aloesin and alpha-linolenic acid can also act as a weak lightening agent by decreasing the presence of tyrosinase. Niacinamide helps by inhibiting the melanosome transfer from melanocytes to keratinocytes and stimulates exfoliation. Soybean trypsin inhibitor from soy has been shown to even skin discoloration by interfering with the phagocytosis of melanosomes by keratinocytes. Antioxidants and physical blockers will also function as whitening agents through protection from UVR and ROS stimulation of melanocytes to produce melanin. Acai, bisabolol, and curcumin may also have benefits in hyperpigmentation. In observation of several mechanisms of action, multiple categories can be used to provide optimal results. Emphasizing the importance of strict adherence to treatment protocols, including appropriate sun protection, will help the patient realize benefits in light of the lessened and evenly distributed melanin throughout the skin.

OILY SKIN

With the exception of isotretinoin, there is a deficiency of efficacious oral treatments available for excess sebum and oily skin. Vitamin A and its derivatives are effective in creating a drying effect and may be continued with lower doses for further benefits. Niacinamide demonstrates a reduction in sebum, along with promoting exfoliation. Soy and its effective constituent genistein are also effective in reducing oil production, possibly through their antiandrogen effects.

DRY SKIN

Xerosis is frequently seen with the lack of exfoliation; certain skin conditions; harsh environments, including wind, low humidity, and extreme temperatures; and aggressive cleansers or chemicals. An approach to treatment and prevention of dry skin from the inside out is addressed by enhancing the skin barrier to prevent water loss and the addition of humectants to draw moisture in. Vitamin B_5, also known as pantothenic acid, functions as both a humectant and supporter of the skin barrier to prevent skin dehydration. Hyaluronic acid is the best know humectant for the skin. Niacinamide strengthens the barrier function by increasing ceramides, long-chain fatty acids, and cholesterol in the stratum corneum and thus decreasing TEWL. Orally administered vitamin E, curcumin, and CoQ10 may also decrease the skin's insensible water loss. Through exfoliation, barrier, and hydration support, one can lock in moisture and lessen the symptoms of dry skin.

ANTI-INFLAMMATORY AGENTS

Skin inflammation is a physiological response to infection and injury, correlated with the aging process and often indicated by redness, swelling, warmth, and irritation. As an adjuvant to topical applications, nutraceuticals with anti-inflammatory characteristics, including allantoin, bisabolol, curcumin, EGCG, ellagic acid, French maritime pine bark, niacinamide, resveratrol, and silymarin, can greatly enhance the healing and lessen the inflammatory symptoms commonly associated with acne and rosacea. The antioxidants beta-carotene, vitamin A, ascorbic acid, vitamin E, lutein, selenium, and zeaxanthin have been shown to have a negative correlation with inflammatory markers, as detailed in one study. Because inflammation commonly involves ROS, antioxidants can also play a potential role in alleviating and preventing the inflammatory response.

THE MARKETPLACE

"Natural" products, with their perceived safety and association with luxury compared with synthetic chemicals, are more frequently sought by health-conscious consumers. Many of the active ingredients in these preservative-free, holistic treatments are highly processed through chemical and manipulative processing and protected by preservatives that are reclassified as other ingredients. A patient's mentality of equating high price with quality leads to high expectations of overpriced products containing rare, exotic, or expensive ingredients with unsubstantiated efficacy. Ecologically minded consumers are also interested in purchasing products with biodegradable or no packaging and with ingredients that are organic, from non–genetically modified organisms, and nontoxic to the environment. These values and perceptions of consumers are likely to affect the skin health nutraceutical marketplace.

FUTURE DIRECTIONS

The future of nutraceutical research will likely lead to isolating active components from botanicals, creating advanced delivery systems, and allowing for increased potency, additional therapeutic applications, and enhanced results. Further studies will elucidate detailed information on biologically active ingredients, giving rise to greater detail to their pharmacokinetics and mechanisms of action. Whereas nutraceuticals can promote their capacity to enhance skin appearance, claims of detailed improvements in skin function are presently available only to products classified as pharmaceuticals in the United States. With further isolation of the active components within nutraceuticals, detailed studies on their effectiveness are likely to narrow the gap between nutraceuticals and pharmaceuticals.

PRODUCTS

The current skin health marketplace for nutraceuticals is large, although few products are well formulated specifically for the skin. Many companies marketing nutraceuticals make unsubstantiated claims that promise unrealistic results. With numerous nutraceuticals available, the onerous task of selecting the appropriate supplement can be confusing to consumers and practitioners alike. A recent survey shows that most nutraceuticals have one or only a few ingredients. To receive noticeable benefits, many ingredients with multiple mechanisms of action are required. As with most supplements, palatability and convenience are important to consumers. Studies have shown that patients do not like to consume multiple capsules and tablets throughout the day, leading to noncompliance and early discontinuation. An optimal oral supplement is complete, compatible, consumable, and complementary to topical treatments and procedures. Copackaging with other products will help lead patients toward a multifaceted approach to skin heath, addressing the needs of the risk-averse populations that seek a less invasive but therapeutic approach and those who are looking to maximize their current regimen.

CONCLUSION

Historical records and current use of botanicals for healing wounds and skin disorders has led us to the isolation, research, and application of their bioactive constituents. By selecting specific categories of nutraceuticals, we can enhance our patient's current regimen with oral supplements, including antioxidants, anti-inflammatory agents, skin-lightening ingredients, and constituents that address oily or dry skin. By considering all of our options in the array of treatments, including topicals, procedures, and nutraceuticals, we can select the most effective and unique combination in achieving an optimal outcome for each and every patient.

REFERENCES

1. Dodge T, Litt D, Kaufman AJ. Influence of the Dietary Supplement Health and Education Act on consumer beliefs about the safety and effectiveness of dietary supplements. *Health Commun.* 2011;16(3):230-244.

2. Hass DJ, Lewis JD. Quality of manufacturer provided information on safety and efficacy claims for dietary supplements for colonic health. *Pharmacoepidemiol Drug Saf.* 2006;15(8):578-586.

3. Crowley R, FitzGerald LH. The impact of cGMP compliance on consumer confidence in dietary supplement products. *Toxicology.* 2006;221(1):9-16.

4. Hussain SP, Hofseth LJ, Harris CC. Radical causes of cancer. *Nat Rev Cancer.* 2003;3(4):276-285.

5. Duan J, Duan J, Zhang Z, Tong T. Irreversible cellular senescence induced by prolonged exposure to H_2O_2 involves DNA-damage-and-repair genes and telomere shortening. *Int J Biochem Cell Biol.* 2005;37(7):1407-1420.

6. Berson DS. Natural antioxidants. *J Drugs Dermatol.* 2008;7(7 Suppl):7-12.

7. Liu RH. Health benefits of fruit and vegetables are from additive and synergistic combinations of phytochemicals. *Am J Clin Nutr.* 2003;78:517S-520S.

8. Hsu S. Green tea and the skin. *J Am Acad Dermatol.* 2005;52(6):1049-1059.

9. Krinsky NI. The antioxidant and biological properties of the carotenoids. *Ann N Y Acad Sci.* 1998;854:443-447.

10. Palozza P, Krinsky NI. Antioxidant effects of carotenoids in vivo and in vitro: an overview. *Methods Enzymol.* 1992;213:403-420.

11. Aggarwal BB, Sung B. Pharmacological basis for the role of curcumin in chronic diseases: an age-old spice with modern targets. *Trends Pharmacol Sci.* 2009;30:85-94.

12. Zhou H, Beevers CS, Huang S. The targets of curcumin. *Curr Drug Targets.* 2011;12:332-347.

13. Sawai H, Okazaki T, Yamamoto H, et al. Requirement of AP-1 for ceramide-induced apoptosis in human leukemia HL-60 cells. *J Biol Chem.* 1995;270(45):27326-27331.

14. Kasai K, Yoshimura M, Koga T, et al. Effects of oral administration of ellagic acid-rich pomegranate extract on ultraviolet-induced pigmentation in the human skin. *J Nutr Sci Vitaminol (Tokyo).* 2006;52(5):383-388.

15. Bae JY, Choi JS, Kang SW, et al. Dietary compound ellagic acid alleviates skin wrinkle and inflammation induced by UV-B irradiation. *Exp Dermatol.* 2010;19:e182-e190.

16. Hseu YC, Chou CW, Senthil Kumar KJ, et al. Ellagic acid protects human keratinocyte (HaCaT) cells against UVA-induced oxidative stress and apoptosis through

the upregulation of the HO-1 and Nrf-2 antioxidant genes. *Food Chem Toxicol.* 2012;50:1245-1255.

17. Chen D, Wan SB, Yang H, et al. EGCG green tea polyphenol and their synthetic analogs for human cancer prevention and treatment. *Adv Clin Chem.* 2011;53:155-177.

18. Wang Y, Ho CT. Polyphenolic chemistry of tea and coffee: a century of progress. *J Agric Food Chem.* 2009;57:8109-8114.

19. Kuriyama S, Shimazu T, Ohmori K, et al. Green tea consumption and mortality due to cardiovascular disease, cancer, and all causes in Japan: the Ohsaki study. *JAMA.* 2006;296(10):1255-1265.

20. Jung JY, Han CR, Jeong YJ, et al. Epigallocatechin gallate inhibits nitric oxide-induced apoptosis in rat PC12 cells. *Neurosci Lett.* 2007;411:222-227.

21. Elmets CA, Singh D, Tubesing K, et al. Cutaneous photoprotection from ultraviolet injury by green tea polyphenols. *J Am Acad Dermatol.* 2001;44:425-432.

22. Zhao J, Jin X, Yaping E, et al. Photoprotective effect of black tea extracts against UVB-induced phototoxicity in skin. *Photochem Photobiol.* 1999;70:637-644.

23. Korać B, Buzadzić B. Doxorubicin toxicity to the skin: possibility of protection with antioxidants enriched yeast. *J Dermatol Sci.* 2001;25(1):45-52.

24. Wei H, Saladi R, Lu Y, et al. Isoflavonegenistein: photoprotection and clinical implications in dermatology. *J Nutr.* 2003;133(11 Suppl 1):S3811-S3819.

25. Thornfeldt C. Cosmeceuticals containing herbs: fact, fiction, and future. *Dermatol Surg.* 2005;31:873-880.

26. Baumann LS. Cosmeceutical critique: soy and its isoflavones. *Skin Allergy News.* 2001;32:17.

27. Shegokar R, Mitri K. Carotenoid lutein: a promising candidate for pharmaceutical and nutraceutical applications. *J Diet Suppl.* 2012;9(3):183-210.

28. Mohammed D, Crowther JM, Matts PJ, et al. Influence of niacinamide containing formulations on the molecular and biophysical properties of the stratum corneum. *Int J Pharmacol.* 2013;441(1-2):192-201.

29. Marini A, Grether-Beck S, Jaenicke T, et al. Pycnogenol effects on skin elasticity and hydration coincide with increased gene expressions of collagen type I and hyaluronic acid synthase in women. *Skin Pharmacol Physiol.* 2012;25(2):86-92.

30. Berson DS. Natural antioxidants. *J Drugs Dermatol.* 2008;7(7 Suppl):7-12.

31. Girish C, Pradhan SC. Hepatoprotective activities of picroliv, curcumin, and ellagic acid compared to silymarin on carbon-tetrachloride-induced liver toxicity in mice. *J Pharmacol Pharmacother.* 2012;3(2):149-155.

32. Polyak SJ, Morishima C, Lohmann V, et al. Identification of hepatoprotective flavonolignans from silymarin. *Proc Natl Acad Sci U S A.* 2010;107(13):5995-5999.

33. Velussi M, Cernigoi AM, DeMonte A, et al. Long-term (12 months) treatment with an anti-oxidant drug (silymarin) is effective on hyperinsulinemia, exogenous insulin need and malondialdehyde levels in cirrhotic diabetic patients. *J Hepatol.* 1997;26(4):871-879.

34. Quinzii CM, Area E, Naini A, et al. Treatment of CoQ(10) deficient fibroblasts with ubiquinone, CoQ analogs, and vitamin C: time- and compound-dependent effects. *PLoS One.* 2010;5(7):e11897.

35. McDaniel DH, Neudecker BA, DiNardo JC, et al. Idebenone: a new antioxidant. Part I. Relative assessment of oxidative stress protection capacity compared to commonly known antioxidants. *J Cosmet Dermatol.* 2005;4(1):10-17.

36. Kishimoto Y, Saito N, Kurita K, et al. Ascorbic acid enhances the expression of type 1 and type 4 collagen and SVCT2 in cultured human skin fibroblasts. *Biochem Biophys Res Commun.* 2013;430(2):579-584.

37. Patel V, Khanna S, Roy S, et al. Natural vitamin E alpha-tocotrienol: retention in vital organs in response to long-term oral supplementation and withdrawal. *Free Radic Res.* 2006;40(7):763-771.

38. Fuchs J, Kern H. Modulation of UV-light-induced skin inflammation by D-alpha-tocopherol and L-ascorbic acid: a clinical study using solar simulated radiation. *Free Radic Biol Med.* 1998;25(9):1006-1012.

39. Asgari MM, Chren MM, Warton EM, et al. Supplement use and risk of cutaneous squamous cell carcinoma. *J Am Acad Dermatol.* 2011;65(6):1145-1151.

40. Park J, Boo J. Isolation of resveratrol from vitis viniferae caulis and its potent inhibition of human tyrosinase. *Evid Based Complement Alternat Med.* 2013;2013:645257.

41. Buonocore D, Lazzeretti A, Tocabens P, et al. Resveratrol-procyanidin blend: nutraceutical and antiaging efficacy evaluated in a placebo controlled, double-blind study. *Clin Cosmet Investig Dermatol.* 2012;5:159-165.

42. Baxter RA. Anti-aging properties of resveratrol: review and report of a potent new antioxidant skin care formulation. *J Cosmet Dermatol.* 2008;7:2-7.

43. La VC. Association between Mediterranean dietary patterns and cancer risk. *Nutr Rev.* 2009;67(Suppl 1):S126-S129.

44. Feart C, Samieri C, Rondeau V, et al. Adherence to a Mediterranean diet, cognitive decline, and risk of dementia. *JAMA.* 2009;302:638-648.

45. Aggarwal BB, Bhardwaj A, Aggarwal RS, et al. Role of resveratrol in prevention and therapy of cancer: preclinical and clinical studies. *Anticancer Res.* 2004; 24:2783-2840.

46. Bournival J, Quessy P, Martinoli MG. Protective effects of resveratrol and quercetin against MPP(+)-induced oxidative stress act by modulating markers of apoptotic death in dopaminergic neurons. *Cell Mol Neurobiol.* 2009;29:1169-1180.

47. Bastianetto S, Zheng WH, Quirion R. Neuroprotective abilities of resveratrol and other red wine constituents against nitric oxide-related toxicity in cultured hippocampal neurons. *Br J Pharmacol.* 2000;131:711-720.

48. Subbaramaiah K, Chung WJ, Michaluart P, et al. Resveratrol inhibits cyclooxygenase-2 transcription and activity in phorbol ester-treated human mammary epithelial cells. *J Biol Chem.* 1998;273:21875-21882.

49. Stahl W, Sies H. Bioactivity and protective effects of natural carotenoids. *Biochim Biophys Acta.* 2005;1740(2):101-107.

50. Rühl R. Induction of PXR-mediated metabolism by beta-carotene. *Biochim Biophys Acta.* 2005;1740(2):162-169.

51. Faulks RM, Southon S. Challenges to understanding and measuring carotenoid bioavailability. *Biochim Biophys Acta.* 2005;1740(2):95-100.

52. Dimitrov NV, Meyer C, Ullrey DE, et al. Bioavailability of beta-carotene in humans. *Am J Clin Nutr.* 1988;48(2):298-304.

53. Mathews-Roth MM. Plasma concentrations of carotenoids after large doses of beta-carotene. *Am J Clin Nutr.* 1990;52(3):500-501.

54. Sonneveld E, van der Saag PT. Metabolism of retinoic acid: implications for development and cancer. *Int J Vitam Nutr Res.* 1998;68:404-410.

55. Green A, Williams G, Neale R, et al. Daily sunscreen application and betacarotene supplementation in prevention of basal-cell and squamous-cell carcinomas of the skin: a randomised controlled trial. *Lancet.* 1999;354(9180):723-729.

56. Moon TE, Levine N, Cartmel B, Bangert JL. Retinoids in prevention of skin cancer. *Cancer Lett.* 1997;114(1-2):203-205.

57. Tangrea JA, Edwards BK, Taylor PR, et al. Long-term therapy with low-dose isotretinoin for prevention of basal cell carcinoma: a multicenter clinical trial. Isotretinoin-Basal Cell Carcinoma Study Group. *J Natl Cancer Inst.* 1992;84(5): 328-332.

58. Levine N, Moon TE, Cartmel B, et al. Trial of retinol and isotretinoin in skin cancer prevention: a randomized, double-blind, controlled trial. Southwest Skin Cancer Prevention Study Group. *Cancer Epidemiol Biomarkers Prev.* 1997;6(11):957-961.

59. Cassidy PB, Fain HD, Cassidy JP, et al. Selenium for the prevention of cutaneous melanoma. *Nutrients*. 2013;5(3):725-749.

60. Rafferty T, Norval M, El-Ghorr A, et al. Dietary selenium levels determine epidermal Langerhans cell numbers in mice. *Biol Trace Elem Res*. 2003;92(2):161-172.

61. Fritz H, Kennedy D, Fergusson D, et al. Selenium and lung cancer: a systematic review and metaanalysis. *PLoS One*. 2011;6(11):e26259.

62. Suadicani P, Hein HO, Gyntelberg F. Serum selenium level and risk of lung cancer mortality: a 16-year follow-up of the Copenhagen Male Study. *Eur Respir J*. 2012;39(6):1443-1448.

63. Hurst R, Hooper L, Norat T, et al. Selenium and prostate cancer: systematic review and meta-analysis. *Am J Clin Nutr*. 2012;96(1):111-122.

64. Sharma AK, Amin S. Post SELECT: selenium on trial. *Future Med Chem*. 2013;5(2):163-174.

65. Matsugo S, Bito T, Konishi T. Photochemical stability of lipoic acid and its impact on skin ageing. *Free Radic Res*. 2011;45(8):918-924.

66. Tsuji-Naito K, Ishikura S, Akagawa M, Saeki H. α-Lipoic acid induces collagen biosynthesis involving prolylhydroxylase expression via activation of TGF-β-Smad signaling in human dermal fibroblasts. *Connect Tissue Res*. 2010;51(5):378-387.

67. Okawa T, Yamaguchi Y, Takada S, et al. Oral administration of collagen tripeptide improves dryness and pruritus in the acetone-induced dry skin model. *J Dermatol Sci*. 2012;66(2):136-143.

68. Aggarwal BB, Shishodia S, Takada Y, et al. TNF blockade: an inflammatory issue. *Ernst Schering Res Found Workshop*. 2006:161-186.

69. Anilkumar TV, Muhamed J, Jose A, et al. Advantages of hyaluronic acid as a component of fibrin sheet for care of acute wound. *Biologicals*. 2011;39(2):81-88.

70. Sakai S, Yasuda R, Sayo T, Ishikawa O, Inoue S. Hyaluronan exists in the normal stratum corneum. *J Invest Dermatol*. 2000;114(6):1184-1187.

71. McGill CR, Green NR, Meadows MC, Gropper SS. Beta-carotene supplementation decreases leukocyte superoxide dismutase activity and serum glutathione peroxidase concentration in humans. *J Nutr Biochem*. 2003;14(11):656-662.

72. Shimogaki H, Tanaka Y, Tamai H, Masuda M. In vitro and in vivo evaluation of ellagic acid on melanogenesis inhibition. *Int J Cosmet Sci*. 2000;22:291-303.

73. Brown MS, Goldstein JL. Drugs used in the treatment of hyperlipoproteinemias. In: Goodman Gilman A, Rall TW, Nies AS, et al., eds. *Goodman and Gilman's The Pharmacological Basis of Therapeutics*. 8th ed. New York: Pergamon; 1990:893-894.

74. Konda S, Geria AN, Halder RM. New horizons in treating disorders of hyperpigmentation in skin of color. *Semin Cutan Med Surg*. 2012;31(2):133-139.

75. Lee J, Jun H, Jung E, et al. Whitening effect of alpha-bisabolol in Asian women subjects. *Int J Cosmet Sci*. 2010;32(4):299-303.

76. Thanos SM, Halliday GM, Damian DL. Nicotinamide reduces photodynamic therapy-induced immunosuppression in humans. *Br J Dermatol*. 201;167(3):631-636.

77. Fowler JF Jr, Woolery-Lloyd H, Waldorf H, Saini R. Innovations in natural ingredients and their use in skin care. *J Drugs Dermatol*. 2010;9(6 Suppl):72-81.

78. Wu J. Anti-inflammatory ingredients. *J Drugs Dermatol*. 2008;7(7 Suppl):13-16.

79. Draelos ZD. Skin lightening preparations and the hydroquinone controversy. *Dermatol Ther*. 2007;20(5):308-313.

80. Ward A, Brogden RN, Heel RC, et al. Isotretinoin: a review of its pharmacological properties and therapeutic efficacy in acne and other skin disorders. *Drugs*. 1984;28(1):6-37.

81. Fowler JF Jr, Woolery-Lloyd H, Waldorf H, Saini R. Innovations in natural ingredients and their use in skin care. *J Drugs Dermatol*. 2010;9(6 Suppl):72-81; quiz 82-33.

82. Surjana D, Damian DL. Nicotinamide in dermatology and photoprotection. *Skin Med*. 2011;9(6):360-365.

83. Tanno O, Ota Y, Kitamura N, Katsube T, Inoue S. Nicotinamide increases biosynthesis of ceramides as well as other stratum corneum lipids to improve the epidermal permeability barrier. *Br J Dermatol.* 2000;143(3):524-531.

84. Draelos ZD, Ertel K, Berge C. Niacinamide-containing facial moisturizer improves skin barrier and benefits subjects with rosacea. *Cutis.* 2005;76(2):135-141.

85. Soma Y, Kashima M, Imaizumi A, et al. Moisturizing effects of topical nicotinamide on atopic dry skin. *Int J Dermatol.* 2005;44(3):197-202.

86. Tanno O, Ota Y, Kitamura N, et al. Nicotinamide increases biosynthesis of ceramides as well as other stratum corneum lipids to improve the epidermal permeability barrier. *Br J Dermatol.* 2000;143(3):524-531.

87. Verdier-Sévrain S, Bonté F. Skin hydration: a review on its molecular mechanisms. *J Cosmet Dermatol.* 2007;6(2):75-82.

88. Staiger C. Comfrey: a clinical overview. *Phytother Res.* 2012;26(10):1441-1448.

89. Braga PC, Dal Sasso M, Fonti E, Culici M. Antioxidant activity of bisabolol: inhibitory effects on chemiluminescence of human neutrophil bursts and cell-free systems. *Pharmacology.* 2009;83(2):110-115.

90. Rhodes LE, Darby G, Massey KA, et al. Oral green tea catechin metabolites are incorporated into human skin and protect against UV radiation-induced cutaneous inflammation in association with reduced production of pro-inflammatory eicosanoid 12-hydroxyeicosatetraenoic acid. *Br J Nutr.* 2013;28:1-10.

91. Al-Okbi SY. Nutraceuticals of anti-inflammatory activity as complementary therapy for rheumatoid arthritis. *Toxicol Ind Health.* 2012; Oct 26 [Epub ahead of print].

92. Geronikaki AA, Gavalas AM. Antioxidants and inflammatory disease: synthetic and natural antioxidants with anti-inflammatory activity. *Comb Chem High Throughput Screen.* 2006;9(6):425-442.

93. Jialal I, Singh U. Is vitamin C an anti-inflammatory agent? *Am J Clin Nutr.* 2006;83(3):525-526.

94. Song JH, Murphy RJ, Narayan R, Davies GBH. Biodegradable and compostable alternatives to conventional plastics. *Philos Trans R Soc Lond B Biol Sci.* 2009;364(1526):2127-2139.

95. Wong VW, Levi B, Rajadas J, et al. Stem cell niches for skin regeneration. *Int J Biomater.* 2012;2012:926059.

96. Johnson JL, Lowell BC, Ryabinina OP, et al. TAT-mediated delivery of a DNA repair enzyme to skin cells rapidly initiates repair of UV-induced DNA damage. *J Inv Dermatol.* 2011;131(3):753-761.

97. Salmela MT, MacDonald TT, Black D, et al. Upregulation of matrix metalloproteinases in a model of T cell mediated tissue injury in the gut: analysis by gene array and in situ hybridisation. *Gut.* 2002;51(4):540-547.

98. Dixon KM, Tongkao-On W, Sequeira VB, et al. Vitamin D and death by sunshine. *Int J Mol Sci.* 2013;14:1964-1977.

99. D'Orazio J, Jarrett S, Amaro-Ortiz A, Scott T. UV radiation and the skin. *J Mol Sci.* 2013;14:12222-12248.

100. Bikle DB, Elalieh H, Welsh J, et al. Protective role of vitamin D signaling in skin cancer formation. *J Steroid Biochem Mol Biol.* 2013;136:271-279.

101. Bailey RL, Dodd KW, Goldman JA, et al. Estimation of total usual calcium and vitamin D intakes in the United States. *J Nutr.* 2010;140:817-822.

102. Institute of Medicine, Food and Nutrition Board. *Dietary Reference Intakes for Calcium and Vitamin D.* Washington, DC: National Academy Press; 2010.

103. Wolpowitz D, Gilchrest BA. The vitamin D questions: how much do you need and how should you get it? *J Am Acad Dermatol.* 2006;54(2):301-317.

104. Webb AR, Kline L, Holick MF. Influence of season and latitude on the cutaneous synthesis of vitamin D3: exposure to winter sunlight in Boston and Edmonton will not promote vitamin D3 synthesis in human skin. *J Clin Endocrinol Metab.* 1988;67:373.

105. Davis CD. Vitamin D and cancer: current dilemmas and future research needs. *Am J Clin Nutr.* 2008;88:565S-569S.

106. Reichrath J. Skin cancer prevention and UV-protection: how to avoid vitamin D-deficiency? *Br J Dermatol.* 2009;161(Suppl 3):54-60.

107. Cranney A, Horsley T, O'Donnell S, et al. Effectiveness and safety of vitamin D in relation to bone health. *Evid Rep Technol Assess (Full Rep).* 2007;(158):1-235.

108. U.S. Department of Agriculture, Agricultural Research Service. Website: www.ars.usda.gov.

DR. ZEIN OBAGI'S PERSONAL PHILOSOPHY ON SKIN HEALTH

CHAPTER

14

A PHILOSOPHY BASED ON SCIENCE, CLINICAL EXPERIENCE, AND PREVENTION

This chapter presents Dr. Zein Obagi's personal approach to treating, repairing, and maintaining skin health throughout a person's lifetime because every stage of life has special needs and requires a particular strategy. The philosophy that guides this approach stems from the realization that most current skin care and cosmetic products revolve around an outdated philosophy of the need for "skin moisturization." Such moisturizing products are popular because they provide instant gratification—they make the skin temporarily feel smooth, calm, and well hydrated. However, the continued application of these kinds of products slows down the rate of natural exfoliation and disrupts the barrier function, leading to further dryness, which then leads to continued use of the same or more potent moisturizing products. In the end, dependence or "moisturizer addiction" develops. This phenomenon is seen almost exclusively in women; men, who generally do not use such products, rarely complain of dry or sensitive skin.

Similarly, most current medical skin care products on the market to treat specific skin diseases are of limited value because they address only the disease, the skin's surface, and the symptoms. They do not improve skin quality and often lack proper use guidelines.

Nevertheless, moisturizers and other cosmetic and medical skin care products are heavily promoted not only to patients but also to physicians, many of whom ignore the lack of real efficacy and base their product recommendations on invalid studies, promotional items, and gifts given by the sponsoring companies. In recent years, the U.S. Food and Drug Administration (FDA) placed stricter limits on the value of promotional items that manufacturers are permitted to give physicians. However, the undue influence persists, in the form of consulting fees, speaking fees, and clinical study funding that companies give physicians who help promote their products.

Box 14.1

Dr. Zein Obagi's Innovations

- The new ZO Systems of products that provide medical and nonmedical systems of products (ZOSH and ZOMD)
- New approaches to preventing skin problems
- New approaches to treating skin problems while simultaneously restoring skin health
- Added new principles to expand the benefits and maintain the results of any treatment
- A range of effective procedures and products that allow physicians to improve the skin of every patient

---

Ensuring that consumers have access to safer, more effective skin care products requires patient education and perhaps further regulation of drug and cosmetic companies—or at least more stringent enforcement of existing laws that prohibit misleading marketing tactics. While awaiting the implementation of these, this chapter will focus on the innovations shown in Box 14.1 that provide true skin benefits. The new ZO Systems include a program for Skin Health Restoration (ZO Skin Health, or ZOSH) and a program for medical treatment (ZO Medical, or ZOMD) within the scope of Skin Health Restoration.

DEVELOPMENT OF ZO SKIN HEALTH

In 1983, Dr. Zein Obagi played a pioneering role in introducing the science of skin health, beginning with the definition of healthy skin and proceeding to defining the principles and designing treatment protocols that help in treating specific skin disease, while simultaneously restoring skin health. Nu-Derm, the first product system developed around these concepts, debuted in 1987 and was distributed by Worldwide Products, Inc. In 1997, a group of investors purchased Worldwide Products and renamed the company Obagi Medical, Inc. This company went public in 2006. Soon after, Dr. Obagi left the company because the direction and objectives of Obagi Medical, Inc. did not agree with his vision and intentions. He devoted his time to expanding the science of skin health by emphasizing the concept of prevention and expanded and enhanced his already popular treatment protocols. These efforts led to the creation of his new company, ZO Skin Health, Inc. His concept of taking the time to address the root of the problem, unusual in the world of "quick fixes," ensures that a dermatologist can help every patient who walks into his or her office, with or without a medical skin disease or problem, restore the health of the patient's skin, and thereby prevent the recurrence of skin problems.

The Obagi name remains the trademark for Obagi Medical, Inc., allowing the company to put this name on many products they produced independently, *without Dr. Obagi's involvement*. To avoid any confusion, the initials ZO (from Zein Obagi) are used to differentiate the system of new products from those of Obagi Medical, Inc. However, in the end, any product that now

Box 14.2

Issues and Observations with Nu-Derm Use

■ Certain patients improved dramatically but others only mildly.

■ Sometimes, after 2 to 3 months of improvement, patients experienced no further improvement despite continuous use.

■ Some patients continued to suffer from anticipated reactions; their skin could not build the needed tolerance.

■ In some cases, the system made pigmentation problems worse.

carries the family name Obagi *alone* has currently no relationship with Dr. Zein Obagi. Only the ZO brands represent Dr. Obagi's formulations and his expanded treatment and prevention protocols.

Patients found the Nu-Derm system easy to use, and many of them achieved highly satisfactory initial results. However, the original Nu-Derm protocols have raised several issues (Box 14.2).

The boom in Internet sales of copycat and other skin care products created additional challenges. In particular, when pharmaceutical and cosmetic companies began selling their products online, patients could directly purchase many medical products at lower prices and without medical supervision that they previously received from their doctors. Primary examples of this phenomenon include hydroquinone (HQ), tretinoin, and even isotretinoin, all of which patients can purchase from websites owned by physicians, pharmaceutical companies, and commercial companies, apparently driven by a profit motive rather than patient safety. As we know, isotretinoin carries so many risks that patients must not use it outside of the FDA-mandated iPledge risk management program. Somewhat similarly, unsupervised use of retinoids and HQ can cause skin irritation and photosensitivity that can worsen skin pigmentation problems and possibly cause ochronosis, a severe and sometimes permanent pigmentation disorder.

Solving the Issues Encountered with Nu-Derm Use

Clinical observation, retrospective analysis, and the advances in the pathophysiology of skin helped in expanding the principles of skin health, while adjustment of product formulations and the creation of more effective treatment protocols helped to solve many of the problems and issues encountered with Nu-Derm use.

The author's research made it clear that the approach to skin health should change to incorporate the new objectives and principles (Box 14.3). To meet these, the new ZO System of products was designed to include both a medical line, ZO Medical (known as ZOMD) and a preventive nonmedical line, ZO Skin Health (known as ZOSH). These products were formulated to provide the already established skin health principles (correction, stimulation, and bleaching and blending) and several new principles (Table 14.1). This makes the ZO Systems one of the most advanced, effective, and comprehensive systems in skin treatment, skin health restoration, skin conditioning, and maintenance and prevention.

The ZO Medical line in particular offers several advantages (Box 14.4).

Box 14.3

New ZO Skin Health Principles and Objectives

These new principles must be incorporated with the original principles—correction, stimulation, bleaching and blending—to provide:

1. Skin barrier function repair
2. DNA protection and repair
3. Elimination of chronic skin inflammation
4. Stabilization of the epidermis, dermis, and melanocytes (increasing skin tolerance and resistance to harmful stimuli)
5. Providing skin resistance to beneficial medical topical agents
6. Long-term maintenance

Comparing ZOMD to Nu-Derm (Table 14.2) will help physicians who are familiar with Nu-Derm to compare and switch to ZOMD if they elect to do so. Table 14.3 shows a comparison of Nu-Derm and ZOMD product names and principles/steps.

ZEIN OBAGI'S SKIN HEALTH PRINCIPLES: CLINICAL APPLICATIONS

One of the reasons that Dr. Obagi left Obagi Medical Products is that the company created separate or independent disease-driven skin treatment systems to treat specific skin diseases or conditions with no apparent regard to overall skin health. In contrast, ZOSH products embody the principle that, unless one restores overall skin health, the effects of disease-specific treatments will be limited and brief. Any skin disease occurs within the larger context of the skin's overall health. Restoring the natural balance and processes that govern skin health can resolve a wide variety of diseases and conditions, not vice versa.

TABLE 14.1   Product Lines Formulated to Meet the ZO Principles

Product Line	Principle/Objective	Contents
ZOSH (Nonmedical)	Preventing skin deterioration, and maintaining skin health	1. A daily basic skin care program 2. A preventive step can be added to the basic program to prevent any specific problem (acne, sun damage, discoloration, and signs of skin aging). For use as needed in any stage of life.
ZOMD	Treating medical skin problems while simultaneously restoring skin health	1. A program for patients with a skin disease 2. Disease-specific agents can be added to be used at specific concentrations, for specific lengths of time
ZOSH (Nonmedical)	Maintenance	1. A program for patients who have completed a course of treatment 2. Topical agents are used for maintaining skin health and treatment results

Box 14.4

Advantages of the New ZO Medical Line

- New state-of-the-art formulations and effective penetration
- Enhanced protocols to increase compliance and rate of treatment success
- Airtight packaging (no oxidation and related loss of efficacy)
- Larger product sizes (economical)
- No public Internet or black-market sales allowed (it is sold only to physicians)
- Expanded treatment applications, including medical and nonmedical conditions
- Support through continuous medical education and manuals by Dr. Obagi and a select faculty of distinguished physicians
- Frequent infusion with more innovative products to broaden the application of product benefits
- Near-constant formulation updates and enhancements to reflect ongoing advances and evolving knowledge of skin care and skin health

What is unique about ZOSH and ZOMD is that these two systems generally follow similar principles. This makes the ZO Systems easy to administer, whether a patient is transitioning from a medical approach to maintenance or from basic skin care and prevention to a medical program. The only difference between the medical and nonmedical systems is that the medical approach uses certain topical agents in treating skin medical problems, whereas the

Table 14.2   Similarities and Differences of Nu-Derm and ZOMD

Principles/Steps	Nu-Derm (Obagi Medical Products)	ZOMD
Cleanser	Yes	Yes
Toner (pH balance)	Yes	Yes
Stimulating scrub	**No**	Yes
Sebum control	**No**	Yes
Epidermal stabilization	**No**	Yes
Exfoliation	Yes	Yes
Bleaching (HQ-based)	Yes	Yes
Bleaching (non-HQ-based)	No	Yes
Melanocyte control (non-HQ-based)	**No**	Yes
Stimulation	Yes	Yes
Dermal stabilization	**No**	Yes
Moisturizers	**Yes**	No
Hydration and calming	No	**Yes**
Sun protection		
Standard	Yes	**No**
Triple-action	**No**	Yes

TABLE 14.3   Comparison of Product Names and Principles/Steps

Principle/Step	Nu-Derm (Obagi Medical Products)	ZOMD
Cleanser	Foaming gel Gentle wash	Oilacleanse Normacleanse Foamacleanse
Toner (pH balance)	Nu-Derm Toner	Balatone
Stimulating scrub	None	Vitascrub
Sebum control	None	Cebatrol
Epidermal stabilization	None	Ossential Daily Power Defense
Exfoliation	Exfoderm	Glycogent
Bleaching (HQ-based, 4%)	Clear	Melamin
Melanocyte control (non-HQ-based) and stabilization	None	Brightenex
Bleaching (non-HQ-based)	None	Brightalive
Stimulation	Tretinoin	Tretinoin
Dermal stabilization and texture repair	None	Ossential Advanced Radical Night Repair Retamax Ossential Growth Factor Serum Plus
Moisturization	Nu-Derm Action	None
Hydration and Calming	None	Ommerse Renewal Crème Ommerse Overnight Recovery Crème Restoracalm
Sun protection	Healthy Skin Protection Multiple products	Oclipse–M Broad Spectrum Tinted Sunscreen SPF 50 Oclipse–C Broad Spectrum Sunscreen SPF 50
Sun protection plus HQ	Sun Fader	None

nonmedical program does not. Following the ZO Skin Health principles moreover allows physicians to create treatment programs geared to a patient's specific medical condition, tolerance, motivation level, and desired results—while avoiding the pitfalls of traditional disease-driven dermatological treatments that fail to restore overall skin health.

ZO NONMEDICAL AND MEDICAL SYSTEMS: PRINCIPLES, OBJECTIVES, AND STEPS

The following section provides a step-by-step guide for ZOMD and ZOSH regimens.

ZO Skin Health Principles and Steps:

1. **Getting skin ready.** This is a step to make skin receptive to the steps that follow. This step is to be used indefinitely. The objectives of preparing skin are as follows:

- Enable the skin to function properly and reduce inflammation
- Enhance penetration of active ingredients used in medical or non-medical regimens to increase their effectiveness
- Prevent and control acne, rosacea, shaving bumps, skin pigmentation problems, enlarged pores, and improve rough, damaged skin texture

The agents used in these steps are cleansers, mechanical stimulation and exfoliation, and sebum control.

2. **Epidermal stabilization.** This step is used in both medical and non-medical regimens. The objectives are to help in barrier function repair and in DNA protection and repair and to calm inflammation. These are accomplished by the product Ossential Daily Power Defense.

3. **Dermal stabilization.** This step is also known as dermal stimulation. The objectives are to provide anti-aging benefits and improve both epidermal and dermal skin texture. Dermal stimulation uses retinol in one of two ways:
   - Mild: Ossential Growth Factor Serum Plus (little to no anticipated reactions)
   - Strong: Ossential Advanced Radical Night Repair and Retamax (both are associated with anticipated reactions)

4. **Hydration and calming.** The objectives are to enhance the therapeutic benefits and provide maximal comfort when using any ZO Program. This step does not weaken the efficacy of the basic skin care preventive or treatment programs. Formulations used for hydration and calming perform the following functions:
   - Increase skin tolerance
   - Reduce irritation and inflammation
   - Enhance hydration from within
   - Improve patient compliance

   The products used in this step are Ommerse Renewal Crème, Ommerse Overnight Recovery Crème, and Restoracalm.

5. **Ultraviolet (UV) protection.** The objective of this step is to protect the skin from damaging UV rays. Both the medical and nonmedical systems use the same formulation (Oclipse) to provide the necessary protection from UV light. The ZO System of photoprotection uses a triple-defense mechanism for protection from UVA, UVB, and high-energy visible light because it goes beyond the sun protection factor (SPF) offered by traditional chemical or physical sunscreens. UV protection is an indispensable part of any skin care regimen.

6. **Non-HQ bleaching and non-HQ blending.** The objective of this step is to decrease melanin production and reduce melanocyte activity through an HQ-free formulation. This helps to avoid photosensitivity that is associated with HQ bleaching and improves the appearance of epidermal discoloration. For bleaching, the Brightalive and C-Bright 10% active vitamin A formula is used when treatment with HQ has been completed, is contraindicated, or is no longer indicated. For non-HQ blending, Brightenex for the face and Brightamax for the body are used in the AM to stabilize melanocytes and help in restoring an even color tone. These products contains retinol, melanin inhibitors, and antioxidants in a natural, patented Oleosome technology that releases active

ingredients gradually. ZO Medical Brightenex use is associated with initial anticipated reactions of redness and exfoliation, which can last 2 to 3 weeks. The effects of Brightenex are enhanced by using Retamax and Ossential Advanced Radical Night Repair in the dermal stabilization step for both facial and nonfacial skin, such as that on arms, legs, and hands.

ZO Medical Treatment and ZO Skin Health Restoration: Principles, Objectives, and Steps

1. **Correction.**
   - Preparing skin (as with ZOSH)
   - Bleaching (HQ)
   - Exfoliation: the objective is to improve texture and accelerate treatment response.
   - Epidermal stabilization: The objective is to strengthen skin, increase patient compliance, and accelerate treatment results. Epidermal stabilization is an *essential* part of any nonmedical or medical treatment programs and should be maintained indefinitely.
2. **Stimulation and blending.** The objective is to restore even skin color tone with minimal bleaching effects because it increases the ability of keratinocytes to evenly absorb any melanin that is produced by melanocytes. Blending is accomplished by a mixture of tretinoin and HQ. Blending (non-HQ-based approach) is accomplished using Brightenex after discontinuing HQ-based blending (when continued use of HQ is no longer indicated). HQ-based and non-HQ-based approaches to blending are shown in Box 14.5.
3. **Stimulation.** The objective is to repair the dermis and provide more even color tone. Keep in mind that stimulation using tretinoin alone repairs the dermis and provides minimal blending. More effective blending can be achieved by tretinoin and HQ (step 2). Therapeutic stimulation requires tretinoin (Table 14.4) and should be completed in a maximum of 5 months (three keratinocyte maturation cycles [KMCs]) (see Chapter 2). Continuing tretinoin use beyond this point can be self-defeating because it will lead to continuous reactions without additional therapeutic benefits. After stopping tretinoin, further stimulation can be obtained by using retinol (in the proper concentration and formulation) in daily skin care and in preventive, maintenance, and anti-aging regimens. If needed, patients can return to treatment with tretinoin alone or mixed with HQ (blending) for an appropriate time period, then resume their long-term retinol stimulation.
4. **Hydration and calming.** The objective is the same as previously discussed for ZOSH.
5. **UV protection.** The objective is the same as previously discussed for ZOSH, and the same formulation (Oclipse) is used to provide the necessary protection from UV light. Box 14.6 shows the triple-defense mechanism for protection from UVA, UVB, and high-energy visible light.

ZOSH and ZOMD formulations provide the skin with numerous benefits (Box 14.7) that many other skin care products do not address because

Box 14.5

Blending:

Hydroquinone (HQ)- and Non-HQ-Based Approaches

THE HQ PLUS TRETINOIN APPROACH

HQ blending should be used for a limited period of time and discontinued when any of the following conditions occur:

- Treatment is completed
- Worsening of pigmentation is seen
- No further improvement is seen
- Anticipated reactions do not subside
- Resistance to HQ develops
- HQ side effects are noted:
  - Photosensitivity
  - Ochronosis
  - Allergy
- The patient is on maintenance

THE NON-HQ APPROACH

Non-HQ blending is an alternative to HQ blending in the following circumstances:

- HQ (bleaching and blending) treatment is complete
- No further improvement is observed from using HQ (resistance develops)
- HQ side effects are noted

The non-HQ blending steps are as follows:

- Brightenex: AM
- Retamax or Ossential Advanced Radical Night Repair: PM
- ZO 3-Step Peel, when indicated and especially during maintenance

most other products focus on superficial skin improvement and not on skin health.

ZO Systems can be used by patients of all skin types. The physician can design nonmedical or medical programs that are suitable for any individual and any medical or nonmedical problem. Any ZO Program can be designed to be aggressive, moderate, or mild, depending on the patient's needs, motivation, and type of skin problem. Certain formulations in both ZOSH and

TABLE 14.4   Stimulation: Type and Agents

Therapeutic (Medical Treatment)	Nontherapeutic (Nonmedical Care)
Tretinoin	Retamax
Tretinoin + hydroquinone	Ossential Advanced Radical Night Repair
	Ossential Growth Factor Serum Plus

Box 14.6

Triple-Action Ultraviolet Light Protection by the ZO System

Action 1 is achieved by epidermal stabilization (Ossential Daily Power Defense) applied in AM to strengthen the skin. This formula will increase skin defenses and tolerance of ultraviolet (UV) light by suppressing inflammation, enhancing DNA protection, and repairing and stabilizing melanocytes to provide "all-day benefits." This step makes the ZO System of photoprotection better than that of any traditional chemical or physical sunblocks (see action 3).

Action 2 is achieved by incorporating natural melanin with physical blockers in one formulation. The melanin creates a barrier or umbrella on the skin surface that protects the skin's natural melanin from UV light for "all-day protection."

Action 3 uses zinc and titanium dioxide as physical blockers to offer extra protection. As such, they are typically used in other sunscreens and can only protect the skin for 2 to 3 hours at most. Studies have shown that people rarely reapply these types of sunblocks frequently enough to achieve adequate protection. That is another reason that ZO UV protection is better than that of other ordinary sunscreens.

ZOMD are potent and will induce anticipated skin reactions for a period of time before skin builds the necessary tolerance.

ZO SYSTEMS ANTICIPATED REACTIONS

Physicians and patients should keep in mind that the more aggressive the program that is chosen, the stronger the initial skin reactions and the deeper the benefits will be. Most reactions disappear within 3 to 6 weeks, followed

---

Box 14.7

Unique Benefits of ZO Systems

- Anti-inflammatory
- DNA repair and protection
- Strengthening and repair of skin barrier function
- Cellular activation and stabilization
- Calming and hydrating without the damage caused by typical moisturizers

Box 14.8

Anticipated Reactions

Most reactions disappear within 3 to 6 weeks, followed by the development of a robust tolerance and restored barrier function, along with visible improvement of the skin.

by the development of a robust tolerance and restored barrier function, along with visible improvement of the skin (Box 14.8). To maximize results, treatment programs with ZO products require at least three KMCs (5 months) to achieve the best results.

Nonmedical-basic skin care and prevention programs also can be made aggressive, moderate, or mild by using certain formulations of retinol. When properly educated by their physicians, patients can choose and control the strength of their own nonmedical programs, which includes knowing when and how to stop skin reactions.

Most ZO products come with airtight pumps. The number of pumps applied determines the strength of the program (Box 14.9).

Additionally, the physician should educate patients about the importance of skin reactions. During treatment, these reactions are normal and expected, and they show that effective repair is taking place. The more significant a reaction a patient can tolerate, the faster and deeper the repair will be during the uncomfortable stage of treatment (repair stage). Keep in mind that most ZOMD formulations are approximately four to five times stronger than those in the ZO nonmedical (ZOSH) program and thus can cause stronger reactions.

Furthermore, the more skin damage a patient has, the more reactions the patient's skin will experience. These reactions stop only when skin becomes strong and healthy. One must eliminate the old, damaged skin to make room for new, healthy skin. ZO formulations that induce anticipated reactions include those shown in Box 14.10.

When starting patients on a ZO System, inform them about which formulations can cause reactions, mark those products, and tell the patients how to minimize or stop reactions when needed. To minimize anticipated reactions, the physician can take one of the steps listed in Box 14.11.

Box 14.9

With any product, the number of pumps determines the strength of the program:

- 4 pumps: ideal for the aggressive approach
- 2 to 3 pumps: ideal for the moderate approach
- 1 to 2 pumps: ideal for the mild approach

Box 14.10

ZO Formulations that Induce Anticipated Reactions

- Ossential Advanced Radical Night Repair
- Retamax
- Brightenex
- Glycogent
- Aknetrol

Box 14.11

Reducing Reactions

- Identify the products that are responsible for the reaction.
- Stop use of the products causing the reaction and allow use of one of the hydrating and calming formulations instead. Reactions usually disappear within 4 days.
- Reduce the frequency and amount of the reaction-causing product that is being applied.
- Reduce the concentration of such products by mixing them with one of the hydrating and calming formulations (Ommerse Renewal Crème, Ommerse Overnight Recovery Crème, or Restoracalm).
  - Ossential Advanced Radical Night Repair cannot be mixed with a hydrating and calming formulation. Patients can reduce the strength of Ossential Advanced Radical Night Repair by applying a hydrating and calming product first.
- After reactions are resolved, the program can be started again at a strength that can be tolerated.

GUIDELINES FOR USING THE ZO SKIN HEALTH AND ZO MEDICAL SYSTEMS

The commonly encountered skin problems and their treatment according to the principles of ZO Skin Health and ZO Medical are shown in Table 14.5. Studying and remembering when to use which particular steps and how to apply the principles that guide them will go a long way toward meeting the needs of a variety of patients. But do not try to memorize individual product names because these names may change. You should, however, memorize skin health principles and steps of application because they will not change. Also remember that the standard duration for applying medical agents present in some of the principles is three KMCs (5 months) to achieve maximal benefits. The only exception involves preparing the skin for a procedure (skin conditioning). Here, use each principle for one to three cycles before the procedure, depending on skin type and the time required to treat and control any active disease. After the procedure, have

TABLE 14.5   Steps and Principles of ZO Systems in Clinical Application

ZO System	Main Objective	Principles: Order and Emphasis
ZOSH	Daily skin care: the basic program	1. Getting skin ready 2. Epidermal stabilization 3. Dermal stabilization 4. Hydration and calming 5. Photoprotection
ZOSH	Early signs of photodamage and nonspecific discoloration	1. Correction 2. Epidermal stabilization 3. Stimulation Emphasis on: • Barrier function repair • DNA repair • Epidermal or dermal stabilization
ZOMD	Photodamage, no discoloration	1. Correction 2. Epidermal stabilization 3. Stimulation Emphasis on: • Barrier function repair • DNA repair • Epidermal or dermal stabilization
ZOMD	Pigmentation problem (with discoloration): The hydroquinone (HQ) approach	1. Correction (preparing skin, HQ-based bleaching, exfoliation) 2. Blending (tretinoin + HQ) Emphasis on: Bleaching and blending
	Pigmentation problem (with discoloration): The non-HQ approach Emphasis on:	1. Correction (Preparing skin, non-HQ-based bleaching or non-HQ-based blending) 2. Melanocyte stabilization 3. Epidermal stabilization 4. Stimulation (non-HQ-based blending) Emphasis on: Non-HQ-based blending
ZOMD	Acne, rosacea, seborrhea	1. Correction 2. Disease-specific topical agents 3. Epidermal stabilization 4. Stimulation (when no pigmentation problems are present) 5. Blending (when pigmentation problems are present) Emphasis on improving texture through: • Exfoliation • Epidermal stabilization • Dermal stabilization
ZOSH	Prevention	Emphasis on what needs to be prevented: 1. Aging: strong dermal stabilization 2. Acne: • Getting skin ready • Epidermal stabilization 3. Skin sensitivity, dryness: • Epidermal stabilization • Dermal stabilization (mild) • Hydration and calming

patients resume skin conditioning for one to three more KMCs until the skin returns to normal.

In the ZOMD regimen, it is also important to remember that using HQ for pigmentation problems (bleaching and blending) provides fast, but short-lived,

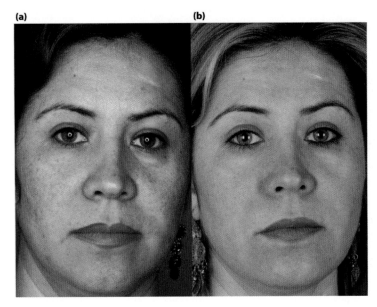

ZOSH Program

- Preparing skin: wash, scrub, oil control
- Non-HQ blending and melanocyte stabilization: Brightenex (AM)
- Barrier repair: Ossential Daily Power Defense (AM)
- Barrier repair: Retamax (PM)
- Photoprotection

FIGURE 14.1 (a) The patient had skin classified as original white. She was diagnosed as having early photodamage and nonspecific discoloration. (b) Six months later. The patient was treated with a nonmedical, non-HQ program.

results. Conversely, the non-HQ approach (blending) is slower but provides lasting results. For this reason, when treating skin pigmentation problems, start with the HQ approach, in the following order:

- Bleaching: up to 5 months, then switch to the non-HQ approach
- Blending: up to 6 or 7 months, then switch to the non-HQ approach

Application of the Principles: Patient Results
Patients suffering from early photodamage and nonspecific discoloration can be treated successfully with ZOSH alone (Figure 14.1) or ZOSH plus a ZO Retinol Stimulation Peel or a ZO 3-Step Peel (Figures 14.2 to 14.5). The

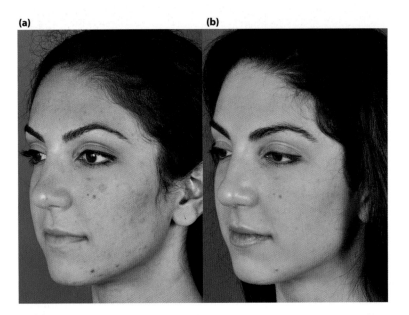

ZOSH Program

- Preparing skin: wash, scrub, oil control
- Non-HQ blending: Brightenex (AM)
- Barrier Repair: Ossential Daily Power Defense (AM)
- Retamax (PM)
- Photoprotection

FIGURE 14.2 (a) The patient had skin classified as deviated white (dark) and medium thick. She was diagnosed as having early photodamage and lentigo solaris. (b) Six months later. The patient was treated with a ZOSH program, during which she had two treatments with a ZO 3-Step Peel.

ZOSH Program

- Preparing skin: wash, scrub, toner

- Barrier repair: Ossential Daily Power Defense (AM)

- ZOSH Advanced Radical Night Repair (PM)

- Hydration and calming

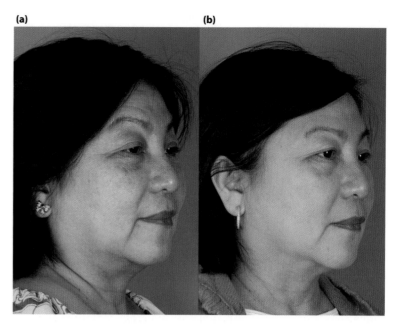

(a) **(b)**

FIGURE 14.3   (a) The patient had skin classified as deviated Asian (medium), thick, and dry. She was diagnosed as having mild aging changes, photodamage, and discoloration. (b) One year later. The patient was treated for 6 months with a ZOSH program, during which she had one ZO Retinol Stimulation Peel. The photograph shows the patient on the same ZOSH program during maintenance at one year.

resolution of the black patient's discoloration and rough texture (see Figure 14.5) is notable given the greater difficulty in treating these problems in patients with black skin.

The ZOMD program was used to treat the patients shown in Figures 14.6 to 14.11. The patient shown in Figure 14.6 had skin classified as complex

ZOSH Program

- Preparing skin: wash, scrub, oil control

- Non-HQ blending: Brightenex (AM)

- Barrier repair: Ossential Daily Power Defense (AM)

- Retamax (PM)

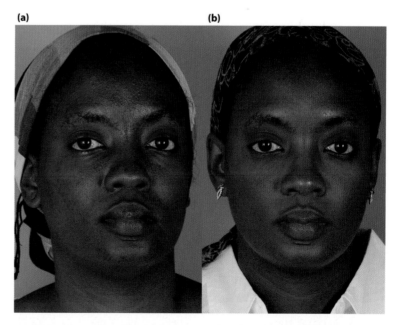

(a) **(b)**

FIGURE 14.4   (a) The patient had skin classified as original black, medium thick, and very oily. She was diagnosed as having rough texture, postinflammatory hyperpigmentation, comedones, and rosacea. This patient's skin demonstrates the negative inflammatory effects of sebum. (b) Six months after treatment with a basic ZOSH program with emphasis on epidermal and melanocyte stabilization, reduction of sebum, and elimination of chronic inflammation. The patient also underwent two treatments with the ZO Retinol Stimulation Peel. This patient is also an ideal candidate for treatment with ZO Medical and isotretinoin. This aproach was deferred because she did not want to have any reactions.

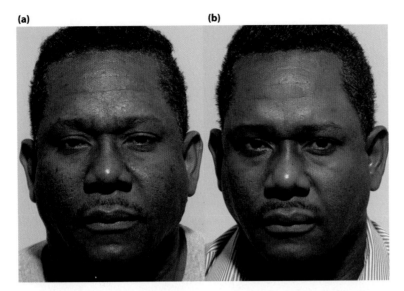

ZOSH Program

- Preparing skin: wash, scrub, oil control
- Non-HQ blending: Brightenex (AM)
- Barrier repair: Ossential Daily Power Defense (AM)
- Retamax (PM)

FIGURE 14.5 (a) The patient had skin classified as original black, thick, and very oily. He was diagnosed as having large pores, rough texture, postinflammatory hyperpigmentation, and pseudofolliculitis barbae. (b) Six months later. The patient was treated with ZOSH, with emphasis on epidermal and melanocyte stabilization and sebum reduction (topical Cebatrol from ZOMD and systemic isotretinoin, 20 mg/day for 5 months). He also had three treatments with the ZO Retinol Stimulation Peel.

and displayed postinflammatory hyperpigmentation and deep acne scars. Although his complex skin type is considered difficult to treat, it can be improved by aggressive and properly performed procedures (peels, laser, the ZOMD program). Another patient with deviated skin type (Figure 14.7) suffered from acne that did not respond to traditional acne treatment; however, she responded well to the ZOMD program and isotretinoin.

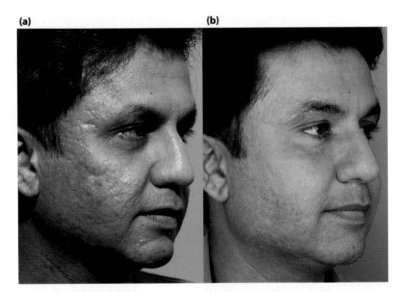

ZOMD Program

- Preparing skin: wash, scrub, oil control
- Bleaching: Melamin (4% HQ) (AM and PM)
- Exfoliation: Glycogent (AM)
- Barrier repair: Ossential Daily Power Defense (AM)
- Blending: Tretinoin 0.1% + Melamix (4% HQ) (PM)
- Retamax (PM)

FIGURE 14.6 (a) The patient had skin classified as complex, thick, and oily. He was diagnosed as having deep acne scars (stretchable and nonstretchable). (b) One year later. The patient was treated with a ZOMD program and had a medium-depth ZO Designed Controlled Depth Peel. Six months later, he had CO_2 fractional laser treatment. His skin was treated with ZOMD (hydroquinone-based) for 5 months before and after each procedure. Procedures were performed after 6 weeks of the ZOMD program. He received isotretinoin, 20 mg daily for 5 months after the second procedure.

ZOMD Program

- Preparing skin: wash, scrub, oil control

- Acne control: Aknetrol (benzoyl peroxide) (AM)

- Bleaching: Melamin (4% HQ) (AM and PM)

- Barrier repair: Ossential Daily Power Defense (AM)

- Blending: tretinoin 0.1% plus Melamix (4% HQ) (PM)

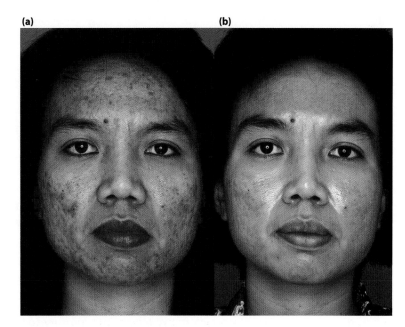

FIGURE 14.7 (a) The patient had skin classified as deviated Asian (medium), thick, and oily. She was diagnosed as having severe cystic acne, postinflammatory hyperpigmentation, and acne scars. She was unresponsive to traditional treatments attempted by multiple dermatologists (topical agents and antibiotics). (b) Eighteen weeks later. The patient was treated with HQ-based ZOMD, hydroquinone, and benzoyl peroxide. She had aggressive correction and stimulation and used isotretinoin for 5 months. She is currently on a ZOSH maintenance program.

The patient with rosacea and PIH was treated successfully with the ZOMD program, isotretinoin, and Invisapeel (Figure 14.8). The patient with rosacea and PIH (Figure 14.9) was successfully treated with an HQ-based ZOMD program along with isotretinoin, whereas the patient with melasma (Figure 14.10) was effectively treated with an HQ-based ZOMD program and a ZO Controlled Depth Peel to the immediate reticular dermis (IRD). Figure 14.11 shows a patient with deviated Asian skin and seborrheic dermatitis, lentigines, seborrheic keratosis, and PIH successfully treated with a ZO Medical program, hyfrecation, and a ZO Controlled Depth Peel to the papillary dermis (PD) level.

PHILOSOPHY ON MOISTURIZERS

The stratum corneum, the outermost layers of the epidermis, forms the skin's all-important barrier function. This barrier, consisting of dead cells called corneocytes, is enveloped by water, lipids, and protein. It maintains normal hydration, prevents penetration of infectious and toxic agents, and regulates electrolyte balance. One significant process that occurs in the stratum corneum is constant renewal through exfoliation. In healthy skin, natural exfoliation is an orderly process in which individual or small groups of corneocytes detach from neighboring cells, drop off, and are replaced by younger cells from the deeper layers. The time it takes for keratinocytes to form, mature, and exfoliate from the stratum corneum is known as the KMC and takes an average of 6 weeks (see Chapter 2). A normal cycle allows the skin to maintain an effective barrier function and healthy water content. It also allows

---

Box 14.12

Undesirable Effects of Habitual Moisturizer Use

CELLULAR EFFECTS

■ Natural skin surface exfoliation of dead corneocytes weakens or ceases.

■ The dead cells accumulate, leading to reduced basal cell mitosis and decreased cellular activity.

■ The water-lipid-protein balance in the stratum corneum is disturbed.

■ The natural delivery of nutrients and water from within the epidermis and dermis is reduced.

■ The barrier function is damaged.

CLINICAL EFFECTS

■ Change in skin texture from suppression of natural skin exfoliation (roughness, dullness, and even accelerated aging)

■ Drier, weaker, and sensitive skin (acquired dryness)

■ Intolerance to products and procedures (acquired sensitivity)

■ Dependence on external moisture supply (addiction)

---

skin hydration and transepidermal water loss to be regulated from within the body. In diseased and damaged skin, however, the barrier function may be impaired, causing xerosis or dry skin.

Recently, a new cause has emerged for dry and sensitive skin—the use of moisturizers. Excessive moisturization of the skin surface slows down the rate of natural exfoliation, thus altering the water, lipid, and protein balance and weakening the skin's barrier function. This leads to strong acquired dryness and sensitivity that lead to increased moisturizer use and, eventually, to an addiction to moisturizers. Box 14.12 shows the undesirable effects of habitual moisturizer use.

EFFECTS OF FACIAL MOISTURIZERS

Moisturizer advertisements perpetrate a big lie—that moisturizers can prevent or decrease skin aging. Facial moisturizers are among the most popular over-the-counter skin care products. Some simply offer increased hydration, whereas others promise repair benefits, such as anti-aging effects, skin firming, and anti-wrinkle activity. The most prevalent claim identifies "dry, thirsty skin" as the major offender in aging or problematic skin. Moisture must be "restored" through external means—through use of special hydrating cleansers, moisturizing foundations, moisturizers to complement the foundations, and so on—or a woman's youth and beauty will be lost forever. The acceptance of these marketing claims has been so widespread that even dermatologists and plastic surgeons recommend use of facial moisturizers to their patients. Scientific evidence to support these marketing claims is invariably not available.

Box 14.13

The Truth about Moisturizers

■ The advertising of moisturizers perpetrates a big lie—that moisturizers prevent or decrease skin aging.

■ Over-the-counter moisturizers do not penetrate below the stratum corneum and never reach deeper into the epidermis.

■ Occasional use of moisturizers can help reduce temporary skin dryness and irritability from prolonged exposure to wind, cold, or heat that tend to dehydrate skin surface, but they should not be used routinely.

True Effects of Moisturizers

Most moisturizers consist of variable percentages of water, lipid, and protein and work by hydrating the skin surface. They do not replace natural hydration to all skin layers. Moisturizer products merely comfort skin, improve surface texture by hydration (artificial smoothing), or plump the surface of skin, leading to a very temporary improvement of wrinkles. They provide a short-lived feeling of skin smoothness and fast gratification and are well tolerated. The "extra" ingredients in moisturizers, such as anti-aging, whitening, and nutritional benefits, are false and not supported by science.

Keep in mind that there is no guarantee that any moisturizer will live up to all of its claims or even contain its advertised ingredients. Moisturizers are considered cosmetics, so the FDA regulates them in a more lenient manner than it does drugs. This means that these products do not need to undergo the same rigorous testing for safety and effectiveness before going to market that prescription drugs require. The popularity of moisturizers with women is a likely result of aggressive marketing by manufacturers and the desire for a quick solution to dryness and signs of aging. But these products do not and cannot live up to their claims because they do not penetrate below the stratum corneum to have any measurable effect, and they inevitably disappoint their users.

Perhaps moisturizer users do not have the patience or inclination to explore the scientific validity of advertising claims, or they simply want to believe that there is a simple answer, a magic formula to erase signs of aging. A program of Skin Health Restoration takes time and patience, and the woman must be

Box 14.14

Moisturizer Addiction

■ By keeping the stratum corneum at a high level of moisture saturation, moisturizers slow down the rate of stratum corneum exfoliation.

■ After constant application, skin becomes dependent on the moisturizers, and constant use is required—that is, an addiction develops.

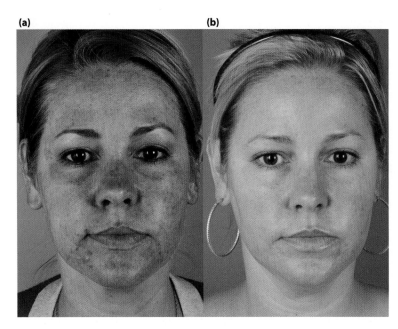

(a) **(b)**

ZOMD Program

- Preparing skin: wash, scrub, oil control

- Exfoliation: Glycogent (AM)

- Bleaching: Melamin (4% HQ) (AM and PM)

- Barrier repair: Ossential Daily Power Defense (AM)

- Blending: Tretinoin 0.1% plus Melamix (4% HQ) (PM)

The Invisapeel was applied three times a week, left on for 3 hours, and then washed off.

FIGURE 14.8 (a) The patient had skin classified as white, medium thick, and very oily skin. She was diagnosed as having rosacea, rough texture, and postinflammatory hyperpigmentation. (b) She was treated with an HQ-based ZOMD program and isotretinoin, 20 mg/day for 5 months. Invisapeel was applied to accelerate and improve results.

willing to renounce the possibility of a quick solution with a moisturizer. Box 14.13 presents the truth about moisturizers. Box 14.14 explains moisturizer addiction.

Skin Sensitivity from Moisturizer Use

The habitual use of facial moisturizers eventually dehydrates skin and creates acquired dryness. In addition, habitual use leads to acquired skin sensitivity

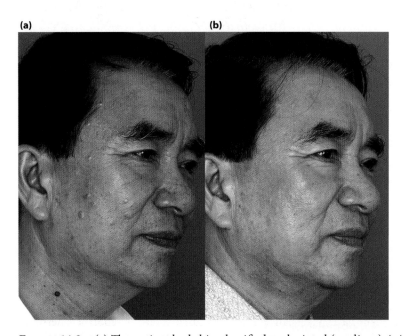

(a) **(b)**

ZOMD Program

- Preparing skin: wash, scrub, oil control

- Exfoliation: Glycogent (AM)

- Bleaching: Melamin (4% HQ) (AM and PM)

- Barrier repair: Ossential Daily Power Defense (AM)

- Blending: tretinoin 0.1% plus Melamix (4% HQ) (PM)

The Invisapeel was applied three times a week, left on for 3 hours, and then washed off.

FIGURE 14.9 (a) The patient had skin classified as deviated (medium) Asian, thick, and very oily. (He was diagnosed as having rosacea, sebaceous gland hyperplasia, and seborrheic dermatitis. (b) One year later. He was treated for 5 months with a non-HQ-based ZOMD program and used isotretinoin, 20 mg/day. Electrodessication was performed to treat the sebaceous gland hyperplasia. One ZO 3-Step Peel was also performed.

ZOMD Maintenance Program

- Preparing skin: wash, scrub, oil control

- Non-HQ blending: Brightenex (AM)

- Barrier repair: Ossential Daily Power Defense (AM)

- Retamax (PM)

- ZO 3-Step Peel planned two to three times per year, if melasma reappeared

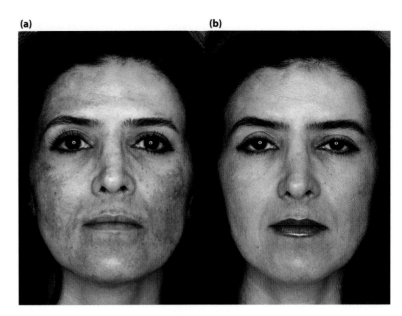

FIGURE 14.10　(a) The patient had skin classified as deviated white (dark), medium thick, and oily. She was diagnosed as having melasma (epidermal and dermal) based on Dr. Zein Obagi Skin Stretch Test. (b) One year later. The patient was treated for 5 months with aggressive HQ-based ZOMD treatment and one ZO Controlled Depth Peel to the immediate reticular dermis.

because of the damaging effects on skin barrier function. It should be noted that "skin sensitivity" is not a true sensitivity disorder, which can be seen with certain cases of skin disease or genetic disorders, but is in fact skin weakness or intolerance. Eliminating the so-called skin sensitivity necessitates discontinuation of the very products that are promoted as a solution to skin

ZOMD Program (Aggressive)

- Preparing skin: wash, scrub, oil control

- Bleaching: Melamin (4% HQ) (1 gram, AM and PM)

- Exfoliation: Glycogent (AM)

- Barrier repair: Ossential Daily Power Defense (AM)

- Blending: tretinoin 0.1% and Melamix (4% HQ) (PM)

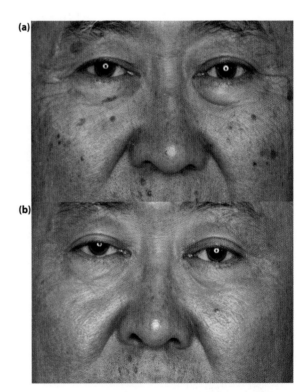

FIGURE 14.11　(a) The patient had skin classified as deviated (medium) Asian. He was diagnosed as having seborrheic dermatitis, lentigines, dermatosis papulosa nigra (DPN), and postinflammatory hyperpigmentation. (b) Six months later. By week 6 of his ZO Medical program, one session of hyfrecation had been performed on the DPNs. By week 12, the patient had undergone a ZO Controlled Depth Peel to the papillary dermis. He followed the same ZOMD program for another 6 weeks and was then started on ZOSH maintenance.

sensitivity—moisturizers—and the beginning of a commitment to skin barrier function repair that will effectively increase skin tolerance and prevent sensitivity. However, conditioned as they are to the desirability of gentle, nonirritating products, many patients will complain about the anticipated reactions that are part of barrier function repair. Dermatologists must spend time reassuring patients that the temporary burning and stinging are desirable reactions that lead to skin tolerance and improved function. It may be too much to expect all patients to eliminate habitual use of moisturizers and accept the anticipated reactions, but one by one, the mindset of patients in these areas may be changed.

Recommendations

In the ZO skin conditioning and Skin Health Restoration programs, certain products have been created to calm and hydrate the skin (the hydration and calming principle—using Ommerse Renewal Crème, Ommerse Overnight Recovery Crème, or Restoracalm). These agents are to be used only when needed for soothing the skin while it is undergoing the correction and stimulation processes. This includes the short period of time during which a patient desires to reduce the normal skin reactions to tretinoin and alpha-hydroxy acids for a *short period* of comfort or for social events. In addition, use of certain hydrators is permitted in patients with atopic dermatitis, asteatosis of old age, or the dry skin type (see Zein Obagi Skin Classification System in Chapter 4), which cannot become properly hydrated because of genetic influence. In these cases, the ZO calming and anti-inflammatory hydrators can be used long term while normal skin barrier functions are being repaired.

Remember that skin does not feel dry and moisturizers are not needed when skin cell functions are intact. Correction and stimulation eventually returns natural hydration from within, especially in the stratum corneum, which often eliminates the need for moisturizers. The cycle of moisturizer addiction can be broken when patients are informed about the damage that excessive moisturizer use can cause and can see the improvements in their skin after Skin Health Restoration.

A SELECTION OF CLINICAL CASES

The following cases were chosen to illustrate Dr. Zein Obagi's approach to using ZO Skin Health (ZOSH) and ZO Medical (ZOMD) principles and products in his treatments. The appropriate treatment and maintenance steps are outlined, and careful consideration is given to the ZO Peels discussed in Chapters 9 and 10. With each case, the patient's skin health is analyzed, which includes the skin's surface texture, color, tolerance, hydration level, and presence or absence of clinical disease. A suitable treatment and maintenance plan then follows.

PATIENT 1: MELASMA

SKIN CLASSIFICATION

Color: original Asian
Thickness: medium
Oiliness: oily
Laxity: minimal
Propensity for atypical healing*: none

PATIENT HISTORY

The patient in Figure 15.1 intermittently used prescription-strength hydroquinone (HQ) for bleaching and blending purposes for 3 years without any medical supervision. After two visits with her initial dermatologist, she began purchasing these HQ products online. Her skin improved minimally at the beginning, but with subsequent ongoing "self-medication," her melasma worsened. She concurrently received four intense pulsed light (IPL) treatments and several exfoliative procedures with glycolic acid. The patient reported that the IPL caused her melasma to worsen and that the exfoliative procedures provided no improvement. She was in good overall health, with no history of allergies. She was currently taking the oral contraceptive pill and had previously used topical antibiotics for acne that commenced at age 12 years.

---

*Propensity for atypical healing is explained in Chapter 4.

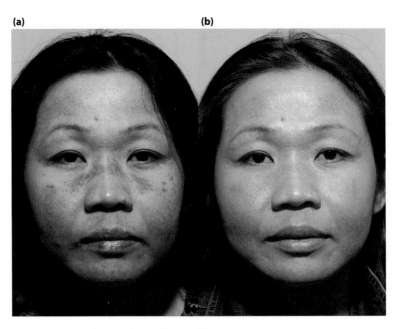

Figure 15.1 Patient 1 before (a) and after (b) treatment.

DIAGNOSIS

The patient was diagnosed with dermal and epidermal melasma (based on Dr. Zein Obagi Skin Stretch test results), rosacea, oily skin, and subjective skin sensitivity.

OVERALL SKIN HEALTH

The patient's skin was uneven in color (melasma), rough in texture, weak in tolerance, and normally hydrated, and active skin disease (rosacea) was present.

TREATMENT PLAN

The treatment plan consisted of an overall approach to restore complete skin health. It emphasized reversing the patient's melasma and rosacea, while also reducing the skin's sensitivity through barrier function repair (Table 15.1).

The following key points were explained to the patient:

- Her skin diagnosis and the appropriate planned course of treatment.
- Skin improvement is expected to occur gradually.
- Reactions (redness, dryness, exfoliation) are anticipated during the early stages of treatment. It is important to continue with the program despite the appearance of these signs so that the skin will build tolerance to the program. Explanation was also given on how to control these reactions when required. She was further advised that the stronger these reactions, the better her results would be, and the faster her skin conditions would improve.
- A long-term maintenance regime will be required after she has finished the treatment because there is no permanent cure for melasma or rosacea.

TABLE 15.1   Patient 1: Treatment Plan

Step	Duration
Start ZOMD program	Six weeks of medical skin conditioning
ZO Controlled Depth Peel to the papillary dermis (PD) More than one procedure may be needed*	Eight to 10 days of healing
After healing, add isotretinoin and restart the ZOMD program	Five months of treatment
Multiple treatments with the ZO 3-Step Stimulation Peel can be performed during this period†	
ZO Maintenance Program	As directed by physician

*In the future, a second ZO Controlled Depth Peel to the PD, a pigment laser procedure, or a CO_2 fractional laser procedure may be required.

†The ZO 3-Step Stimulation Peel will help to exfoliate the pigmentation at a faster rate while also providing dermal benefit for improvement of rough texture.

The ZOMD treatment products used by the patient for skin conditioning are shown in Table 15.2.

Treatment Preparation and Course

After 6 weeks of using the ZOMD treatment steps for skin conditioning, the patient consented to undergo a ZO Controlled Depth Peel to the papillary dermis (PD). In preparation for this peel, the patient was:

- Instructed to stop both the exfoliation (Glycogent) and blending (Melamix, tretinoin) steps 4 days before the peel. The purpose of this was to arrest any remaining anticipated reactions.
- Told about the postpeel healing stages and their duration
- Provided with written home-care instructions and product supplies
- Questioned about herpes simplex virus history and, if needed, provided with the appropriate prophylaxis

The patient underwent a ZO Controlled Depth Peel to the PD as scheduled, and her skin healed fully within 8 days. By postpeel day 10, she restarted application of the ZOMD products. She proceeded gradually, following the same steps that she had used for initial skin conditioning. As tolerated, she increased the program strength until the desired aggressive approach was achieved.

After her skin had healed from the peel, isotretinoin, 20 mg/day, was introduced to treat her rosacea simultaneously. Isotretinoin was specifically chosen instead of photodynamic therapy because the latter is contraindicated in patients who have both melasma and rosacea. Of note, the patient fulfilled the isotretinoin risk management program requirements before beginning treatment. One month later, a single ZO 3-Step Peel was performed to improve her skin's texture. Treatment was completed within 6 months, and a maintenance program was then recommended (Table 15.3).

Treatment Notes

- HQ used for bleaching (Melamin) purposes should be discontinued in all patients after 5 months. This is to avoid inducing photosensitivity and HQ resistance.

TABLE 15.2   Patient 1: ZOMD Products Used for Treatment

Step	Product	Application	Comment
Skin preparation			
Cleanse	Oilacleanse	AM and PM	Oily skin cleanser for all pigmentation problems. It is used to boost epidermal renewal and deeply cleanse pores.
Scrub	Vitascrub	Once daily	
Oil control	Cebatrol	AM and PM	For both chemical and mechanical exfoliation, enhanced epidermal renewal, and deep pore cleansing
			This sebum-reducing astringent provides deep pore cleansing, antibacterial activity, and anti-inflammatory benefits. It may cause a stinging sensation.
Epidermal exfoliation	Glycogen	AM, 2 pumps (½ gram)	For epidermal exfoliation and renewal and to further enhance the penetration of other agents. (Glycogent was given to this patient to address the rosacea. It is not used routinely in melasma treatment.) Glycogent causes a stinging sensation.
Bleaching	Melamin (4% hydroquinone [HQ])	AM and PM, 4 pumps for each application as follows: Treat the entire face. Focus product application on severely affected areas. Decrease the amount of product applied to nonaffected areas.	HQ for skin bleaching combined with anti-inflammatory agents. The patient previously used HQ for 3 years to bleach her skin. Intermittently, she also used HQ with tretinoin, but she stopped this combination once anticipated reactions began to appear. At the time of the initial consultation with the patient, there was no evidence of HQ resistance. The melasma HQ treatment protocol was therefore selected to provide both bleaching and blending effects.
Epidermal stabilization	Ossential Daily Power Defense	AM and PM, 3 pumps	For barrier function renewal, anti-inflammatory activity, DNA repair and protection, antioxidant benefit, and melanocyte stabilization, and to increase the skin's resistance to ultraviolet light.
Blending	Melamix (4% HQ) plus tretinoin (0.1%)	AM and PM In milder cases, only blending can be performed and only at PM. With each application, freshly mix together: Melamix (2 pumps) and tretinoin (1 gram) (size of 1 inch of regular toothpaste)	HQ and tretinoin, when combined in this penetration-enhancing formula, generate a blending effect. Blending offers both dermal stimulation and the restoration of an even skin tone without any bleaching effect. This mixture causes strong anticipated reactions (redness, dryness, and exfoliation). Anti-inflammatory and barrier repair agents are added to the formula to calm these reactions. As with bleaching, the mixture is to be applied to the entire face, focusing application on severely affected areas.
Controlling reactions	Ommerse Daily Renewal Crème Ommerse Overnight Recovery Crème Hydrafirm (eye cream)	AM and PM, as needed	Anti-inflammatory, nourishing agents to be used only occasionally. They are given to calm the skin during the reaction phase.
Sun Protection	Oclipse Broad Spectrum Tinted Sunscreen SPF 30 or Oclipse-C Broad Spectrum Sunscreen SPF 50	AM, reapply as needed	A comprehensive sunscreen with physical blocks (UVA/UVB), fractionated melanin (high-energy visible light), and antioxidants.

TABLE 15.3 Patient 1: Products Used for Maintenance

Step	Product	Application
Skin preparation	Oilacleanse Vitascrub Cebatrol	Maintained
Exfoliation	Glycogent	Discontinued
Bleaching	Melamin (4% HQ)	Discontinued
Non-HQ melanocyte stabilization, blending	Brightenex (no bleaching effects)	AM, 3 pumps
Epidermal stabilization	Ossential Daily Power Defense	Maintained AM only, 3 pumps
Blending	Melamix (4% HQ) Tretinoin (0.1%)	Discontinued
Stimulation	Retamax	PM, 3 pumps
Hydration	Ommerse Daily Renewal Crème	
	Ommerse Overnight Recovery Crème Hydrafirm	Maintained, but optional AM and PM, as needed
Ultraviolet protection	Oclipse Broad Spectrum Tinted Sunscreen SPF 30 or Oclipse-C Broad Spectrum Sunscreen SPF 50	Maintained AM, reapply as needed

- Blending (Melamix, tretinoin) can continue for 7 to 8 months. It should be applied PM but only during the early phases of maintenance. The blending step should be replaced by Retamax for long-term stimulation and stabilization. Alternatively, if patients require blending beyond 7 or 8 months, they may alternate between blending one night and retinol stimulation (Ossential Advanced Radical Night Repair or Retamax) the following night.

Treatment Results

This patient achieved outstanding results on program completion. Her skin now fulfilled all the criteria for skin health, including a smooth skin surface, even color throughout, strong tolerance, natural hydration, and no active clinical disease.

The patient will continue with the previously detailed maintenance regimen, and she will be placed in ZO Skin Health Circle to receive ongoing observation and service. However, despite the use of a maintenance program, it is possible for melasma and rosacea to return. This can occur a year or more after initial successful treatment. She was informed of this possibility on her initial consultation, and as such, the physician cannot rule out further need for bleaching, blending, exfoliation, or use of isotretinoin.

PATIENT 2: SOLAR ELASTOSIS

SKIN CLASSIFICATION

Color: light white
Thickness: medium
Oiliness: normal
Laxity: moderate
Propensity for atypical healing: none

PATIENT HISTORY

The patient in Figure 15.2 was highly motivated to improve her appearance. Fifty-five years of sun exposure had created classic solar elastosis marked by leathery texture, yellowish color, and deep, firm wrinkles and furrows that failed to improve on stretching. Of note, she had a positive past history for cold sores but was otherwise in good overall health.

DIAGNOSIS

Solar elastosis, acquired skin sensitivity, and skin dehydration.

OVERALL SKIN HEALTH

The patient's skin was even in color, displayed a rough texture, and was sensitive with poor hydration (due to moisturizer overuse).

TREATMENT PLAN

This patient primarily required a deep resurfacing procedure such as a CO_2 fractional laser or a medium-depth ZO Designed Controlled Depth Peel. However, with her initial poor skin health, she was neither able to benefit nor tolerate such a procedure. Her skin needed strengthening before undergoing any resurfacing. The primary aim was to repair her skin's barrier function and restore natural hydration to the epidermis and dermis. This can be accomplished by nonmedical skin conditioning (ZOSH) for 6 to 8 weeks (Table 15.4). It is essential for the skin to be properly hydrated before the CO_2 fractional laser procedure or the ZO Controlled Depth Peel is performed in order to obtain an even response and uniform results.

(a)   (b)

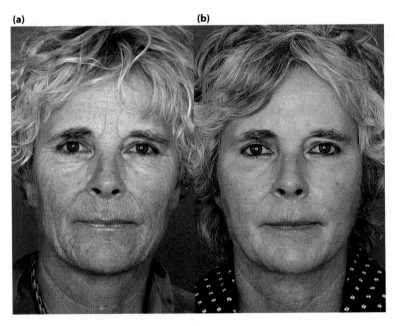

FIGURE 15.2   Patient 2 before (a) and after (b) treatment.

TABLE 15.4 Patient 2: Treatment Plans

Step	Product	Application	Comment
	Treatment Plan to Eliminate Skin Sensitivity		
Skin preparation	Offects Hydrating Cleanser	AM and PM	Cleanser for normal to dry skin that hydrates and rejuvenates without disrupting the moisture barrier
	Offects Exfoliating Polish	Once daily or less, as tolerated	Exfoliating scrub to increase epidermal turnover and promote healthy circulation
	Balatone	AM and PM	A calming, pH-balancing toner used to invigorate dry, weak skin
Epidermal stabilization	Ossential Daily Power Defense	AM, 2 to 3 pumps	To repair skin's barrier function
Dermal stabilization	Ossential Growth Factor Serum Plus	PM, 2 to 3 pumps	To stimulate dermal activity and hydration
Hydrating and calming	Ommerse Daily Renewal Crème Ommerse Overnight Recovery Crème	AM and PM, as needed	Anti-inflammatory nourishing agents to be used only occasionally to calm the skin during the reaction phase
Sun protection	Oclipse Broad Spectrum Tinted Sunscreen SPF 30 or Oclipse-C Broad Spectrum Sunscreen SPF 50	AM, reapply as needed	Comprehensive sunscreen with physical blocks (UVA/UVB), fractionated melanin (high-energy visible light), and antioxidants
Stabilization	Ossential Advanced Radical Night Repair	PM, 2 to 3 pumps Begin by using once weekly, and gradually increase until tolerated nightly.	High-potency retinol for aggressive anti-aging and dermal stimulation
	Treatment Plan for Skin Conditioning		
Skin preparation Cleanse Scrub Oil control	Oilacleanse Vitascrub Cebatrol	AM and PM Once daily AM and PM	
Epidermal stabilization	Ossential Daily Power Defense	AM, 2 to 3 pumps	
Stimulation (blending)	Melamix (4% HQ) Tretinoin 0.1%	PM With each application, freshly mix together: Melamix (2 pumps; ½ gram) and tretinoin (1 gram)	Blending offers aggressive dermal stimulation and the restoration of an even skin tone without any bleaching effect.

Treatment Course

Because the patient reported having skin sensitivity, her treatment plan was divided into two parts: 1) eliminating skin sensitivity using ZO Skin Health (ZOSH) (nonmedical) and 2) conditioning her skin to prepare it for needed procedures and managing skin after the procedure. The treatment choice for eliminating skin sensitivity consisted of epidermal stabilization using Ossential Daily Power Defense and dermal stabilization using Ossential

Growth Factor Serum Plus, with the addition of Ossential Advanced Radical Night Repair to be used gradually until it is tolerated as a nightly application. This would indicate the elimination of skin sensitivity and moisturizer addiction. ZOMD skin conditioning was started at that time to prepare skin for the procedure.

It is important to note that the patient's skin-conditioning program (ZOMD) did not include bleaching (Melamin) because she had no pigmentation problems. However, blending using tretinoin plus HQ was used at PM as a general repair to control skin melanocytes, to maintain even color tone, and to prevent potential postinflammatory hyperpigmentation (PIH).

Selecting the Appropriate Procedure

Considering this patient's skin type and her clinical presentation—light white skin of medium thickness, solar elastosis, and textural problems (a leathery feel with unstretchable wrinkles)—one of several resurfacing procedures could be used:

1. **Phenol peel.** In expert hands, this peel produces exceptional results. However, it is not recommended because it will thin the skin and result in permanent hypopigmentation or depigmentation.
2. **Standard dermabrasion.** This too is a very effective procedure when properly performed. However, today many dermatologists consider it obsolete.
3. **CO_2 laser resurfacing.** This is an effective procedure when performed in the correct manner. However, this choice carries a high rate of complications.
4. **CO_2 fractional laser resurfacing.** This procedure is currently quite popular. It is ideal for improving textural problems of the skin (unstretchable wrinkles and scars). Patients may require one to three of these procedures, depending on the skill and aggressiveness of the physician.
5. **ZO Designed Controlled Depth Peel (medium depth).** This peel could also be a viable and effective option for this patient. As with CO_2 fractional laser resurfacing, she may require one to three peels, depending on the practitioner's skills.

In many appropriate cases, combining the ZO Controlled Depth Peel with a CO_2 fractional laser provides synergistic results. In such scenarios, the peel is performed first, reaching at least the immediate reticular dermis (IRD) (observing for frost with no visible pink background). Immediately after, during the same treatment session, a CO_2 fractional laser is used to efface the remaining indurated wrinkles or scars.

Procedure Choice for This Patient

After the patient began a treatment protocol that consisted of 6 weeks of skin conditioning (ZO Skin Health Restoration) using ZOMD she had one ZO Designed Controlled Depth Peel that reached the PD, IRD, and upper reticular dermis (URD). After healing, she resumed her ZO regimen for a further 12 weeks. She later began the maintenance program as a member of the ZO Skin Health Circle. Her post-treatment photo was taken 1 year after initial treatment.

Overall, this case highlights the importance of eliminating skin sensitivity before peels or fractional resurfacing procedures. Skin conditioning (ZO Skin Health Restoration) is essential before these procedures because it helps restore even skin hydration. This is crucial because water is the chromophore for both the CO_2 laser and the trichloroacetic acid (TCA) procedure. If the skin is poorly hydrated, the laser will cause severe burns and lead to serious complications. Similarly, TCA cannot coagulate skin proteins in poorly hydrated skin, and no frost or only a thin frost will form. This can mislead the physician into applying more TCA in an attempt to achieve a frost and may cause severe, deep, caustic burns and other complications. Achieving properly hydrated skin before a procedure avoids all these problems and ensures a safer outcome with more even results.

PATIENT 3: PHOTODAMAGE

SKIN CLASSIFICATION

Color: normal white
Thickness: thick
Oiliness: oily
Laxity: minimal
Propensity for atypical healing: none

PATIENT HISTORY

The patient in Figure 15.3 endured many years of extensive sun exposure without adequate protection. This resulted in repeated sunburns. She presented to the clinic eager to improve the large brown spots and freckling throughout her face. One year prior, a basal cell carcinoma had been removed from the

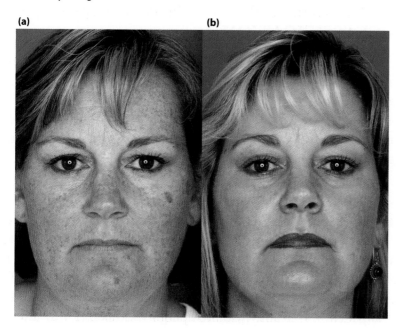

(a)   (b)

FIGURE 15.3   Patient 3 before (a) and after (b) treatment.

left side of her chin. The patient was otherwise healthy with no allergic history or prior cold sores.

DIAGNOSIS

Severe photodamage, actinic keratoses, lentigines, freckles, oily skin.

OVERALL SKIN HEALTH

The patient's skin showed roughness, oiliness, discoloration (freckles and lentigines), mild sensitivity, poor hydration, and severe photodamage with actinic keratosis on a background of prior basal cell carcinoma.

TREATMENT PLAN

The patient required a combination of ZOMD creams and a ZO Controlled Depth Peel to the IRD. The moderate protocol for skin conditioning was selected as the appropriate program. This regimen was used before and after the peel (Table 15.5). The objectives were to repair damaged DNA and provide total epidermal renewal, with dermal stimulation.

Maintenance

This patient's maintenance program was designed with an emphasis placed on stabilization of the epidermis, the melanocytes, and the dermis (Table 15.6).

PATIENT 4: ACNE SCARS

SKIN CLASSIFICATION

Color: dark white
Thickness: thick
Oiliness: oily
Laxity: minimal
Propensity for atypical healing: none

PATIENT HISTORY

The patient in Figure 15.4 has a history of severe acne during adolescence. Her disease left various scars, primarily on the bilateral cheeks. Several physicians refused to perform deep resurfacing procedures because of her dark skin color. The patient was healthy with no allergies and no prior history of cold sores.

TABLE 15.5 Patient 3: ZOMD Products Used for Treatment and Skin Conditioning

Step	Products	Application	Comment
Skin preparation	Oilacleanse	AM and PM	Oily skin cleanser for all pigmentation problems
	Vitascrub	Once daily	A chemical and mechanical exfoliant to improve the patient's skin texture and enhance epidermal renewal
	Cebatrol	AM and PM	Oil reduction step particularly important when treating pigmentation disorders
Epidermal exfoliation	Glycogent	AM, 2 to 3 pumps	An exfoliative lotion for texture repair and a faster rate of pigmentation improvement
Bleaching (HQ approach)	Melamin (4% HQ)	AM and PM, 4 pumps	HQ used to bleach the skin and reduce the excess pigment production
Epidermal stabilization	Ossential Daily Power Defense	AM and PM, 3 pumps	Barrier restoration, ultraviolet (UV) protection, and melanocyte stabilization
Blending	Melamix (4% HQ) Tretinoin (0.1%)	PM With each application, freshly mix together: Melamix (2 pumps) and tretinoin (1 gram)	Blending is used to provide a more even skin tone while aggressively causing dermal stimulation.
Hydration and calming	Ommerse Daily Renewal Crème, Ommerse Overnight Recovery Crème	AM and PM, as needed	Used occasionally to calm and nourish the skin during the reaction phase.
UV protection	Oclipse Broad Spectrum Tinted Sunscreen SPF 30 or Oclipse-C Broad Spectrum Sunscreen SPF 50	AM and reapplication	Sunscreen with physical blocks (UVA/UVB), fractionated melanin (high-energy visible light), and antioxidants Because of her photosensitivity, she is susceptible to the damaging effects of UV rays and requires a robust approach in sun protection. By combining Ossential Daily Power Defense use with either of these two sunscreens, she is protecting her skin both internally and externally. This provides comprehensive photoprotection and, invariably, better overall skin health.

DIAGNOSIS

Acne scarring (icepick scars, stretchable and depressed scars), and PIH.

OVERALL SKIN HEALTH

The patient's skin was rough in texture, oily, discolored (PIH), and tolerant, with no active disease and normal hydration.

TREATMENT PLAN

The goal was to prescribe an aggressive ZOMD skin-conditioning program for 6 to 8 weeks, and then perform a resurfacing procedure. A few supportive

TABLE 15.6 Patient 3: Products Used for Maintenance

Step	Product	Application
Skin preparation	Oilacleanse Vitascrub Cebatrol	Maintained
Exfoliation	Glycogent	Discontinued
Bleaching	Melamin (4% HQ)	Discontinued
Non-HQ melanocyte stabilization	Brightenex	AM, 3 pumps
Epidermal stabilization	Ossential Daily Power Defense	Maintained AM only, 3 pumps
Blending	Melamix (4% HQ) Tretinoin (0.1%)	Discontinued
Stimulation	Retamax	PM, 3 pumps
Hydration	Ommerse Daily Renewal Crème Ommerse Overnight Recovery Crème	Maintained, but optional AM and PM, as needed
Ultraviolet protection	Oclipse Broad Spectrum Tinted Sunscreen SPF 30 or Oclipse-C Broad Spectrum Sunscreen SPF 50	Maintained AM, reapply as needed

procedures would also be necessary during this period to address the different types of scars. After she had healed from the procedure, she was to continue with the ZOMD program, and isotretinoin would be added simultaneously for 3 to 5 months.

Treatment Note

This patient and several others mentioned in this book used the original Nu-Derm system. Although the patient's response to Nu-Derm was good, restoration of skin to normal health took longer because of certain factors

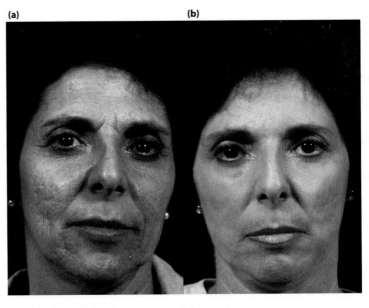

FIGURE 15.4 Patient 4 before (a) and after (b) treatment.

that were not recognized 20 years ago when Nu-Derm was introduced. Had the ZOMD program been used instead, it would have resulted in faster healing and more permanent skin health. Table 15.7 shows a comparison of the Nu-Derm system used by this patient and what could have been used with ZOMD.

Treatment Course

The patient underwent a ZO Designed Controlled Depth Peel with varying depths throughout her face, including the PD, IRD, and URD. The patient's skin healed completely within 12 days. Postoperatively, she suffered from strong PIH for 2 months, which did not respond to bleaching and blending. However, a good response followed when sebum was reduced through the addition of isotretinoin, 20 mg/day for 3 months. Supportive procedures performed during

TABLE 15.7 Comparison of the Nu-Derm System Used by the Patient and the ZOMD Program

Nu-Derm		ZOMD	
Program Previously Used for This Patient		**New Program**	
The Steps		*The Steps*	
SKIN PREPARATION			
Oily skin cleanser	Foaming Gel	Oilacleanse	Remove impurities
Surface skin scrub	NA	Vitascrub	Mechanical stimulation and exfoliation (skin renewal)
Sebum control	NA	Cebatrol	Exfoliate, anti-inflammatory
pH balance "all"	Toner	Balatone Dry, sensitive skin	Calming
CORRECTION			
Target	Nu-Derm	ZOMD	Objective
Epidermal repair	Exfoderm	Glycogent	Renew the epidermis through exfoliation
Bleaching	Clear	Melamin (4% HQ)	Reduce melanin production
Epidermal stabilization: for barrier function and DNA repair	NA	Ossential Daily Power Defense	Anti-inflammatory, ultraviolet (UV) protection and melanocyte stabilization, barrier function renewal, DNA repair
STIMULATION (NONHYDROQUINONE)			
Target	Nu-Derm	ZOMD	Objective
Epidermis and dermis	Tretinoin	Tretinoin	Stimulate epidermal and dermal repair
Blending (Stimulation plus Hydroquinone)			
Target	Nu-Derm	ZOMD	Objective
Epidermis, dermis, melanin	Tretinoin plus Blender (4% HQ)	Tretinoin plus Melamix (4% HQ)	Stimulate and restore even color
Skin texture	N/A	Advanced Radical Night Repair, Retamax (after blending has been accomplished)	Improve texture and provide anti-aging benefits
REACTION CONTROL/HYDRATION AND CALMING			
Target	Nu-Derm	ZOMD	Objective
Reactions	Action (will weaken the treatment)	Restoracalm (will not weaken the treatment)	Calming, hydrating, and anti-inflammatory

the initial conditioning period included punch excision for icepick scars and scar subcision. A total of 10 icepick scars were punched out and allowed to heal naturally. Afterward, only slight depressions were left, which were later corrected with a peel. Two other depressed scars on the right cheek were subcised 1 month before the peel. With this technique, a special needle was used to lift the base of the scars and break up the fibrous attachments.

This patient used the Nu-Derm system. Here, a comparison will be made between Nu-Derm and the new approach of ZOMD. For skin preparation, the Nu-Derm system uses a cleanser (Foaming Gel) for general oily skin cleansing in addition to a toner for all patients. Both of these steps provided weak epidermal renewal and sebum control. It took years to learn that certain steps need to be added to skin preparation to achieve the desired objectives, such as mechanical exfoliation (ZO Medical Vitascrub) and sebum control (ZO Medical Cebatrol), both of which are essential. Oilacleanse, a cleanser for oily skin with additional anti-inflammatory benefits and acantholytic activity, is also used for ZOMD. Vitascrub is used to renew the epidermis through mechanical exfoliation and deep pore cleansing. Cebatrol provides sebum control to reduce skin inflammation. The ZOMD toner would not be selected for this patient because it is reserved for dry and sensitive skin.

Regarding the principle of epidermal correction, the Nu-Derm system uses Exfoderm for exfoliation and Clear (4% HQ) for bleaching. Similarly, ZOMD uses Glycogent for exfoliation and Melamin (4% HQ) for bleaching. However, ZOMD has introduced an additional component to the correction stage that strengthens skin and improves tolerance (Ossential Daily Power Defense). This novel addition provides epidermal stabilization, repairs the barrier function, controls inflammation, and repairs damaged DNA.

For stimulation, the Nu-Derm system uses only tretinoin and, for blending, tretinoin with Blender. The Nu-Derm system does not provide a non-HQ bleaching or blending option. Comparatively, for stimulation, ZOMD offers HQ blending in treatment and non-HQ (blending and bleaching) in maintenance as follows: use tretinoin for stimulation during treatment and retinol (in the form of Ossential Advanced Radical Night Repair or Retamax) in maintenance; use tretinoin mixed with 4% HQ for blending during treatment and a non-HQ bleaching product, Brightalive, C-Bright 10% vitamin C; and use non-HQ blending, Brightenex, with the added benefits of melanocyte stabilization during maintenance.

The Nu-Derm system uses a moisturizer to control reactions, which weakens the treatment program. Instead of a moisturizer, the ZOMD system uses Restoracalm, which provides a wide range of benefits and does not counterproductively weaken the treatment program.

PATIENTS 5 AND 6: OCHRONOSIS

Table 15.8 provides skin classification data for patients 5 and 6; Table 15.9 provides skin health data for patients 5 and 6; and Table 15.10 provides diagnostic data for patients 5 and 6.

TABLE 15.8   Patients 5 and 6: Skin Classification

	Patient 5	Patient 6
Color	Asian	Black
Thickness	Medium-thick	Thick
Oiliness	Oily	Oily
Laxity	Minimal	Minimal
Propensity for atypical healing	None	None

TABLE 15.9   Patients 5 and 6: Skin Health

	Patient 5	Patient 6
Texture	Rough	Rough
Color	Discolored	Discolored
Tolerance	Normal	Very sensitive
Hydration	Normal	Normal
Disease	Postinflammatory hyperpigmentation, ochronosis on face	Ochronosis on face, neck, and chest

TABLE 15.10   Patients 5 and 6: Diagnosis

Patient 5	Patient 6
Superficial ochronosis, postinflammatory hyperpigmentation, and depigmentation following CO_2 fractional laser	Deep ochronosis, contact dermatitis with severe irritation, and sensitivity

PATIENT HISTORY

Patient 5

The patient in Figure 15.5 is a physician who for several years was treating herself with HQ for melasma. She presented to the clinic with increased pigmentation periorally. Prior treatment in a different clinic with a CO_2 fractional laser led to PIH and focal depigmentation but produced no improvement of the ochronosis.

Patient 6

After years of using HQ (4%), the pigmentation of the patient in Figure 15.6 worsened. She progressed to using 8% HQ, 10% HQ, Triluma (fluocinolone, HQ 4%, and tretinoin 0.05%), and other compounded products prescribed by several physicians. She also received glycolic acid peels and used multiple Mesoestetic Cosmelan peels (azeleic acid and kojic acid, among other ingredients). Her condition only worsened.

TREATMENT PLAN FOR PATIENT 5

The treatment plan for patient 5 consisted of two programs: program A and program B.

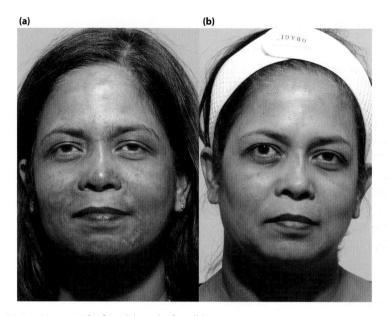

FIGURE 15.5   Patient 5 before (a) and after (b) treatment.

Program A

Program A consisted of 4 months of a non-HQ ZOMD program with dermal stabilization to overcome HQ resistance and to stabilize melanocytes. Program A included the principles shown in Table 15.11. After program A, the patient's skin improved slightly, but the ochronosis failed to improve. The patient then began program B.

Program B

Before undergoing CO_2 fractional laser, the patient's skin was conditioned for 6 weeks with an HQ-based bleaching and blending regimen. Preparation of the skin was generally the same as shown for program A, but a few additional agents were added. Glycogent was used AM and PM (2 pumps) for exfoliation. Brightenex was stopped, and instead, Melamin (4% HQ) was used for bleaching, AM and PM. Blending was accomplished with tretinoin (1%, 4 pumps) and Melamix (2 pumps) used PM. Blending replaced Ossential Advanced Radical Night Repair.

Her entire face was treated with a CO_2 fractional laser, and this provided significant improvement after healing had occurred. Later, a QsNd-YAG 1,064-nm laser was used over the areas that had not fully cleared from the CO_2

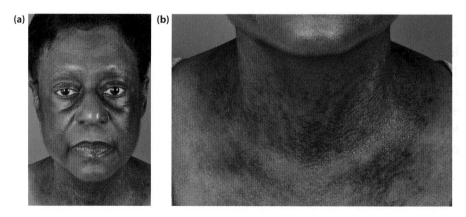

FIGURE 15.6   Patient 6 before (a) and after (b) treatment.

TABLE 15.11   Program A for Patient 5

Step	Products	Application
Skin preparation	Oilacleanse	AM and PM
	Vitascrub	Once daily
	Cebatrol	AM and PM
Blending and melanocyte stabilization (nonhydroquinone)	Brightenex	AM, 3 pumps
Barrier repair and epidermal stabilization	Ossential Daily Power Defense	AM and PM, 3 pumps
Dermal stimulation and stabilization	Ossential Advanced Radical Night Repair	PM, 2 to 3 pumps
Hydration and calming	Ommerse Daily Renewal Crème Ommerse Overnight Recovery Crème	AM and PM, as needed
Sun protection	Oclipse-C Broad Spectrum Sunscreen SPF 50	AM, reapply as needed

fractional laser treatment. A ZO Controlled Depth Peel to the level of the PD was further performed to even-out facial tone. By the end of all treatments, the patient showed complete clearance of the mild ochronosis, so the HQ-based approach (program B) was discontinued, and a non-HQ-based maintenance program was started.

TREATMENT PLAN FOR PATIENT 6

The treatment plan for patient 6, with severe ochronosis and sensitivity, made use of a non-HQ ZOSH approach. This program included preparing the skin with Offects Hydrating Cleanser, AM and PM; Balatone, AM and PM; epidermal stabilization with Ossential Daily Power Defense, AM and PM; mild dermal stabilization with Ossential Growth Factor Serum Plus, PM; Hydration and Calming with Ommerse Daily Renewal Crème and Ommerse Overnight Recovery Crème, AM and PM; and sun protection with Oclipse-C Broad Spectrum SPF 50, AM.

   While on this non-HQ-based program, the patient showed increased tolerance and improved sensitivity. Her ochronosis was not treated because it was extremely deep, and unfortunately, the damage was permanent.

Treatment Note
It is imperative that HQ use be discontinued for a period of 3 to 4 months. This eliminates the skin's resistance to HQ, allows proper melanization, and reduces photosensitivity. It is important to recognize ochronosis, but it is not a sign of an allergy to HQ. If required, HQ can be used again in these patients for skin conditioning, but only when following the appropriate guidelines as outlined previously.

INDEX

Page numbers followed by *f* indicate figures; those followed by *t* indicate tables.

S

U